MEDICAL GUIDES TO COMPLEMENTARY AND ALTERNATIVE MEDICINE

Medical Hypnosis

MEDICAL GUIDES TO COMPLEMENTARY AND ALTERNATIVE MEDICINE

Medical Hypnosis
An Introduction and Clinical Guide

Roberta Temes, PH.D.

Private Practice, Medical Hypnosis, Brooklyn, New York
Clinical Assistant Professor, Department of Psychiatry, SUNY Health Science Center, Brooklyn, New York

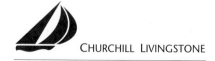

CHURCHILL LIVINGSTONE

A Division of Harcourt Brace & Company
New York Edinburgh London Philadelphia San Francisco Tokyo

CHURCHILL LIVINGSTONE
A Division of Harcourt Brace & Company

The Curtis Center
Independence Square West
Philadelphia, Pennsylvania 19106

Library of Congress Cataloging-in-Publication Data

Medical hypnosis: an introduction and clinical guide / [edited by]
Roberta Temes.—1st ed.

p.   cm.

ISBN 0–443–06010–X

1. Hypnotism—Therapeutic use.   I. Temes, Roberta.
    [DNLM: 1. Hypnosis.   WM 415 M489 1999]

RC495.M43 1999   615.8′512—dc21

DNLM/DLC   98-25700

MEDICAL HYPNOSIS
An Introduction and Clinical Guide   ISBN 0–443–06010–X

Churchill Livingstone® is a registered trademark of Harcourt Brace &
Company. ⤳™ is a trademark of Harcourt Brace & Company.

Printed in the United States of America

Last digit is the print number: 9 8 7 6 5 4 3 2 1

Contributors

Ann Damsbo, Ph.D.
Private Practice, San Diego, California
Psychotherapy

Dabney Ewin, M.D.
Clinical Professor of Surgery and Psychiatry, Tulane Medical School, New Orleans, Louisiana; Clinical Professor of Psychiatry, Louisiana State University School of Medicine, New Orleans, Louisiana
Hypnosis in the Emergency Room

Larry Goldman, M.D., F.A.C.O.G., F.A.S.C.H., F.F.S.C.H.
Private Practice, Fort Myers, Florida; Past President, Florida Society of Clinical Hypnosis, Past Chairman, Department of OB-GYN, Lee Memorial and Gulf Coast Hospitals, Fort Myers, Florida
Hypnosis in Obstetrics and Gynecology

Melvin A. Gravitz, B.A., M.A., Ph.D.
Clinical Professor of Psychiatry and Behavioral Sciences, George Washington University Medical School, Washington, D.C.; Independent Practice of Clinical and Forensic Psychology and Hypnosis, Washington, D.C.
Medical Hypnosis: A Historical Perspective

Howard Hall, Ph.D., Psy.D.
Assistant Professor of Pediatrics, Department of Pediatrics, Case Western Reserve University, Cleveland, Ohio; Attending, Rainbow Babies and Children's Hospital, Cleveland, Ohio
Hypnosis and Pediatrics

Rodger Kessler, B.S., M.A., Ph.D.
Clinical Psychologist, Berlin Family Health and Central Vermont Medical Center, Montpelier, Vermont
Hypnotic Preparation in Anesthesia and Surgery

Elvira V. Lang, M.D.
Associate Professor, The University of Iowa College of Medicine, Iowa City, Iowa; Director, Vascular and Interventional Radiology, The University of Iowa Hospitals and Clinics, Iowa City, Iowa
Hypnosis in Radiology

Dorothy Larkin, B.S.N., M.A., Ph.D. Cand.
Instructor, College of New Rochelle Graduate Program Holistic Nursing, New Rochelle, New York; Past President, NY Milton H. Erikson Society for Psychotherapy and Hypnosis
Nursing

Eleanor Laser, Ph.D.
Private Practice, Lincolnwood, Illinois
Hypnosis in Radiology

Alexander A. Levitan, M.D., M.P.H.
Formerly Clinical Associate Professor, University of Minnesota, Minneapolis, Minnesota; Consulting Oncologist, Unity Hospital, Fridley, Minnesota
Oncology

Karen N. Olness, M.D.
Professor of Pediatrics, Family Medicine, and International Health, Case Western Reserve University, Cleveland, Ohio; Director, International Child Health, Rainbow Babies and Children's Hospital, Cleveland, Ohio
Contemporary Context: Psychoneuroimmunology

Samuel Perlman, M.A., D.D.S.
Private Practice, New Rochelle, New York
Dentistry

Gerard Sunnen, M.D.
Associate Clinical Professor of Psychiatry, New York University–Bellevue Medical Center, New York, New York
What Is Hypnosis?

Roberta Temes, Ph.D.
Private Practice, Medical Hypnosis, Brooklyn, New York; Clinical Assistant Professor, Department of Psychiatry, SUNY Health Science Center, Brooklyn, New York
Welcome to Hypnosis

Marcia J. Wagaman, M.D.
Formerly Clinical Assistant Professor, University of South Florida, Tampa, Florida; Asthma and Allergy Centre and Private Practice; St. Petersburg, Florida
Hypnosis and Its Usefulness in Managing Patients with Respiratory Problems

Thomas Whalen, M.D.
Director of Surgical Preparation, Anesthesia Associates of New Mexico, Albuquerque, New Mexico
Hypnotic Preparation in Anesthesia and Surgery

Foreword

Poised as we are on the cusp of a millennium, we are witnessing the slow, steady reentry of mind or consciousness into medicine.

Some people find this development surprising, because for most of this century it appeared as if we might be able to develop a system of medicine that was wholly objective and material in nature. The contributions of this effort have been magnificent; they speak for themselves and need no defense. In this process, however, consciousness or mind was confined to the sidelines. Its absence has been deeply missed, because it has led to the neglect of the qualities we find utterly precious not just health care but in life in general—a belief in the causal power of our own minds and the value we attribute to experiences such as love, empathy, caring, and compassion.

When we *have* paid attention to the mind as a factor in health during the 20th century, its role has been largely pathologized—e.g., mental *illness,* psychosomatic *disease.* Even the placebo response has been viewed pejoratively as an obstacle that must be overcome in clinical research. As if this were not a sufficient level of disrespect of consciousness, many researchers and theorists have essentially defined the mind out of existence by equating it with the physical brain or by relegating it to the status of an epiphenomenon of the brain. According to these views, consciousness is an unnecessary concept at best and a harmful illusion at worst. Thus, for generations of modern scientists, "mind" has become merely a metaphor for the electrochemical activity of the brain—neurotransmitters acting on receptor sites in "a computer made of meat," to borrow Marvin Minsky's dramatic image.

The vast, sprawling literature of the field of clinical hypnosis decisively challenges the notion that the mind is merely a "ghost in the machine" because hypnotic phenomena show that mental activities can bring about robust physical changes that no ghost could possibly achieve. Hypnosis demonstrates, in the most straightforward way, that consciousness is not effete and not simply along for the ride; it must be accorded respect. This is a magnificent contribution because it opens a window for the restoration of meanings, purposes, goals, and values in health, without which any concept of healing is limited and ultimately unfulfilling.

Philosopher John Searle has bluntly asserted that, at our present state of knowledge, *no one knows* what consciousness is, and we need to explore all sorts of ideas to find out. I am convinced that experts in the field of clinical hypnosis have something vital to contribute to this vigorous discussion, which is gathering a degree of steam not seen in generations.

Still, many health care professionals have antiquated views about hypnosis and are hesitant to explore it. Some continue to associate hypnosis with stage tricks and the seance chamber and believe it has no place in the clinic or hospital. To those who harbor such thoughts, read on; you are about to encounter empirical evidence that will surely elicit your critical respect. As a nudge to open-mindedness, I urge you to consider emerging developments from several areas of science that point toward new ways of thinking about the nature of the mind.

Mathematician and cognitive scientist David Chalmers, for example, has recently suggested that consciousness may be *fundamental* in the universe, perhaps on a par with matter and energy—neither derivable from, nor reducible to, anything else, including the brain. This view attributes causal power to consciousness, perhaps the sort of mental power often described in the annals of clinical hypnosis. Chalmers' view does not stand alone; similar ideas have been advanced by scholars from fields as diverse as quantum mechanics, psychology, systems theory, and more. We do not know, of course, which if any of these theories will carry the day. But the fact that they are being offered by respected authorities should allay any intellectual or emotional doubts we might experience about exploring the phenomena in the chapters that follow.

In addition to answering questions, this book raises them. What is the precise mechanism—if the word is even appropriate—of hypnosis? What are the intervening variables between the *experience* of hypnosis and what happens "downstream" in molecules, cells, tissues, and organs? How can something that feels so ethereal and immaterial as a thought have such dramatic effects on the material body? What is the nature of the actual linkage between mind and body? Some of these questions will be answered by further research; others, particularly the precise nature of the mind-body connection, are more difficult—*so* difficult they "make our brain hurt," as one researcher has lamented, when we try to grasp them. They confront us with the mystery of being, over which humans have eternally puzzled.

Some mysteries are so dark and impenetrable they can be threatening, and we turn away. Is this why medical hypnosis, after captivating clinicians in the 19th century, nearly faded from our medical radar screen? Was it more comfortable to focus on a material approach that emphasized the concrete and visible? Does the resurgence of hypnosis indicate that we've gotten our nerve up to confront the great unknowns once again? I like to think this is the case—that our profession has become mature, wise, and courageous enough to face the deepest mysteries of our own minds once more.

This book is first and foremost a guide for clinicians, who will be more interested in the practical aspects of hypnosis than its philosophical implications. But in the material ahead, let us keep one eye trained on the larger view. Hypnosis confronts us with the question of *who we are*—the nature of our mind, and thus our origins and destiny. Why is it important to bear these issues in mind? If we neglect the philosophical and the spiritual sides of life, medical science can degenerate into a utilitarian materialism that is lethal to the human spirit. A profusion of studies show that human health withers in the absence of a perceived sense of meaning and purpose in life. Medicine, therefore, should ideally nourish as well as cure. In order to do so, it needs a continual infusion not just from science but also from the domains of philosophy, religion, and spirituality. The field of clinical hypnosis is caressed by *both* the empirical and the spiritual because of the central role of consciousness in hypnotic phenomena. If we fail to keep this larger picture in mind, hypnosis is likely to become a mere tool, which, however useful it may be, will not fulfill its potential contributions to human welfare.

I wish to express my admiration for the contributors to this fine volume, and to Dr. Roberta Temes and Dr. Marc Micozzi for assembling them. When the history of our medical age is written, the explorers of hypnosis will, I believe, occupy a high place. If so, the honor will be fitting; for what territory is worth greater attention than our own mind and its potential to heal?

Larry Dossey, M.D.
Executive Editor, *Alternative Therapies in Health and Medicine*

Preface

When 12-year-old Karen opened her mouth during an outpatient preoperative procedure, she had every intention of cooperating with the otolaryngologist. As the instruments entered her throat, however, Karen realized that no matter what her intention was, inevitably her jaws would clamp down on the hands that were to cure her. The doctor could not complete his work, Karen was disappointed in herself, surgery was scheduled for Wednesday, and I did not know how in the world to help my daughter.

A colleague at the mental health center where I was then employed listened to my tale and offered a solution. "Why don't I try hypnotizing Karen to easily keep her mouth open and feel no discomfort?" John suggested. I brought Karen into work with me the following day, sat on the couch next to her while John spoke to her for about 10 minutes, and wondered if it was doing any good. I knew nothing about hypnosis back then, in the 1970s; it was never mentioned in my classes or written about in my textbooks.

On Wednesday morning Karen breezed through the preoperative procedure and eagerly went off to the operating room. I became a believer. I began my conversion to hypnosis by reading books, taking classes, attending conferences, and participating in workshops. For the last two decades I have practiced hypnosis, lectured about it, and created hypnosis audiotapes.

Physicians use hypnosis to help patients in many ways: to control pain, prepare for surgery, quit smoking, stick to a particular food program, and accomplish all the amazing feats described by the authors of the chapters that follow.

Dr. Gerard Sunnen begins this text by introducing us to theories of hypnosis and describing the physiologic and cognitive effects of hypnosis on the human body and mind. Dr. Sunnen's poetic writing elucidates the metaphysics of hypnosis.

Next, Dr. Mel Gravitz presents an historic overview of hypnosis, which reminds us that hypnotic techniques have been used for centuries. He tells us that 200 years ago mesmerism was used as an anesthetic during a mastectomy.

Dr. Karen Olness presents the latest research in the mind/body linkage. Her careful analyses of the published studies and her own investigations show no signs of the hyperbole so common in the popular press. Instead, we read of the earnest travails of scrupulous scientific examination and along the way we learn that intentional immunomodulation by humans is possible.

In their exhaustive review of the literature, Drs. Rodger Kessler and Thomas Whalen present evidence that the hypnotically prepared patient does better than the nonhypnotized patient before, during, and after surgery.

When you read about Dr. Dabney Ewin's Emergency Room technique for repairing a dislocated shoulder you will wish you could be an eye witness to this procedure.

Dr. Larry Goldman makes childbirth sound like fun and offers several easy-to-follow hypnosis scripts to be used during pregnancy, labor, and delivery. Dr. Howard Hall describes the range of hypnotic interventions with children and includes detailed case studies from both his practice and his family. Drs. Elvira Lang and Eleanor Laser, recognizing the limits of intravenous conscious sedation, have trained all their radiology suite personnel, not only the nursing and medical staff, in the uses of hypnosis. Their case examples are illuminating. No aborted MRIs in that unit; even claustrophobic patients remain calm.

Dr. Al Levitan describes the usefulness of hypnosis when treating the patient who has cancer.

Contained within Dr. Marcia Wagaman's precise analysis of the role of hypnosis in the treatment of respiratory disorders is a serious warning to physicians about what *not* to say to the hypnotized patient who has asthma.

Dr. Samuel Perlman presents evidence that a trip to the dentist is akin to a trip to the beach. You will enjoy and probably practice his description of the 20-second handshake induction.

Dorothy Larkin's chapter will make you wish that every nurse in every hospital was trained in the conversational hypnotic techniques she so aptly illustrates.

Dr. Ann Damsbo writes about the ways in which she uses hypnosis in her psychotherapy practice and in her personal life.

Hypnosis is nonpharmacologic, noninvasive, and relatively inexpensive. The authors cited above have demonstrated that it can effectively and positively influence our health. It is only a matter of time before every medical center will advocate and every medical school will teach hypnosis.

ROBERTA TEMES, PH.D.

Series Editor's Preface

Hypnosis has been in and out of vogue as a psychotherapeutic technique, and the use of hypnosis as part of the practice of psychiatry is not the subject of this volume. As a volume in the series Medical Guides to Complementary and Alternative Medicine, this text focuses on the use of hypnosis as an adjunct or complement (or in a supportive role) to medical specialty practices, thus addressing the practice of clinical hypnosis.

As the application of hypnosis to medicine became more scientific, there were efforts to objectively determine the susceptibility of an individual to hypnotic suggestion without having to explain or understand the "mechanism of action." Susceptibility scales such as the Stanford Hypnotic Susceptibility Scale (Wutzenhoffer and Hilgard, 1959) and the Hypnotic Induction Profile (HIP) (Spiegel and Spiegel, 1978) were developed to predict outcome on the basis of variables easily ascertained in the clinical setting. As experience accumulated, it became recognized that most people are more or less susceptible to hypnosis for the uses described in this book.

However, the concept of susceptibility scales or indices remains an important one as applied to complementary and alternative therapies. We know that not all individuals benefit to the same extent from the various complementary therapies, such as acupuncture, various "mind-body" techniques, and meditation. However, if favorable outcomes can be predicted on the basis of objectively ascertained clinical variables, such therapies would be of great assistance in providing appropriate care for different individuals for different conditions, thereby reaffirming the principle of individuality in complementary and alternative medicine while maintaining a generalizable practice.

The development of clinical hypnosis in this way may provide a guide to other, more recently integrated complementary and alternative therapies.

MARC S. MICOZZI, M.D. PH.D.

Contents

Part One
THE MIND/BODY CONNECTION

1. Welcome to Hypnosis 3
   Roberta Temes

2. What Is Hypnosis? 7
   Gerard Sunnen

3. Medical Hypnosis: A Historical Perspective 21
   Melvin A. Gravitz

4. Contemporary Context:
   Psychoneuroimmunology 33
   Karen N. Olness

Part Two
HYPNOSIS AND THE MEDICAL SPECIALTY

5. Hypnotic Preparation in Anesthesia and
   Surgery 43
   Rodger Kessler
   Thomas Whalen

6. Hypnosis in the Emergency Room 59
   Dabney Ewin

7. Hypnosis in Obstetrics and Gynecology 65
   Larry Goldman

8. Hypnosis and Pediatrics 79
   Howard Hall

9. Hypnosis in Radiology 95
   Elvira V. Lang
   Eleanor Laser

10. Oncology 107
    Alexander A. Levitan

11. Hypnosis and Its Usefulness in Managing Patients
    with Respiratory Problems 115
    Marcia J. Wagaman

Part Three
HYPNOSIS AND OTHER HEALTH CARE PROFESSIONS

12. Dentistry 131
    Samuel Perlman

13. Nursing 141
    Dorothy Larkin

14. Psychotherapy 151
    Ann Damsbo

    Index 159

part one

The Mind/Body Connection

Welcome to Hypnosis

Roberta Temes

INTRODUCTION

Hypnosis may very well be the original mind/body therapy. It is a tool that can be used in the practice of medicine as an adjunct therapy in the treatment of disease. Like the surgeon's scalpel, hypnosis is only as good as the professional who uses it.

As Gerard Sunnen will explain in Chapter 2, scholars ponder the exact definition of hypnosis. Most agree that hypnosis is a state of awareness that permits the patient to accept suggestions without censoring them. In 1993, the Division of Psychological Hypnosis of the American Psychological Association defined hypnosis as a procedure wherein changes in sensations, perceptions, thoughts, feelings, or behavior are suggested. Dr. Milton Erickson (1901–1980), one of the pioneers of hypnotherapy and the founder and first president of the American Society of Clinical Hypnosis, defined hypnosis as a natural, everyday experience of unconscious learning via successful communication. (See his book, *Healing in Hypnosis,* Irvington, NY, 1983.) Dr. Herbert Spiegel defines hypnosis as the condition that occurs when the patient feels as if he is floating, feels as if he is simultaneously "here" and "there" (i.e., achieves dissociation), and is able to maintain focused concentration while being open to suggestions. Most clinicians also agree that during hypnosis the patient increases his ability to absorb specific thoughts, feelings, or imagery and decreases his interest in extraneous matters. A hypnotized patient is alert, but his mind easily will accept information that he might normally reject, critique, or intellectually dispute. Hypnotized patients can return to their regular state whenever they want. Usually, however, they enjoy the hypnotic state so much that they have no desire to open their eyes and end the hypnosis and, therefore, remain hypnotized until the hypnotist directs them to come back to their original state.

The hypnosis procedure consists of an *induction,* which gets the patient into the trance state, and then the suggestions, sometimes called a *script*, which are spoken to the patient to help achieve the goals of the hypnosis session. An induction can be accomplished in a minute or two, or may extend for a longer period of time. The script can also take just a few minutes. Thus the entire hypnotic procedure may be extremely brief. Many hypnotists vary their inductions and their suggestions to suit the needs of the patient.

Every person has an innate talent for hypnosis and the extent of that talent is unknown until an actual hypnosis session is conducted. In their 1978 book, *Trance and Treatment,* Drs. Herbert and David Spiegel say that patients fit along a continuum, from those who are extremely easy to hypnotize to those who barely go into a trance. Those people who are highly hypnotizable are usually passionate and emotional. They tend to be trusting and respond well to direct suggestion. On the other end of the scale are the patients who are reasonable and enjoy using their intellectual and analytic skills They do best when treated in a collegial fashion and given ample explanations. The ability to experience hypnosis has no correlation with IQ or with a strong or a gullible mind. The ability to be hypnotized does seem to be correlated with a fixed biological marker—the white of the eye that is visible when a patient rolls his eyes upward—the eye-roll sign. Some hypnotists administer a hypnosis susceptibility scale, such as the Spiegels' *hypnotic induction profile,* to assess the patient's hypnotizability before beginning a session with a new patient. Other hypnotists use scales of hypnotizability only when conducting research. Induction styles and scripts vary. Some hypnotists use an *eye-fixation* induction, instructing the patient to stare at a particular object (hence the popularized swinging pendulum) until the eyes close. Cooperative patients do best with a *basic induction,* which usually includes progressive relaxation as well as information about the altered feelings experienced during hypnosis.

Extremely rigid, critical patients do well with a *confusion induction.* The confusion technique rapidly goes from topic to topic and is so disconcerting and ambiguous that the patient eventually stops struggling to make sense of the hypnotist's puzzling words and simply relaxes and goes with the program. Patients who expect hypnosis to do "magic" may be reassured if their induction includes an *arm levitation* suggestion, such as, "your mind can control your body so easily that now, as you think about it, your arm will become so light that it will automatically rise upward; it will lift all by itself." These patients also appreciate the opportunity to experience an altered sensation, perhaps a suggestion to smell a particular food or to hear a certain piece of music. These are people who need discernible evidence that some-

thing unusual is occurring; for them hypnosis must become an observable phenomenon.

While under hypnosis, compliant patients may respond best to the *authoritative suggestion:* "Read this book." For other patients, the *direct suggestion,* which is slightly less authoritative, will be more effective: "Please read this book." An *indirect suggestion* is often extremely beneficial: "Many physicians are interested in reading this book; you, too, might enjoy reading it."

Dr. Milton Erickson, whose scripts often included metaphors and anecdotes, tried to match his words and style to those of the patient. The naturalistic, *Ericksonian* approach, sometimes called the *utilization* approach, makes use of the idiosyncratic aspects of the patient's personality and learning style. The approach casually, yet carefully, incorporates the natural ways and habits of the patient into the hypnotic experience—both the induction and the script. An Ericksonian suggestion is indirect and permissive and might have *embedded suggestions:* "I don't know whether you will decide to begin reading now or later, today or tomorrow. Wouldn't it be interesting if you continued reading this book and enjoying it until it was finished?" Ericksonians prefer indirect suggestions to direct suggestions and do not necessarily use relaxation in the induction or the script.

Some practitioners encourage their patients to use *ideomotor signals* during the hypnotic trance. Such signals help the practitioner know that the patient is following prompts. Ideomotor movements are the subtle muscle movements that occur when a person is thinking or visualizing. The movement is an automatic response to an internal experience, a motor response to an idea. Some people may nod their head, others will blink their eyes, still others may alter their breathing rate. During hypnosis the movement is often robot-like and seems mechanized. Patient and hypnotist may decide before trance which ideomotor signal will be used to communicate during the session, when speaking may seem like too much of an effort. Usually a finger signal is agreed upon and "yes" or "no" are represented by particular finger motions.

Glove anesthesia is a hypnotic technique that allows the patient's hand to become numb and then transfer that numbness to any part of the body the hand will touch, thereby diminishing pain. *Catalepsy* is hypnosis-induced rigidity of the body or particularly designated body parts, usually a limb. *Posthypnotic suggestion* is a technique that instructs the patient to behave in a certain manner at a designated time in the future.

For more information about other terms, methods, and clinical studies, each chapter has an extensive reference list. Also, each of the two national hypnosis societies listed below publish an academic journal. Many cities have Ericksonian societies, as well. Health professionals who wish to incorporate hypnosis into their practices must decide whether to become proficient at hypnosis themselves, like those specialists who have contributed chapters to this book, or whether to refer patients to outside hypnotists. It is best to locate a qualified hypnotist or a training program by contacting a medical school or either of these two national hypnosis societies: Society for Clinical and Experimental Hypnosis (509-332-7555) or American Society of Clinical Hypnosis (847-297-3317).

2

What Is Hypnosis?

Gerard Sunnen

INTRODUCTION

We are witnessing a blossoming sophistication in the science of the mind and especially in the elucidation of how the psyche interrelates with the physical body. It is in this domain that hypnosis finds its rightful niche as a science that deals almost exclusively with mind/body interactions; for this reason, hypnosis has had a fascinating historical trajectory.

Historically, hypnotic phenomena have been interpreted in different ways through the tinted glass of each culture's ideology. In Grecian sleep temples, for example, hypnosis was seen as a sleep state facilitating communication with deities (Zilboorg 1941); in Mesmer's time, it was conceptualized as an agitated condition stemming from the absorption of cosmic forces (Crabtree 1993).

Hypnotic phenomena are not easily measured or quantifiably grasped. They are neither countable bacterial colonies on an agar plate nor hypnotic phenomena capable of precise delineation, as would be a cardiac rhythm. To some extent, they can be measured by any one of many psychological tests gauging suggestibility, hypnotic susceptibility, or the aptitude for imagery (Balthazard 1993, Field 1965, Bowers 1986). These tests may be administered before or after hypnosis. Tests may also center upon physiological parameters expressed through the electroencephalogram (EEG) or the metabolism of cerebral pathways (Graffin 1995). However, the complexity factor in hypnosis resides in that its manifestations tend to be subjective as much as objective, expressing themselves in the context of the global person (Mott 1995).

THE EXPERIENCE OF HYPNOSIS

Although there is fairly good general agreement regarding the psychological and physiological phenomena elicited through hypnosis, rich controversies exist regarding the mechanisms by which they occur (Kirsh 1995).

Participants vary greatly in their experiences during hypnosis (Hilgard 1965, Freundlich 1974). Certain feelings stand out as commonly encountered, whereas others remain idiosyncratic or rare (Twenlow 1982). In clinical situations, some people exit from the hypnotic experience astonished to have felt a state of mind so vastly different from their normal waking state, whereas others talk as if nothing unusual had happened. In the former case, the vivid impact of the experience will serve to facilitate further hypnotic work through the subject's conviction that some tangible phenomenon has indeed taken place. In spite of any novel sensations in the latter case, individuals may, much to their surprise, be able to show a full range of hypnotic phenomena. For example, a severely overweight woman in her thirties, who had a long history of failed attempts at following dietary regimens, came out of her first hypnotic session disappointed. She imagined that she would have experienced a feeling of other-worldliness during trance, whereas in fact, she reported only a slightly enhanced level of relaxation. As treatment continued and suggestions were offered to follow a nutritional plan with ease, she expressed surprise. In spite of the absence of subjective changes during hypnotic sessions, she was able to actualize the message of the suggestions seemingly automatically.

During the deeper stages of hypnotic experience, participants may be asked to talk about or to notice how they feel. The answers are usually spoken in monotone, slowly, and with pauses. A query asked during hypnosis, even if not assiduously answered at the time, makes it easier for more detailed reports to be shared after hypnosis because some degree of observing self-awareness will have been kindled.

Physio-Motor Changes

During hypnosis the motions and the internal workings of the body often feel decelerated. There may be a sense of inertia or a feeling of not desiring to move; if movements are made, they have a tendency to be carried out less frequently, to have reduced range, and to be experienced internally as if made in slow motion. There is frequently a pervasive sensation of comfortable heaviness permeating the neuromusculature. This sensation, which goes hand-in-hand with physiological appeasement, may be looked for and suggested during the induction because its presence tends to convince the participant that some real internal change has indeed transpired.

One of the characteristics of hypnosis is physiological languor, but not all hypnotic phenomena occur in this context (Malort 1984). Although in medical hypnosis we tend to suggest to our patients a global relaxation response, there are hypnotic-like states in which activation rather than relaxation is a prominent feature (Fellows 1993). Certain states are sometimes elicited in the course of religious ceremonials, as is observed in Sufi dancing dervishes (Rouget 1980). In modern clinical practice, suggestions of physical action in the context of psychological relaxation are often utilized. It is possible, for example, to present posthypnotic suggestions for the purpose of enhancing athletic performance, which requires intense concentration and physical effort. The athlete, during trance, visualizes himself actualizing a performance with peak mastery. Once these images are incorporated into memory posthypnotically, they can exert a positive influence upon the performance itself (Liggett 1993, Stanton 1994).

Relaxation and Meditation

Relaxation has both physical and psychological components. Parallel with physiological parameters, the experience is one of repose and calm. Of all the hypnotic phenomena, relaxation is the most easily and consistently observed. In some individuals the relaxation can be extremely pronounced, and it is not infrequent for first-time participants of hypnosis to say that they have never before felt a relaxation level so profound.

This important global response is already present in *neutral hypnosis* (i.e., hypnosis without any overt suggestions or the phase of the hypnotic process following induction and preceding the presentation of suggestions) (Edmonston 1977). By adding proper suggestions, neutral hypnosis can be amplified many times over. Once experienced by the patient, relaxation can, through the techniques of *self-hypnosis* (the process by which a trance is brought on by the participant himself) or posthypnotic suggestion, be applied during situations previously experienced as stressful or anxiogenic.

The feeling of relaxation in hypnosis can range from mild, general deceleration to pervasive peacefulness. In the latter instance, the parts of the mind that contribute to anxiety are quieted.

Physiological Changes Observed in Hypnosis

The literature contains many accounts of physiological changes associated with hypnosis (Sturgis 1990). It is important to note, however, that no physiological variable has been shown to be systematically or regularly associated with hypnosis (Sarbin 1972). Most experiments that purportedly show a correlative relationship to physiological variables fare equivocally on replication or are methodologically imperfect.

The physiological changes observed during hypnosis are greatly influenced by the nature of the suggestions administered. It stands to reason that incentives to relaxation will lead to a different physiological response configuration compared with suggestions centering upon activation in any one of its forms.

It is common to observe cardiac variability during the initial phase of hypnotic induction (DeBenedittis 1994), which may be due to feelings of novelty about the upcoming experience, especially if it is a first experience. This response is followed by a slowing regular rhythm as deeper stages of hypnosis are achieved (Harris 1993).

Reduced bleeding time has been reported in patients undergoing surgical procedures with the assistance of hypnoanesthesia (Bishay 1984). Vasodilation and increased circulation to otherwise poorly perfused areas have also been reported in response to hypoanesthesia instructions (Rossi 1997).

Longitudinal studies on blood pressure reduction through hypnosis have yielded erratic results, depending upon the research approach. However, by means of training in self-hypnosis (Deabler 1973) and especially with the integration of hypnosis with biofeedback support, hypertensive subjects have been able to modulate and even normalize their blood pressure readings (Friedman 1977).

A slowing of the breathing rate can be observed in individuals within the deeper dimensions of the hypnotic experience (Sarbin 1956). Breathing is then more likely to show less amplitude and to be more abdominally expressed. On the other hand, respiratory rate, predictably, is found to increase when cognitions of fear, anger, pain, or muscular activity are elicited (Dudley 1964).

A number of metabolic changes have been reported to take place following hypnotic suggestions. Among them are alterations in blood glucose level, basal metabolic rate, calcium metabolism, and oxygen saturation (Lovett-Doust 1953). There are also reports that the body temperature may be raised or lowered, depending upon the suggestion presented (Margolis 1983).

The hypnotic experience has been approached through many physiological channels, including gastric secretions (Klein 1989), cerebral blood flow (Diehl 1989), cerebral oxygen consumption (Maiolo 1969), and electrodermal activity (Boucsein 1992).

Few endocrine studies have been performed. Release of adrenocorticotropic hormone (ACTH) by the pituitary gland can be affected directly by emotional stimuli, and some researchers have reported a drop in plasma cortisol titers to significantly low levels shortly after hypnotic induction (Sachar 1964). Cutaneous functions have occasionally shown marked sensitivity to hypnotic influence (Burgess 1996).

A sudden change in brain voltage that is initiated by an external stimulus is referred to as an evoked potential (Davic-Jefdic 1993, Jutai 1993). Some experiments seem to show a diminution of visual evoked potentials in hypnosis (Banyai 1981).

Numerous studies have attempted to analyze EEG patterns in hypnosis (DePascalis 1993). Some researchers have found enhancement of theta rhythm after hypnotic induction (Tebecis 1975). EEG measurements comparing neutral hypnosis—which presumably would reflect the physiological essence of the hypnotic state because of the absence of administered suggestions—and the state of wakefulness have interested many researchers. Several studies have shown an augmentation of alpha wave density during hypnosis (Melzack 1975). Others have discovered EEG patterns in neutral hypnosis marked by enhanced delta and theta activity, with concomitant reduction of alpha and beta wave manifestation (Saletu 1987).

Despite the efforts of numerous researchers, the hypnotic condition has not yielded substantive physiological correspondence. Despite the growing sophistication of medical technology, much needs to be accomplished to correlate psychological dynamics with some yet elusive central nervous system alteration. We are nevertheless gently reminded of Freud's futuristic remark that every thought—and presumably every alteration in mental state, including hypnosis—will eventually prove to be accompanied by a specific neurophysiological event.

Anticipatory anxiety is a universal source of stress. Self-reproach, guilt, resentment, and dwelling negatively on the past are also sidestepped, as the mind is asked to confine itself to an experiential grounding in the very present time. There is a moving away from the perceived complexities of the current life situation into self-reflection. Some contemporary theoretical approaches suggest that the frontal lobes of the hypnotized individual act as if they have been distanced from the nervous system (Crawford 1994, Gruzelier 1993). In the construct of this rough neurophysiological model, the frontal lobes, in their psychological correlation with concerns about the past and worries about the future, may function as if they had assumed relative dormancy.

Relaxation is a complex global state involving not only physical and physiological realms but also dimensions touching upon the emotions and thought processes. It is hardly possible for an individual to be fully relaxed and physically at rest and at the same time emotionally disquieted by ruminative feelings, such as resentment or shame or by activated thoughts fueled by worry and unrest. Hypnosis in its relaxing action touches all dimensions of the body and the psyche. In this sense, it can be said that hypnosis is the most potent nonpharmacological relaxing agent known to science.

Descriptions of the subjective experience of the hypnotic trance often include alterations in the perception of time flow and sensations of relative removal from the ties connecting the individual to reality. Yet, during hypnosis, the individual may still feel, with varied intensity, the presence of the hypnotherapist, and with it, a sense of security and resassurance. In hypnosis, the elements of this relationship are closely intertwined with the experience of the trance because part of the patient's psyche is linked to the hypnotist's psyche in a process of dynamic communication, a dyadic alliance (Diamond 1984). The hypnotherapist may communicate with one part of the subject's self, then with another, but there remains an interpersonal bridge, regardless of the clinical approach of the hypnotist, which may be very permissive, choice-giving, and open-ended in the manner that suggestions are presented. Indeed, no matter what the style of the hypnotic process, the structure of the therapeutic relationship imbues its experience.

Self-hypnosis expands the privilege of autonomy (Garver 1984). The link of interpersonal rapport is dissolved as the experience becomes more fully intrapsychic. A more conscious portion of the mind gives suggestions, affirmations, and directives to another, more unconscious part (Sacerdote 1981). According to some authors, the autonomy accompanying self-hypnosis may invite disproportionate wanderings of attention and less task orientation than that observed in the more structured heterohypnosis (Fromm 1990).

Sometimes the individual enters a self-hypnotic state and does not give himself specific suggestions, which may be called *neutral self-hypnosis,* a state marked by relaxation, free-floating imagery, and dream fragments or sequences. In neutral self-hypnosis, the sense of control floats, undirected. In this unstructured trance state, the subject may observe and remember or not observe and not remember.

If we add one ingredient to this self-induced trance state, we have meditation. That ingredient is focused watchfulness.

The meditative trance is similar in quality to the self-hypnotic experience. In meditation, however, the individual starts out with no overt induction process but rather with the resolve to begin and continue the experience and to direct the observing self toward a meditative focus (Sanders 1991). This point of convergence may be a part of the body (e.g., the solar plexus), an imagined or spoken sound (mantra), a meditative image (mandala), or a selected spiritual idea (Naranjo 1971). Meditative focusing is showing ever richer potential in harmonizing the mind/body related dysfunctions (Shapiro 1982).

Time Changes

In the experience of hypnosis, the sense of time is shifted from external to internal events. Consequently, the sensation of time passing is correspondingly stretched because internal events are subjectively slowed (Blakely 1991, Von Kirchenheim 1991). Time feels less insistently present, and it is not uncommon for a participant to estimate the duration of a hypnotic session to have been 30 minutes, when in fact it has been only a few minutes (St. Jean 1988). In other cases, time feels as if it has stood completely still, as if frozen.

Body Image Changes

The experience of how the body feels during the normal waking state is often changed during hypnosis. With eyes closed, the waking subject, when asked to convey the configuration of the body as it is experienced, will usually describe a fairly anatomical rendition, with all the body parts in their respective positions. More precisely, the homunculus in the brain, with its disproportionate emphasis upon head, eyes, and feet, will correspond to the imaginal rendition.

The experience of how the body feels during the normal waking state is often changed during hypnosis. Without directive suggestions, the body may feel heavy, as if pushing into the cushions of the chair; or the body may feel lighter, as if floating. At times the body will feel larger, expanded, and macroscopic, as if filling the entire room. Rarely, it may feel microscopic (Gill 1959, Freundlich 1974).

Changes in Thinking Processes

Along with physiological slowdown, the flow of thoughts is likely to show variability in its velocity and direction. In any given day or moment, the course of our *thinking current,* the rate at which one thought follows others, varies. It may be faster in the evening than in the early morning. In depression, it is likely to be slowed down. In hypomania and in psychostimulant intoxication, it will be accelerated.

What is the relationship of the flow of thought to the experience of being aware of oneself? Is it ever possible to be devoid of thoughts and still be acutely conscious? In hypnosis, the flow of thoughts sometimes is reported to stop completely. At the same time, the individual is alert and aware, is not depressed, and knows that thoughts have ceased coming to mind. Often, there is a sense of amazement that awareness of one's awareness is exquisitely preserved, when all the while thoughts have desisted in manifesting themselves (Ludwig 1972).

When the current of thought is slowed, its structure is also likely to be changed. *Trance logic* refers to mental mechanisms in which logically incongruous ideas can coexist without clashing (Orne 1959). A student of mathematics, for example, came out of his hypnotic experience with a feeling of wonderment. During his hypnotic session he said he had felt, however fleetingly, the concept of infinite distance and endless time. After hypnosis, he talked about the experience as an everlasting revelation that, in spite of his efforts, his rational self could not experientially retrieve.

Emotional Changes

Although the word emotion most directly conveys the idea of a feeling, it is in fact a conglomerate body of processes involving the autonomic nervous system and many psychological associations (Bryant 1989).

Although it is possible in hypnosis to quell emotions as in deep relaxation, it is also possible to enhance certain feeling states. Sometimes, during a hypnotherapeutic situation, a solitary feeling may be presented to the patient for contemplation and amplification. A demoralized individual, for example, may be asked to center solely upon a sensation of optimism. For some participants this can be difficult because they may need to have an actual memory trace or a contextual milieu for this feeling. In this situation, a specific life event can be resurrected, one that was associated with happiness, feelings of self-confidence, and situational mastery. These feelings, once recreated, can be then hypnotically intensified so that they may exert their posthypnotic ego-strengthening influence.

An interesting feature of hypnotically induced feelings is that they tend to persist beyond the hypnotic session. This phenomenon draws associations to Papez's description of how emotions reverberate in the limbic system (Papez 1937). For example, a chronically depressed patient at age 54 could not recall any instance during his life when he experienced feelings of happiness. Then, during one of his sessions, he retrieved the memory of walking as a small boy with his uncle in the countryside, not far from some railroad tracks. A train whistled in the distance and he started imitating its sound and running in a skipping way. He remembered feeling happy then, if only for a few evanescent moments. In hypnosis, he was asked to invite those same feelings into his awareness, to then amplify them through meditative focusing. The ability to experience feelings of joy and freedom became progressively easier, and he gradually started to integrate them into his everyday life, coloring his existence with more joyfulness.

Changes in Imagination

To some degree, the ability to create mental images is present in everyone. It is most pronounced in dreams when the messages flowing from the sense organs are drastically reduced and awareness is shifted to the ever-ongoing inner mental life. In the waking state, the effer-

vescence of mental images surfaces in daydreams. The imagery of daydreams is complex, under partial volitional control, and uniquely expressed in everyone; they may contain visual impressions, feelings, some aesthetic sensations, the interplay of dialogue, and intricate scenarios. Daydreams may be so engrossing that coming back to reality feels shocking.

Clinically, it is important to know the style of imagery used by our patients. In hypnotic induction and in treatment, the stimulation of imagery, in any one of its modalities, provides an important vehicle for progress. It makes little sense, for example, to reduce relaxation by suggesting a sense of heaviness in the body musculature when someone much more naturally responds to suggestions of warmth (i.e., the image of lying down in heated sand), or to more visual scenes (i.e., seeing oneself in a verdant garden or a sunbathed beach) (Kroger 1976).

The ability to create, intensify, and sustain images is enhanced in hypnosis (Hammond 1990). In certain participants, this faculty can be activated to such a degree that the sense of reality recedes and imagery takes precedence. We then have a situation in which the processes of wakefulness coexist with the processes of imagery formation. Further along this continuum, imagery can be so intensely vivid that it is referred to as a *hallucination:* With eyes open, the participant is able to see an object or a person as if it were there. Conversely, the participant might also not see an object that really is there, a *negative hallucination.*

Imagery is turned into a therapeutic tool in hypnosis. Images constructed by the patient can, through their real representations or the symbol they convey, point in the direction of creative insight, enhanced self-perception, personal growth, and problem resolution. Through their influence, they have been found to exert important therapeutic effects (Porter 1978, Sheikh 1978).

Hypnotic Effects Upon the Senses

Every second, in the uncharted leap of body to mind, billions of sensory inflow signals become actualized sensations. A hand dipped in the icy water of a wintry lake, for example, will send signals via the lateral spinothalamic tract to nuclei in the thalamus, then on to the postcentral gyrus. Somewhere along the way, feelings of cold will be created. This raw sensation can, however, be modified by other areas of the mind. The sudden startle of a flight of birds in our wintry scene will shift patterns of perception, and the feeling of cold will momentarily be overridden.

Hypnosis mobilizes this ability to move into or away from sensory experience. Sensations can be made to expand or recede. For example, a participant may be convinced to feel pain more distant, less insistent, less sharp and more diffuse, less lancinating and more soothingly warm, or anesthetizingly cold. The process by which this is done can be learned by the patient for therapeutic gain. The stroke victim can be taught to home in on awareness of the vestiges of sensory inputs in an affected limb, in order to make it more functional with time (Appel 1992, Warner 1988). The child accident victim can be guided to veer away from the insistent annoyance of uncomfortable casts to aid in the quality and speed of recovery.

Memory Changes

As dreams dramatically show, the distant and detailed memories of childhood years can be vividly brought back to us as adults. The nervous system stores every experience. New experiences are recorded in its substance, in a sequenced series of bioexperiential events requiring, for their integrity, the proper functioning of short, intermediate, and long-term memory mechanisms.

Many memories, although indelibly present, do not gain entrance to consciousness because they are connected to too much anxiety or psychic pain. Others are cast aside because, in the priority of things, they have little relevance. Conversely, some memories impinge too insistently upon daily life experience and may be disruptive. With effort, one can push for the retrieval of a forgotten detail or, as in suppression, one can consciously coax into oblivion an uncomfortable fact.

The ability of the mind to modulate access to personal memory stores is itself a malleable quality. In the hypnotic state, the individual may be asked to move away from present reality and to rekindle the remembrance of an event (Dinges 1992, Schacter 1996). This phenomenon of enhanced recall is called *hypermnesia*.

In the phenomenon of posthypnotic amnesia, the subject forgets what has transpired during the hypnotic experience (Williamsen 1965). This effect may occur on its own, or may be encouraged by suggestions (Kinnunen 1996). In either case, the elements of the experience usually return to awareness at some point in the future, typically some days after the event.

Age Regression and Revivification

Whereas memory retrieval and hypermnesia involve a coming to the surface of specific events and effects, age regression implies a more complex phenomenon, namely the reliving of a part of the past in the context of the developmental stage of that time (Orne 1951).

For example, an adult subject (it usually has to be a hypnotically talented one), is asked to travel backward to relive some segment of his adolescence. The hypnotist advises, "You are now about 15 years old. Can you talk about what you are doing and how you feel?" The participant begins an inward search and then talks about an event with varying amounts of detail and effect. Why, of all possible remembrances, did he home in on the memory he chose?

In the hypnotherapy situation, if the event is emotionally charged, the participant may be asked to act as if he is on the side lines, as an observer, in order to reduce the possible affectual impact and its possible disruptive effects. In complete age regression, the episode is relived in all its immediacy and intensity. We are reminded of Penfield's patients who, when cortically stimulated, could actually re-experience segments of their past in their proper sequence (Penfield 1950). With further regression, the expressions, verbal intonations, and the emotional responses of the period re-emerge, turning back developmental time. Regressed to infancy, there may be drooling, monosyllables, and sometimes, amazingly, a Babinski reflex (Raikov 1982). Clinically, age regression and revivification find usefulness in the clarification, release, and reintegration of repressed affect in preparation for conflict resolution and psychological liberation.

"ANESTHESIA AWARENESS" AND ITS RELATION TO HYPNOSIS

The phenomenon of the possible preservation of portions of awareness during chemical anesthesia is not strictly a mainstream feature of hypnosis. However, it presents fascinating theoretical questions and research directions into the dynamics of awareness as they relate to various mental states. The crucial connective thread between hypnosis and anesthesia comes from data suggesting that events occurring during anesthesia may be retrieved by the use of hypnosis (Edwin 1990), and that the process of anesthesia itself may be beneficially influenced by hypnotic intervention (Erickson 1994).

It has been assumed for decades that a patient in the moderate or even deeper levels of chemical anesthesia was in a state of other-worldliness and had relinquished all semblance of consciousness. Some authors (Crile 1947), however, began to study the relationship between anesthesia and awareness and described instances in which the coexistence of the two were not necessarily incompatible.

Recent studies have increasingly focused upon hypnotic recollection of the anesthesia experience (Rossi 1988). Although consciously, many of the patients have little or no memory of their surgical experience, some (especially highly hypnotizable ones) are able to reconnect with these buried memories, in the context of trance.

It has been reasonably established that some patients in such situations are attuned to meaningful communications by the treating personnel (Wilson 1969). This occurrence has prompted hypnotherapists to introduce suggestions to patients awaiting operative procedures; these suggestions are designed to protect the patients against inadvertent negative communications, which may be reacted to, physiologically or psychologically, with nefarious stress reactions. For example, in the event that one of the operating personnel mentions, "there is a lot of blood loss here," the patient may respond with a rise in blood pressure and increased heart rate, promoting cardiac instability. In such a situation, affirmative hypnotic suggestions can act not only as a protective buffer but also as an activator to positive adaptation mechanisms, making successful negotiation of the surgical process more likely (Nathan 1987).

CURRENT CONCEPTS OF HYPNOSIS

Although the manifestations and capabilities of hypnosis have received increasing acknowledgment, the essence of its mechanisms remains difficult to define (Chaves 1994). Today, even with the impressive advances in the understanding of psychological mechanisms, theories of hypnosis are remarkably numerous and divergent (Lynn 1991). The search for a unified theory has been elusive. To be integrated, such a theory would have to explain the multitude of hypnotic phenomena, from age regression to anesthesia and from catalepsy to hallucination; it would have to account for the wide ranges of individual manifestations and show the reasons for the striking subjective experiences that are often induced.

Because theories are approximations, it is probable that several of them are concurrently valid, each seeing a portion of a multidimensional process involving psychological, physiological, and social mechanisms. The following theories are important currents of thought regarding hypnotic phenomena.

Physiological Theories

Those who correlate conditions of consciousness with changes in the central nervous system or those who hold that physiological events may precede all mental events look for physical reasons to explain hypnosis (i.e., variations in the EEG, in evoked potentials, in cerebral blood flow, or in neurotransmitter dynamics) (Spiegel 1992). In the future, as the sophistication in noninvasive central nervous system visualization techniques progresses, the most subtle elements of the physiological accompaniments of the hypnotic condition may yield its yet elusive enigmas. Difficulties with this approach have to do partly with the different manifestations of hypnotic states. For example, in passive or in neutral self-hypnosis, in which participants are physiologically slowed down, we would expect readings in all the previously mentioned tests to be different from those taken during active hypnosis, where the participant, eyes open and alert, may be very task-oriented.

Investigations into the function of the reticular activating system, the diffuse thalamic projections, the activities of the frontal lobes, and the limbic system have been inconclusive. We still do not possess sufficient knowledge about the functioning of these areas of the central nervous system as they relate to the creation of normal consciousness, let alone hypnosis.

There are investigators who share Charcot's concepts that hypnosis is based upon physiological disturbances (Guillain 1955) or Pavlov's ideas of cortical alterations of function and the mechanics of energy in psychic activity (Drabovitch 1934, Kraines 1969). For some, the right hemisphere, with its connectedness to imagery and feeling states, is more involved with hypnotic phenomena (Gabel 1988). Others have been impressed by behavioral or anatomical capabilities such as the eye-roll sign (the capacity of the eyes to roll backward into the head) as reliable indicators of hypnotic susceptibility (Spiegel 1978).

Because body and mind are likely to converge at some yet unknown interface of brain function, it is conceivable that hypnosis, at some level, encompasses some tangible bodily functions. The question remains then: If a particular neurophysiological constellation proves to be a characteristic feature of hypnosis, is it an effect of hypnosis or a cause?

Sleep State Theory

Early magnetists were fooled by the resemblance of the hypnotic state to sleep (Gravitz 1991). They assumed that because their subjects were in a state of slumber, hypnosis was indeed a variant of the sleeping state. Yet, they could not resolve the apparent contradiction that their subjects behaved, in many ways, more as if awake than asleep (Darnton 1970).

In recent years, sleep has been increasingly studied and has become more equated with a state of aliveness than one of suspended animation. It has been divided and subdivided into stages, correlated with a variety of dreaming activities, neurohumoral shifts, neurotransmitter metabolism changes, and chronobiological cycles. Sleep is a dynamic, phasic process with, presumably, several functions, some of which are still unclear. Could hypnosis possibly be one of the many sleep stages? Or is hypnosis a sleep stage with some degree of awareness added to it, as in the phenomenon of lucid dreaming, in which the individual, while remaining asleep, attains the awareness that the dream is, in actuality, part of the process of dreaming itself (Tart 1979)?

Pavlov termed hypnosis "partial sleep." In his view, both sleep and hypnosis resulted from the inhibition of certain cerebral areas. In hypnosis, he postulated, the preservation of "sentinel points" or channels of communication accounted for some limited reactivity to surroundings (Pavlov 1923). Some investigators point out that light sleep can become hypnotic-like by means of establishing rapport through response to suggestion, and that, at times, hypnotized individuals have fallen asleep when left undisturbed or given appropriate suggestions. (Greenleaf 1986).

Because hypnosis has some, albeit limited, common denominators to certain sleep states, it is understandable that the functioning of the neurological pathways involved in the physiology of sleep kindles special inquisitiveness. Among these are certain postulated subcortical sleep-regulating nuclei adjoining the third ventricle, the contributions of the reticular formation, selected pontine nuclei, and the neurotransmitter serotonin. Whether these structures and their associated biochemical components are necessarily directly involved in hypnosis is unknown (Levitt 1963). When global physiological measures are considered, however, hypnosis is very close to wakefulness. Reflexes are not altered in hypnosis, whereas in sleep, they are diminished or absent. Moreover, sleep is accompanied by marked modifications in the output of awareness because it is channeled into the environment, whereas in hypnosis, responsiveness to outside stimuli is preserved. In the current analysis, hypnosis appears to be a condition that is neither the usual waking state nor any of the sleep stages.

Hypnosis as a Modified or Special State of Consciousness

The view that hypnosis is a special state of consciousness finds many followers (James 1935, Silverman 1968) who point out that individuals often report experiences outside the realm of their ordinary reality. Many deeply hypnotized participants describe how incredibly relaxed or peaceful their experience was, and how differently they perceived the flow of time, the configuration of their body image, or the experiencing of their awareness (Shor 1962). The usual waking state has a familiar experiential quality. We know it to be there most of our waking hours and, it is argued, we would know of any significant deviation from it.

During hypnosis, this subjective alteration in the personal field of awareness or aliveness is correlated by "state of consciousness" (or state) theorists to depths of hypnosis (Tart 1975, Ludwig 1972). To determine how "deeply" an individual has experienced trance in this system, we would ask for an introspective report, usually with reference to an arbitrary scale (Tart 1979). For example, zero could represent the usual waking state and 10 the deepest trance the participant estimates could be attained.

State theorists posit quantitative (in, for example, the substantivity of consciousness), as well as qualitative changes (certain mental processes may be more or less operational, that is, shift to primary process thinking, alterations in ego mechanisms, or redirection to introspective orientation).

A strong support for the state theory is the occurrence of trance logic that refers to the ability of deeply hypnotized subjects to experience comfortably the coexistence of logically inconsistent perceptions or ideas (Orne 1959). The "ability of the subject to mix freely his perceptions derived from reality from those that stem from imagination and are perceived as hallucinations" cannot be done by imitators (Martin 1996). However, trance logic is also found in dreams, in primary process thinking, and in schizophrenia. How unique is it to hypnosis?

If the waking state is one state of consciousness, albeit the dominant one, and hypnosis is another, we may then ask, how many states are there? Is there a spectrum of states? If so, how does hypnosis fit into it? Is the usual state of consciousness experienced in the same fashion by everyone, or are there significant individual variations?

The school of states of consciousness develops many of its concepts from Eastern philosophies, which have a much longer tradition of interest in these areas (Sheikh 1981). In the Western tradition, states of mind are often equated with neurological and psychiatric conditions having repercussions upon consciousness (i.e., hyperalertness, sedation, stupor, light coma, or deep coma) and part of the problem in defining hypnosis may be semantic: At this time, we may not have developed the terminology to describe the complex and varied conscious mental configuration in the mind's repertory.

Although theorists often put themselves in state and nonstate camps, these divisions may, in the end, be unnecessarily polarizing (Perry 1992). A more integrated view would see hypnotic phenomena as occurring within the context of certain mental sets (state theory) and as capable of being intensified and shaped by many relevant influences, such as social communication, cognitive factors, and interpersonal variables (nonstate theory).

Hypnosis as an Atavistic Phenomenon

This theoretical view holds that hypnosis represents a more primordial style of mentation, a return to an archaic mental functioning, in which suggestion plays an important role (Meares 1972). This primeval mental state is normally superseded, but not replaced, in the waking state by logical, intellectual, and critical faculties. In this model, during the antediluvian periods of their mental evolution, humans functioned much more fully in modes of thought in which nonverbal communication, "hypnotic-like" rapport, and body/mind connectedness were in prominent evidence (Nash 1989).

In the perspective of this theory, several facets of hypnosis may be explained: In many hypnotic inductions, critical faculties are placed at bay by giving monotonous, repetitive suggestions. The prestige of the hypnotherapist is influential, perhaps in the same way as that of important figures long ago in our evolutionary past. Nonverbal communications are well known to occur prominently in hypnosis (Erickson 1959). The participant often reports being able to draw inferences from many subliminal cues and to have increased sensitivity to the meta-meaning and the emotional messages inherent in communications.

In the atavistic hypothesis, depth of hypnosis can be equated to completeness of regression. Spontaneous pseudo-trance or daydreams could represent a mixture of noetic and atavistic processes. Posthypnotic suggestion phenomena, the remarkable action by which instructions given during hypnosis are carried out seemingly automatically at some point in the future, and sometimes in the distant future, are explained by a mechanism of introjection, in which a participant accepts the hypnotist's messages as his own and carries them out as self-fulfilling time-released personal actions.

The atavistic theory is attractive, but it does not adequately account for hypnotic phenomena such as anesthesia and hallucinations.

Psychoanalytically Oriented Theories

Somewhat similar to the atavistic theory, but much more centered on stages of personal development, are psychoanalytically inspired theories of hypnosis that see portions of the participant's psyche as regressing to an infantile ego state, with the hypnotherapist acting as a parental figure (Schilder 1956). The concept of hypnotic rapport becomes imbued with notions of *transference,* the process by which feelings, attitudes, and wishes, originally linked with an important person in one's earlier life, are channeled onto others (Gill 1959).

Freud had difficulty integrating hypnosis into his psychoanalytic theories. He was strongly influenced by the ideas of both Charcot and Bernheim (Bernheim 1897), but came to see hypnotic phenomena through the perspective of transference (Ellenberger 1970). We may ask whether transference, like suggestibility, is a surface manifestation of hypnosis, or a primary ingredient.

Ferenczi believed that hypnosis recapitulated the Oedipal situation (Ferenczi 1909). He also used expressions such as "paternal hypnosis" and "maternal hypnosis" to further describe the nature of the libidinal regression. If the induction was of the authoritarian or commanding type, the subject would associate the hypnotist with a strong father and, if permissive, with the mother. Implied in this view is a gender-oriented element in the hypnotic condition that, barring some claims by occasional subjects who experience erotic feelings in their trance, is not borne out by clinical observations.

In the psychoanalytic view, hypnosis implies a regressed condition in which magical expectations, dependency strivings, and primitive wishes and fears are operational (Schilder 1958, Gruenwald 1982). Because, seen from this perspective, the hypnotist is placed in an omnipotent position, many psychoanalysts have stayed away from its use. Others, however, pointing to the rich potential of the transference condition implied in hypnosis, have integrated its applications within the psychotherapeutic context (Wolberg 1964).

Hypnosis as a Dissociative Condition

To Haule, the concept of dissociation was central to hypnosis (Haule 1986). Dissociation may be defined as a personality trait, characterized by modification of connections between affect, cognition, and perception of voluntary control over behavior, as well as modifications in the subjective experience of affect, voluntary control, and perception (Sanders 1986). In this process, a body of ideas, emotions, and behaviors is capable of splitting off from the personality to express itself with a certain degree of autonomy. This dissociated material, actively separated from awareness, can be brought to manifest itself through the use of certain techniques, among them hypnosis (Bowers 1991).

Automatic handwriting provides a poignant illustration of this phenomenon: The participant, conscious and alert, can watch his hand write out answers to questions or even produce lengthy narratives, as if detached from the supervision of the self. In this situation, there is an observing ego and a dissociated ego that is perceived by the observing ego as acting independently. In clinical situations, these two egos can be seen when the participant, during induction with the arm levitation method, for example, is amazed to feel his arm rising, seemingly by itself, to eventually touch his face, thus signaling the onset of hypnosis.

Although we do not know the precise nature of the mechanisms of dissociation (Counts 1990), either in the central nervous system or in the psychological architecture, this theory describes some but not all of the characteristics of hypnosis. The relationship of hypnotizability to the capacity for dissociation continues to require further elucidation (Frankel 1990).

Ego State Theory

Ego state theory is closely connected to dissociation theory and also to concepts dealing with the phenomenon of multiple personality, psychogenic amnesia, and fugue states.

Ego state theory postulates the existence of networks of personality traits, experiences, feelings and behaviors, which in various degrees of cohesion are bound by common principles (Watkins 1991). Several ego states may coexist as fairly distinct entities within the same individual, and their boundaries are thought to be loosely defined and malleable, in contrast to the more rigidly constructed demarcations found in multiple personality syndromes. In the hypnotic situation, different ego states may be communicated with, for the purpose of bringing about a more global psychological integration (ego state therapy) (Beahrs 1982).

Behavioral Theories

This viewpoint contrasts with state theories of hypnosis, seeking to strip the hypnotic state of its status as a separate entity or as a distinct condition of consciousness. To bolster this position, some authors point out that all the phenomena said to occur in the hypnotic condition can be produced in normal subjects in their normal waking state (Barber 1995).

If, side by side, we observe a hypnotized subject and a simulator responding to the best of their abilities to the suggestions of a hypnotherapist, we may have cause to wonder who is who. Using this behavioral perspective, it is true that there may be difficulties in telling them apart because responses to instructions can be so convincing in both situations. Is hypnosis a more or less consciously determined simulation? A role play? Could hypnosis be the expression of complex behaviors fashioned from perceptions to social cues?

To cut through the argument of outright mimicry, we could, as amply documented by historical examples (the work of Esdaille in particular [Esdaille 1850]), attempt to perform a major operation on the hypnotized individual without recourse to chemical anesthesia. It is likely that the simulator, on approach of the scalpel, will quickly give up the charade. Simulators may, in addition, have difficulties faking the appearance of a Babinski reflex during age regression, or truly experiencing an auditory or visual hallucination.

Simulation is a conscious maneuver. On a more unconscious level, however, some theorists believe (Sarbin 1972) that hypnosis derives from deep motivations to behave like a hypnotized person should. The definition of what constitutes hypnotic behavior can be overtly or subtly communicated by our culture or by the hypnotherapist who presents cues, verbal and nonverbal, to this effect. This definition would explain the varied manifestations of hypnosis in different cultures and during different historical periods, but it would not elucidate the deeper intrapsychic mechanisms presumably needed for their creation.

The drive to behave in ways suggested by the hypnotherapist is related, in this model, to the completeness of the hypnotic rapport. The strength of the motivation to fulfill the hypnotist's expectations has been proven to be remarkably strong in some individuals (task motivation) (Megas 1975). It is felt that the role-taking behavior of the subject may be so complete, profound, and intense that there is total belief in its consistency and validity. The behavior of the hypnotized individual becomes wholly congruent with self-image and the suggested perception of reality assumes such complete self-syntonicity that phenomena, even phenomena involving the deepest mechanisms of perception and the participation of the autonomic nervous system, are spontaneously expressed.

Hemispheric Laterality Theory

It has been long assumed that the brain is an organ whose symmetry implied an equal sharing, by each hemisphere, of its many functions. For centuries, the contributions made by the brain were not realized; yet the Ebers Papyrus (2500 BC) tells of a man who, as a result of head injuries "lost his ability for speech without paralysis of his tongue." Later, Roman physicians described deficiencies in consciousness, perception, and behavior due to cerebral traumas incurred by gladiators. In 1861, Broca described a patient who had lost the "faculty for articulated speech," with the sparing of verbal and written comprehension, as a result of a left hemispheric lesion. In 1874 Wernicke described a different syndrome, loss of verbal comprehension with preservation of elocution, as a sequela of a lesion in the posterior portion of the first temporal gyrus (Gardner 1975).

Since these early findings, the brain "localizationists" have worked to find discrete territories for each of the many faculties expressed by humans. Although successful for purely motor or sensory modalities, this compartmentalizing approach has had many difficulties with the mapping of associational areas and with such psychological dimensions as emotionality, intelligence, and other higher mental functions. This line of research has provided an appreciation for the intricacies and the plasticity of the brain—as seen, for example, in its adaptation to injury—and for the dynamic interrelatedness of both hemispheres as they complement each other.

Sketching some global differences, the left hemisphere in most individuals has more jurisdiction over expressive speech, syntax, writing, reading, arithmetic, and rhythm; the right hemisphere has greater involvement in processing visual patterns, spatial configurations, holistic analyses, melody, imagery, and the proper interpretation of special meaning and metaphors.

It is in this area that hypnosis and hemispheric function meet (Frumkin 1978). Can resistance to induction be considered a manifestation of logical left hemispheric overbearance? By what neurophysiological mechanisms do techniques such as confusion, paradox, *double-bind* (the simultaneous communication of conflicting messages), or *reframing* (changing a person's perspective of events or situations in order to change their meaning), work to circumvent them? How can abilities inherently present in the right or the left hemisphere be best utilized to enhance the effectiveness of therapeutic hypnotic intervention?

HYPNOSIS—QUESTIONS FOR THE FUTURE

The many unresolved issues concerning the nature of hypnosis and the growing sophistication in its exercise make its future promising in numerous areas, from research to clinical practice. At the same time, and this is seen in the increasing volume of papers dealing with hypnosis (Graham 1991), there is widening medical and public acceptance of its therapeutic potential (Fromm 1972). Since its birth as a science, hypnosis has shown a cyclical evolution with fluctuating levels of interest from the scientific community. Today, however, hypnosis appears to be firmly implanted as a medical tool, and its future is likely to witness its progressive maturation in its varied applications to the spectrum of medical practice (Morgan 1992).

Since the early work of Breuer and Freud, hypnosis has found a place in the study of repression, conversion, dissociation, catharsis, and psychogenic amnesia, among other preconscious and unconscious processes. Although relatively abandoned for decades in favor of free association and dream interpretation (Cheek 1995), hypnosis has recently been "rediscovered" for the experimental investigation of conflicts, for the study of ego

homeostasis and enhancement, and for the therapeutic utilization of imagery. Somewhat akin to the population of identified neurotropic molecules that is steadily growing in number, the dynamics of the psychological processes in hypnosis will likely continue to yield ever greater evidence of their variety, complexity, and plasticity. With this knowledge, techniques of hypnotic treatment will become more efficient and more accessible to patients.

There is currently a tendency to integrate different therapeutic modalities in the promise of achieving more efficient individual change. The future of hypnosis will likely witness studies of its usefulness as a facilitator to other therapies, much as hypnobehavioral approaches have already been applied to systematic desensitization, aversion, flooding, assertiveness training, short-term dynamic psychotherapy, and imagery techniques.

As a quintessential facilitator to mind/body communications, hypnosis will continue to become integrated into holistic patient care. Facilitating this integration is research that points to the interconnectedness of all phenomena, mental and physical, in the organism. Psychoneuroimmunology, for example—the science of the interactive relationship between neurophysiological, immune system, and mental functions—continues to demonstrate the potent contribution of the psyche to the function of all biological processes (Vishwanath 1996).

Some medical specialties geared to the management of human factors inherent to novel technologies will invite specialized mind/body disciplines, including hypnosis, to enhance their therapeutic capacity. In space medicine, for example, the possibility of applying hypnotic phenomena to the problems encountered by space mission crews is being explored. Nausea associated with prolonged weightlessness is a particularly disabling problem, poorly controlled by medications. Self-hypnosis has clear potential to modify, and in many cases to abolish space-engendered symptoms without depressing consciousness or creating side effects. It can also assist in the adjustment to new circadian rhythms and in the attainment of deep relaxation designed to make the best of erratic rest periods. It is conceivable, in future missions requiring long travel time, that crew selection will privilege the ability to induce prolonged trances.

In view of these considerations, it is evident that hypnosis presents fascinating opportunities for medical and psychotherapeutic research. Aside from these very tangible promises, the mental mechanisms responsible for the vast array of hypnotic phenomena, once understood, can open rich insights, not only into the most intimate connections of body to mind, but into the nature of consciousness itself.

REFERENCES

Appel P: Performance enhancement in physical medicine and rehabilitation. Am J Clin Hypn 35(1):13–24, 1992

Balthazard C: The hypnosis scales at their centenary: Some fundamental issues still unresolved. Int J Clin Exp Hypn 41:47–73, 1993

Banyai EI, Meszaros I, Greguss AC: Alteration of activity level: The essence of hypnosis or a byproduct of the type of induction? In Adam G, Meszaros I, Banyai EI (eds): Advances in Physiological Sciences, vol 17. Brain and Behavior. New York, Pergamon, pp 457–465, 1981

Barber TX: Hypnosis: A scientific approach. Northvale, New Jersey, Jason Aronson, 1995

Beahrs J: Unity and multiplicity: Multilevel consciousness of self in hypnosis. In Psychiatric Disorder and Mental Health. New York, Brunner Mazel, 1982

Bernheim H: Suggestive therapeutics. New York, Putnam, 1897

Bishay EG, Lee C: Studies of the effects of hypnoanesthesia on regional blood flow by transcutaneous oxygen monitoring. Am J Clin Hypn 27(1):64–69, 1984

Blakely T: Orientation in time: Implications for psychopathology and psychotherapy. Am J Clin Hypn 34(2):100–110, 1991

Boucsein W: Electrodermal Activity. New York, Plenum Press, 1992

Bowers KS: Dissociation in hypnosis and multiple personality disorder. Int J Clin Exp Hypn 39(3):155–176, 1991

Bowers KS, LeBaron S: Hypnosis and hypnotizability: Applications for clinical intervention. Int J Clin Exp Hypn 37:457–467, 1986

Bryant R, McConkey K: Hypnotic emotions and physical sensations: A real-simulating analysis. Int J Clin Exp Hypn 37:305–319, 1989

Burgess P: The use of hypnosis with dermatological conditions. Australian Journal of Clinical and Experimental Hypnosis 24:110–119, 1996

Chaves J: Hypnosis: The struggle for a definition. Contemporary Hypnosis 11:145–146, 1994

Cheek DB: Why did the fathers of psychoanalysis abandon hypnosis? Hypnos 22(4):211–215, 1995

Counts R: The concept of dissociation. J Am Acad Psychoanal 18:460–479, 1990

Crabtree A: From Mesmer to Freud: Magnetic Sleep and the Roots of Psychological Healing. New Haven, Yale University Press, 1993

Crawford H: Brain dynamics and hypnosis: Attentional and disattentional processes. Int J Clin Exp Hypn 42(3):204–232, 1994

Crile GW: Autobiography. Philadelphia, Lippincott, 1947

Darnton R: Mesmerism and the end of the Enlightenment in France. New York, Schocken, 1970

Davic-Jefdic M, Barnes G: Event-related potentials during cognitive processing in hypnotic and nonhypnotic conditions. Psychitria Danubina 5(1–2):47–61, 1993

Deabler H, Fidel E, Dillenkoffer R: The use of relaxation and hypnosis in lowering high blood pressure. Am J Clin Hypn 16:75–83, 1973

DeBenedittis G, Cigada M, Bianchi A: Autonomic changes during hypnosis: A heart rate variability power spectrum analysis as a marker of sympatho-vagal balance. Int J Clin Exp Hypn 42(2):140–152, 1994

De Pascalis V: EEG spectral analysis during hypnotic induction, hypnotic dream and age regression. International Journal of Psychopathology 15(2):153–166, 1993

Diamolnd MJ: It takes two to tango—Some thoughts on the neglected importance of the hypnotist in an interactive hypnotherapeutic relationship. Am J Clin Hypn 27(1):3–13, 1984

Diehl B, Meyer H, Ulrich P: Mean hemispheric blood perfusion during autogenic training and hypnosis. Psychiatry Res 29(3):317–318, 1989

Dinges D, Whitehouse W, Orne E: Evaluating hypnotic memory enhancement (hypermnesia and reminiscence) using multitrial forced recall. Journal of Experimental Psychology 18:1139–1147, 1992

Drabovich W: Fragilité de la liberté et séduction des dictatures. Essai de Psychologie Sociale. France, Mercure de France, 1934

Dudley DL, Holmes TH, Martin CJ: Changes in respiration associated with hypnotically induced emotion, pain and exercise. Psychosom Med 26:46–57, 1964

Edmonston W: Neutral hypnosis as relaxation. Am J Clin Hypn 20:69–75, 1977

Edwin D: Hypnotic technique for recall of sounds heard under general anaesthesia. In Bonke B, Fitch W, Millar K (eds): Memory and Awareness in Anaesthesia. Amsterdam, Swets Zeitlinger, 1990, pp 226–232

Ellenberg H: The Discovery of the Unconscious. New York, Basic Books, 1970

Erickson JC: The use of hypnosis in anesthesia. Int J Clin Exp Hypn 42(1):8–12, 1994

Erickson MH: Further clinical techniques of hypnosis: Utilization techniques. Am J Clin Hypn 2:3–21, 1959

Esdaile J: Mesmerism in India and its practical application in surgery and medicine. London, Longmans Green, 1850

Fellows BJ, Richardson J: Relaxed and alert hypnosis: An experimental comparison. Contemporary Hypnosis 10:49–54, 1993

Ferenczi S: Introjecktion und Vebertragung. JB Psychoanalyse 1:422, 1909

Field PB: An inventory scale of hypnotic depth. Int J Clin Exp Hypn 13:238–249, 1965

Frankel FH: Hypnotizability and dissociation. Am J Psychiatry 147:823–829, 1990

Freundlich B, Fisher S: The role of body experience in hypnotic behavior. Int J Clin Exp Hypn 22:68–83, 1974

Friedman H, Taub H: The use of hypnosis and biofeedback procedures for essential hypertension. Int J Clin Exp Hypn 25:335–347, 1977

Fromm E: Quo vadis hypnosis: Predictions of future trends in hypnosis research. In Fromm E, Shor R (eds): Hypnosis: Research in Developments and Perspectives. New York, Aldine Atherton, 1972

Fromm E, Kahn S: Self Hypnosis. The Chicago Paradigm. New York, Guilford, 1990

Frumkin L, Ripley H, Cox G: Changes in cerebral hemispheric lateralization with hypnosis. Biol Psychiatry 13:741–750, 1978

Gabel S: The right hemisphere in imagery, hypnosis, rapid eye movement sleep and dreaming: Empirical and tentative conclusions. J Nerv Ment Dis 176:323–331, 1988

Gardner E: Fundamentals of Neurology: A Psychophysiological Approach. Philadelphia, W.B. Saunders Co., 1975

Garver R: Eight steps to self hypnosis. Am J Clin Hypn 26(4):232–235, 1984

Gill M, Brenman M: Hypnosis and related states: Psychoanalytic studies in regression. New York, International Universities Press, 1954

Graffin N, Ray W, Lundy R: EEG concomitants of hypnosis and hypnotic susceptibility. J Pers Soc Psychol 50:1004–1012, 1995

Graham KR: Hypnosis: A case study in science. Hypnos 17:78–84, 1991

Gravitz MA: Early theories of hypnosis: A clinical perspective. In Lynn S, Rhue J (eds): Theories of Hypnosis: Current Models and Perspectives. New York, Guilford, 1991, pp 19–42

Greenleaf E: What to do when a patient falls asleep in hypnosis. In Zilbergeld B, Edelstein MG, Araoz DL (eds): Hypnosis: Questions and Answers. New York, Norton, 1986, pp 160–169

Gruenwald D: A psychoanalytic view of hypnosis. Am J Clin Hypn 24(3):185–190, 1982

Gruzelier J, Warren K: Neuropsychological evidence of reductions on left frontal tests with hypnosis. Psychol 23(1):93–101, 1993

Guillain G: JM Charcot (1835–1893). Sa vie et son oeuvre. Masson, Paris.

Hammond DC: Age-progression. In Hammond DC (ed): Handbook of Suggestions and Metaphors. New York, Norton, 1990, pp 515–516

Harris R, Porges S, Clemenson-Carpenter M: Hypnotic susceptibility, mood state and cardiovascular reactivity. Am J Clin Hypn 36(1):15–25, 1993

Haule J: The perceptual alteration scale: A scale measuring dissociation. Am J Clin Hypn 29(2):86–94, 1986

Hilgard ER: Hypnotic Susceptibility. New York, Harcourt Brace, 1965

James W: The Varieties of Religious Experience. New York, Longmans Green, 1935

Jutai J, Gruzelier J, Golds J: Bilateral auditory evoked potentials in conditions of hypnosis and focused attention. Int J Psychophysiol 15(2):167–176, 1993

Kinnunen T, Zamansky H: Hypnotic amnesia and learning: A dissociation interpretation. Am J Clin Hypn 38(4):247–253, 1996

Kirsh I, Lynn SJ: The altered state of hypnosis: Changes in the theoretical landscape. Am Psychol 50:846–858, 1995

Klein K, Spiegel D: Modulation of gastric acid secretion by hypnosis. Gastroenterology 96(6):1383–1387, 1989

Kraines SH: Hypnosis: Physiologic inhibition and excitation. Psychosomatic 10:36–41, 1969

Kroger WS: Hypnosis and behavior modification: Imagery conditioning. Philadelphia, Lippincott, 1976

Levitt E, Brady J: Psychophysiology of hypnosis. In Schneck JM (ed): Psychophysiology of Hypnosis. Indianapolis, Bobbs-Merrill, 1963, pp 314–362

Liggett D, Hamada S: Enhancing the visualization of gymnasts. Am J Clin Hypn 35(3):190–197, 1993

Lovett-Doust JW: Studies in the physiology of awareness: Oximetric analysis of emotion and the differential planes of consciousness seen in hypnosis. Journal of Clinical and Experimental Psychopathology 14:113–126, 1953

Ludwig A: Altered states of consciousness. In Tart C (ed): Altered States of Consciousness. Garden City, Doubleday & Co., 1972, pp 11–24

Lynn S, Rhue J: Theories of Hypnosis: Current Models and Perspectives. New York, Guilford, 1991

Maiolo AT, Porro GB, Granone F: Cerebral hemodynamics and metabolism in hypnosis. Br Med J 1:314–320, 1969

Malort JM: Active–alert hypnosis: Replication and extension of previous research. J Abnorm Psychol 93:246–249, 1984

Margolis CG, Domangue BB, Ehleben MS: Hypnosis in the early treatment of burns: A pilot study. Am J Clin Hypn 26:9–15, 1983

Martin D, Lynn SJ: The hypnotic simulation index: Successful discrimination of real versus simulating participants. Int J Clin Exp Hypn 44(4):338–353, 1996

Meares A: A System of Medical Hypnosis. New York, Julien Press, 1972

Megas JC, Coe W: Hypnosis as role-enactment: The effect of positive information about hypnosis on self role congruence. Am J Clin Hypn 18(2):132–137, 1975

Melzack R, Perry C: Self-regulation of pain: The uses of alphafreedback and hypnotic training for the control of chronic pain. Exp Neurol 46:452–469, 1975

Morgan J, Darby B, Heath B: The future of hypnosis through the remainder of the decade: A Delphi poll. Am J Clin Hypn 34(3):149–157, 1992

Mott T: Hypnotizability testing and clinical hypnosis. Am J Clin Hypn 32:2–3, 1995

Naranjo C, Orenstein R: On the Psychology of Meditation. New York, Viking, 1971

Nash M, Spindler D: Hypnosis and transference: A measure of archaic involvement with the hypnotist. J Clin Exp Hypn 37:129–144, 1989

Nathan RG, Morris DA, Goebel RA: Preoperative and intraoperative rehearsal in hypnoanaesthesia for major surgery. Am J Clin Hypn 29(4):238–241, 1987

Orne M: The nature of hypnosis: Artifact and essence. J Abnorm Psychol 58:277–299, 1959

Orne MT: The mechanisms of hypnotic age regression: An experimental study. Journal of Abnormal and Social Psychology 46:213–225, 1951

Papez JW: A proposed mechanism of emotion. Archives of Neurology and Psychiatry 38:725, 1937

Pavlov IP: Conditioned Reflexes. London, Oxford University Press, 1927

Pavlov IP: The identity of inhibition with sleep and hypnosis. Scientific Monthly 17:603–608, 1923

Penfield W, Rasmussen R: The cerebral cortex of man: A clinical study of localization of function. New York, Macmillan, 1950

Perry C: Theorizing about hypnosis in either/or terms. Int J Clin Exp Hypn 40:238–252, 1992

Porter J: Suggestions and success imagery for study problems. Int J Clin Exp Hypn 26(2):63–75, 1978

Raikov V: Hypnotic age regression to the neonatal period: Comparisons with role playing. Int J Clin Exp Hypn 30:108–116, 1982

Rossi A, Cavatton G, Marotti A: Hemodynamics following real and hypnosis-simulated phlebotomy. Am J Clin Hypn 40(11):368–375, 1997

Rossi EL, Cheek DB: Mind-Body Therapy. New York, Norton, 1988

Rouget G: La Musique et la Trance. Paris, Gallimard, 1980

Sacerdote P: Teaching self-hypnosis to adults. Int J Clin Exp Hypn 29(3):282–299, 1981

Sachar EJ, Fishman JR, Mason JW: The influence of the trance on plasma 17-hydrocorticosteroid concentration. Psychosom Med 26:635–636, 1964

Sanders S: Clinical Self-hypnosis: The Power of Words and Images. New York, Guilford, 1991

Sanders S: The perceptual alteration scale: A scale measuring dissociation. Am J Clin Hypn 29(2):95–102, 1986

Saletu B: Brain function during hypnosis, acupuncture and transcendental meditation. In Taneli B, Perris C, Kemali D (eds): Advances in Biological Psychiatry: Neurophysiological Correlates of Relaxation and Psychopathology, vol 16. Basel, Karger, 1987, pp 18–40

Sarbin TR: Physiological effects of hypnotic stimulation. In Dorcus RM (ed): Hypnosis and its Therapeutic Applications. New York, McGraw-Hill, 1956, pp 1–57

Sarbin TR, Coe WC: Hypnosis: A Social-Psychological Analysis of Influence Communication. New York, Holt Reinhart Winston, 1972

Sarbin T, Slagle R: Hypnosis and psychophysiological outcomes. In Fromm E, Shor R (eds): Hypnosis: Research Developments and Perspectives. Chicago, Aldine Atherton, 1972, pp 185–214

Schacter DL: Searching for memory: The brain, the mind and the past. New York, Basic Books, 1996

Schilder P, Kanders O: The Nature of Hypnosis, part II. New York, International Universities Press, 1956, pp 45–184

Schilder PF: Regression in the service of the ago. New York, International Union Press, 1958

Shapiro D: Overview: Clinical and psychological comparison of meditation with other self-control strategies. Am J Psychiatry 139(3):267–274, 1982

Sheikh A: Eidetic psychotherapy. In Singer J, Pope K (eds): The Power of Human Imagination. New York, Plenum Publishing Corp., 1978

Sheikh AA, Sheikh KS: Eastern and Western Approaches to Healing: Ancient Wisdom and Modern Knowledge. New York, John Wiley & Sons, 1981

Shor RE: Three dimensions of hypnotic depth. Int J Clin Exp Hypn 10:23–38, 1962

Silverman J: A paradigm for the study of altered states of consciousness. Br J Psychiatry 114:1201–1218, 1968

Spiegel D, King R: Hypnotizability and CSF HVA levels among psychiatric patients. Biol Psychiatry 31:95–98, 1992

Spiegel H, Spiegel D: Trance and Treatment: Clinical Uses of Hypnosis. New York, Basic Books, 1978

Stanton H: Sports imagery and hypnosis: A potent mix. Australian Journal of Clinical and Experimental Hypnosis 22(2):119–124, 1994

St Jean R: Hypnotic underestimation of time: Fact or artifact? British Journal of Experimental and Clinical Hypnosis 5(2):82–86, 1988

Sturgis L, Coe W: Physiological responsiveness during hypnosis. Int J Clin Exp Hypn 38(3):196–207, 1990

Tart CT: From spontaneous event to lucidity: A review of attempts to consciously control nocturnal dreaming. In Wolman B (ed): Handbook of Dreams: Research, Theories and Applications. New York, Van Nostrand Reinhold, 1979, pp 226–268

Tart CT: Quick and convenient assessment of hypnotic depth: Self report scales. Am J Clin Exp Hypn 21:186–207, 1979

Tart CT: States of Consciousness. New York, Dutton, 1975

Tebecis AK, Provins KA, Farnbach RW: Hypnosis and EEG. J Nerv Ment Dis 161:1–17, 1975

Twenlow SW, Gabbard G, Jones F: The out-of-body experience: A phenomenological typology based on questionnaire responses. Am J Psychiatry 139:450–455, 1982

Vishwanath R: The psychoneuroimmunology system: A recently evolved networking organ system. Med Hypotheses 47(4):265–268, 1996

Von Kirchenheim C, Persinger M: Time distortion: A comparison of hypnotic induction and progressive relaxation procedures. Int J Clin Exp Hypn 39(2):63–66, 1991

Warner L, McNeil ME: Mental imagery and its potential for physical therapy. Phys Ther 68:516–521, 1988

Watkins J, Watkins H: Hypnosis and ego-state therapy. *In* Keller P, Heyman S (eds): Innovations in Clinical Practice: A Source Book. Sarasota, Professional Resource Exchange, 1991, pp 23–37

Williamsen JA, Johnson HJ, Ericksen CW: Some characteristics of hypnotic amnesia. J Abnorm Psychol 70:123–131, 1965

Wilson J, Turner D: Awareness during caesarean section under general anaesthesia. Br Med J 1:280–283, 1969

Wolberg LR: Hypnoanalysis. New York, Grune & Stratton, 1964

Zilborg G: A History of Medical Psychology. New York, Norton, 1941

3

Medical Hypnosis: A Historical Perspective

Melvin A. Gravitz

INTRODUCTION

The historical origins of the therapeutic method known in modern times as hypnosis can be traced back more than two centuries. It had earlier been known by a variety of terms, including animal magnetism, mesmerism, artificial somnambulism, induced sleep, personal magnetism, and suggestive therapeutics, among others. Although the early nineteenth century name of hypnotism is now considered archaic and was replaced many decades ago by the current name of hypnosis (Gravitz 1997a), not all modern authorities, including this author, agree that these several terms refer to the same process. This chapter generally uses the term *hypnosis.* The changes in nomenclature over the years reflect the progressive changes in our theoretical and conceptual understanding of the fundamental processes underlying the efficacy of the modality. The various theories that evolved over the past two centuries have been discussed elsewhere in detail (Gravitz 1993a).

Whatever the preferred nomenclatures and theories, hypnosis has proven to be a useful treatment method in a wide variety of medical and psychological conditions. Furthermore, when applied by trained and competent health professionals, hypnosis has been observed to be a benign technique in that significant negative side effects are absent; indeed, any uncomfortable side effects that have been reported by patients tend to be transient and insignificant, and most subjects describe the hypnotic experience in positive terms.

This chapter reviews the historical progression of scientific knowledge of what hypnosis is, how it is induced, and where it can be effectively applied in medical treatment. Elsewhere in this volume, the wide range of modern uses in clinical medicine is discussed.

ANCIENT TIMES

Many ancient people used induced trances as healing mediums, including ancient Chinese, Egyptians, Hebrews, Indians, Persians, Greeks, Romans, and others. The founder of Chinese medicine, Wang Tai, who lived more than 4000 years ago, taught his disciples a therapeutic method that was based on manual passes over the body of the patient and simultaneous incantations for cure. Two centuries later, the Hindu Veda described similar procedures, and the Egyptians more than 3000 years ago utilized healing methods that, by their description, are similar to modern-day applications of hypnosis (Gravitz 1993a).

A number of ancient physicians became aware that there was an interrelationship between mental and physical factors in health and illness. As one example, Hippocrates knew that "the soul sees quite well the afflictions suffered by the body." In ancient Greece, Asclepiades (known to the Romans as Aesculapius) eased the pain and suffering of his patients by stroking them with his hands and inducing sleep-like states in them. He was also aware of the importance of attitude and expectancy on the part of his patients. Many temples were dedicated to him, and, while there, patients were expected and indeed required to have trust and faith in the healing process that was being undertaken. In the Hebrew bible, the "laying on of hands" was described as a treatment method, and later the manual touch of important cultural figures came to be regarded as therapeutic. This so-called *royal touch* was utilized by a number of Roman emperors, and in Europe by the time of the Middle Ages, the *royal touch* was widely applied. Even earlier, certain metals, charms, and amulets were utilized, and over the centuries, suggestion, belief, and expectancy began to emerge as important factors in the curative process even though the ancients did not understand the mechanisms that underlay those processes.

Precursors of Mesmerism

Eventually, the important influence of mental forces on health began to be emphasized by a few physicians. In the later 1500s, Heronymous Nymann wrote about the power of the imagination on health and illness (Diethelm 1970). He realized that the effects of certain medications were due to the imagination (i.e., mental forces) rather than to the intrinsic pharmacological qualities of the drug. Through bold conceptual insights such as these, the links between bodily functions, illness, and psychological influences slowly began to be established.

In the 15th century, Petrus Pomponatius and others believed that illness could be cured by magnetic emanations. He applied metallic magnets to parts of the body where a disorder was considered to reside. He astutely observed that "when those who are endowed with this faculty [of magnetism] operate by employing the force of the imagination and the will, this force affects their blood and their spirits" (Vincent 1893).

In the next century, Paracelsus, a noted Swiss-born physician and philosopher, held the belief that magnetic radiation from the earth affected the body in ways that could negatively or positively impact health. Consequently, following a tradition that predated him, he applied mineral magnets to parts of the body that were considered to be the seat of the illness being treated. His logic was that magnetism could cure and readjust the dysfunction of the body's own magnetic properties that had caused the disorder. At the same time, Paracelsus was aware, as was Hippocrates before him, that thought, belief, and will were critical influences upon the process of health and illness.

During the 17th century, Johann Van Helmont maintained that magnetic powers enabled individuals to influence each other. A similar view was held by William Maxwell, the personal physician of King Charles I of England. In his *De Medicina Magnetica,* Maxwell described a system that he termed *magnetic medicine,* in which he believed that human illness could be cured by transferring it via magnetism to animals and plants (Maxwell 1679). He also believed that a *vital spirit* was present in everyone, and by means of this spirit all living things, including plants, animals, and people, were related to each other. Kenelm Digby, who was a contemporary physician, had developed his own theory of so-called sympathetic medicine in which it was assumed that there was an invisible "powder of sympathy" by which wounds could be treated from a distance. He was apparently not aware of the now known importance of expectation and belief in such a process.

Another important healer of the 1600s was Valentine Greatrakes who treated hundreds of persons in England and Ireland by manually stroking the affected parts of the body in which disease or illness lay. His theory was that by stroking the body the illness was first driven into the extremities and then entirely out of the body of the patient. Often, his patients displayed convulsive movements that were similar to what decades later were called the "crisis" (Laver 1978). The importance of belief and confidence underlies the reported effectiveness of Greatrake's many successes. After a while, however, his reputation began to suffer because it was found that his cures were often temporary, and his patients began to lose confidence in his ability to heal them. Once again, faith, belief, and expectancy underlie this sequence of events (Gravitz 1993a).

During those times, magnetic healing acquired both

good and bad connotations because not all medical authorities believed that magnetism was a positive force, and some even attributed the effects of the magnetic treatment to evil forces. An English contemporary, Robert Fludd, maintained that human behavior, including health and illness, was influenced by heavenly bodies (i.e., the planets, the sun, and the stars). This was a time when astrology was regarded as high science, and the belief that planetary forces affected human behavior was very strong.

In the 18th century, the importance of exorcism as a therapeutic method in medicine became prominent through the work of Johann Joseph Gassner. who was a well regarded authority on that religious ritual. Gassner considered that there were two types of illness: the natural, which was appropriate for treatment by physicians, and the preternatural, or spiritual, which belonged under the care of the clergy. The latter disorders were considered to be diabolical in origin and consequently could be treated only by religious methods.

During the 17th and 18th centuries, a widely held belief was that there were atmospheric influences similar to tides which influenced human health. Richard Mead, a prominent English physician, formulated the mathematically derived position that periodic changes in the atmosphere due to planetary forces induced modifications of gravity, elasticity, and air pressure that impacted the human body in health and disease (Mead 1704). Such views persisted into the 19th century. Thomas Forster held that "peculiar states" of the atmosphere affected the mental state of the individual and could even result in what he termed insanity (Forster 1819).

It was Franz Anton Mesmer, however, who merged the above ideas about atmospheric tides, magnetic influences, exorcism, and other factors into a medical treatment system out of which evolved his own views to which he gave the name *animal magnetism.*

MESMER AND HIS TIME

Modern hypnosis is considered to have its primary roots in Mesmer's theories. He lived from 1734 to 1815, and in his day he was strongly influential in his native Germany and then in France where most of his work was done. His therapeutic methodology, soon known as *mesmerism,* quickly spread to other parts of Europe, especially Germany and England, and eventually to the new United States. Born in the town of Iznang in that part of Europe known as Swabia, Franz Anton Mesmer was the son of a forester. In early adulthood, he studied philosophy, law, and astronomy but eventually he turned to medicine and enrolled at the Medical Faculty

of Vienna in Austria from which he graduated in 1776 at the age of 32. In those days it was customary to write a thesis for the degree of doctor of medicine, and he wrote his on the influence of planetary forces on health and illness (Pattie 1994).

Mesmer's dissertation drew heavily from writers who had preceded him, especially Paracelsus, Maxwell, Fludd, and Van Helmont, but his thesis borrowed principally from Mead's 1704 *De Imperio Solis* (Pattie 1994). In this highly technical work, Mesmer theorized that there were tides on the earth and within the human body that responded to the movements of the planets, and illness resulted when such tides were disturbed (Mesmer 1766). The clinical section of his thesis contained a number of cases in which the symptoms were described as varying with the phases of the moon. These included epilepsy, physical appearance, vertigo, paralysis, tremors, hemorrhages, and numerous other disorders.

After completing his medical education, Mesmer began his practice in Vienna, and 2 years later, he married a wealthy widow. That union enabled him to live in great style and to become a patron of music and opera. He played the glass harmonica, an instrument invented by Benjamin Franklin. As a friend of the arts, Mesmer became the sponsor of the young musical genius Wolfgang Amadeus Mozart, and, in gratitude, Mozart dedicated his one-act opera, *Bastien et Bastienne,* to Mesmer.

Based upon his doctoral dissertation, and with the assistance of Maxmillian Hell, who was the Astronomer Royal, Mesmer began to use custom-made shaped, metal magnets. He applied them to parts of his patients' bodies as treatment for their various illnesses. His reputation grew because of the effectiveness of his magnetic treatments, and his influence spread beyond the environs of Vienna to other venues. The first patient on whom he used his magnetic treatment was a young woman, Franziska Oesterlin, whom he treated in his own home in 1773–1774. This patient was afflicted with at least 15 apparently severe symptoms that were periodic in their manifestations, and Mesmer was soon able to predict their occurrence. He then sought to modify their course, after it occurred to him that he could induce an "artificial tide" and then manipulate that by magnetic influence. Consequently, he had his patient swallow a preparation containing iron after which he attached several magnets to her body, one on her abdomen and two on her legs. The patient soon reported that she felt a fluid running downward through her body and all of her symptoms left her for several hours. Mesmer reasoned that these effects on her could not be caused solely by the magnets but must have arisen from an "essentially different agent," such as by a fluid accumulated in his own person that was transmitted to the patient. The magnets were considered to be a means of reinforcing the animal (i.e., biological) magnetism and giving it a direction.

Another historically important early patient of Mesmer's was Maria Therese Paradis, who was 18 years of age when he treated her. When she was 3½ years old she awoke one morning totally blind. The physicians who examined her considered her condition to be hopeless and diagnosed it as an amaurosis (i.e. a blindness due to injury or degeneration of the optic nerve in which there was no visible damage to the eye and is of unknown etiology) (Pattie 1994). She was treated unsuccessfully by the contemporary methods of electric shock, leeches, and diuretics. Maria Therese's parents provided music lessons for their daughter, and she became a talented singer and player of the clavichord and the organ. When she was 11 years old, Maria Therese became a protégée of the empress and received a pension so that she might continue her musical career.

Mesmer treated Maria Therese with animal magnetism, and some improvements were reportedly observed. Indeed, both Mesmer and Maria Therese's father declared that she was now able to see. Mesmer later reported that complications arose when several prominent physicians who had been unable to cure her began conspiring to remove Maria Therese from his care so that he could not present her to the empress as he had planned. Furthermore, they convinced her father that his daughter's pension might be discontinued if she became merely another young musician rather than a blind musical genius. Therese and her mother did not agree with the father's concerns, and the family's discord affected the daughter, who consequently relapsed. The Maria Therese Paradis debacle quickly became a topic for malicious gossip about Mesmer's unorthodox methods and created antagonism within the medical establishment (O'Doherty 1992).

As a result of the Paradis scandal and the blemish on his personal and professional reputation, Mesmer opted to depart Vienna, and he moved to Paris in February, 1778. At that time, the "city of light" was hospitable to a number of new ideas, even those with little scientific foundation. Mesmer, with his unorthodox medical theories and techniques, soon developed a thriving practice once again. Among his clientele were members of the royal court and upper class nobility, yet he also demonstrated a concern for the lower socioeconomic classes and their medical problems. As a result, he set aside 1 day a week for a clinic at which such generally impecunious patients could come for treatment. Because his case load increased and transportation was difficult in those days, Mesmer also made it a practice to visit outlying areas away from Paris where he could treat villagers. Mesmer was a pioneer in the provision of low-cost health care and the concept of traveling medical clinics.

Mesmer was a prolific author (Mesmer 1781). The year following his arrival in Paris, he published his *Mémoir* in which he listed 27 propositions to explain animal magnetism (Mesmer 1779). These can be summarized as four basic principles: (1) A subtle fluid fills the universe and forms a connecting medium between a person, the earth, and the heavenly bodies, and also between people; (2) disease originates from the unequal distribution of this fluid in the human body, while recovery is achieved when the equilibrium is restored; (3) with the help of certain techniques, this fluid can be channeled, stored, and conveyed to other persons; and (4) in this manner, so-called crises can be provoked in persons and disease cured (Ellenberger 1970).

Mesmer continued to maintain his strong belief in the efficacy of animal magnetism and the conviction that he had discovered a revolutionary natural physical fluid that existed everywhere in nature, in all people, and required no medications. In that respect, it was naive for Mesmer to expect that the French medical establishment would welcome him and his different ideas, which included the belief that all previous medication and treatments were now outdated. If the French medical community accepted his ideas, they would then have to abandon all that was traditional to them and all that they had been taught: thus his arrival in Paris was largely unwelcome. Even so, he quickly attracted a number of disciples, some of whom were prominent French physicians of the day, and these devoted followers were soon organized into a large number of so-called Societies of Harmony throughout France and eventually elsewhere in Europe and even in French possessions overseas.

By the time Mesmer arrived in Paris, he had discontinued the application of mineral magnets to his patients' bodies because he concluded they were unnecessary; and his theory had changed so that he believed that the therapeutic fluid of animal magnetism was transmitted directly from him to his patient, and it was this transferred fluid that readjusted the patient's own bodily fluidic imbalance.

Another innovation of Mesmer's in Paris was his use of the *baquet,* a wooden container containing a mix of magnetized iron filings, water, and glass. A number of iron rods protruded. His patients sat in a circle linked to each other by silken cords, and each touched one of the protruding rods. The theory was that magnetic energy from the *baquet* would traverse through the iron rods into the bodies of the patients and by means of the silken cords around the circle create a sort of reverberating circuit.

In Paris, Mesmer also began to utilize self-hypnosis. This development was important because it emphasized the patient's own input to the treatment. Modern-day self-hypnosis for medical problems can be seen as having originated with this innovation that occurred in about 1779 (Gravitz 1994).

Mesmer's reputation in Paris grew because of his success with a number of medical problems that responded to his magnetic treatments. One such problem of the day was pain during childbirth. Mesmer was the first to use his mode of treatment, in about 1784, for the alleviation of such distress. He was criticized for doing so because certain circles in those days believed that women ought to suffer during childbirth and that it was a positive concomitant. But Mesmer persisted, and, as a result, pain relief for obstetrical and surgical procedures dates its origins to that time (Gravitz 1988a).

In addition, Mesmer was aware of the importance of the relationship between magnetizer and patient, which became known as "rapport." He emphasized that the psychological component of rapport was crucial, for he maintained that animal magnetism "must in the first place be transmitted through feeling" (Mesmer 1781). Magnetic rapport referred to the patient's special feelings toward the magnetizer and to the belief that the patient could sense the magnetizer's thoughts. The reverse was recognized as well, and the term *magnetic reciprocity* was employed to describe this construct. A century later, these concepts led to the important therapeutic findings of transference and countertransference, particularly through the seminal work of Sigmund Freud, a Viennese physician.

Mesmer's animal magnetism had as a principal rule of treatment that the patient experience a so-called "crisis" while magnetized. This crisis referred to a series of convulsive contortions in the patient that occurred at the height of the treatment session and left the patient emotionally and physically exhausted but frequently with remission of the presenting symptoms. The crisis was a precursor of what later became known as *catharsis* and *abreaction.* Today we realize that many of the patients seen at that time presented with hysterically based complaints that were hypersuggestive to the expectations of the mesmeric situation (i.e., demand characteristics, in modern terminology), and they believed in the therapeutic value of the crises.

As a result of the controversy surrounding Mesmer and his methodology, King Louis XVI convened two investigative commissions of inquiry that consisted of distinguished members of French medicine and science. One of these commissions was chaired by Benjamin Franklin, who was then the first American diplomatic representative to Paris. After studying animal magnetism and observing the work of a disciple and not of Mesmer himself, both commissions rightly concluded that the magnetic fluid did not exist. Furthermore, they held that imagination was the essential factor responsible for the positive effects of mesmerism, and because

imagination was at that time regarded as unscientific, animal magnetism was considered an unworthy method of treatment (Franklin 1837).

One of the commissioners, however, did dissent from the majority view: In a minority statement, Laurent de Jussieu, an eminent botanist, wrote that the positive effects of mesmerism had been overlooked by the investigators, and he raised the relevant point that imagination itself might be a useful therapeutic force (de Jussieu 1784). In his own reaction to the reports of the commissions, one of Mesmer's associates agreed that imagination played the greatest role in the positive results of mesmerism. "If Mesmer had no secret then, that he has been able to make the imagination exert an influence upon health, would he not still be a wonder doctor? *If treatment by the use of the imagination is the best treatment, why do we not make use of it?*" (Eslon 1784). A hypothesis was established that subsequently led to significant advances in modern medicine and psychotherapy, including the entire field of psychosomatic medicine.

With the publication of the reports of the two commissions, both mesmerism and Mesmer himself soon faded from the scene. Mesmer left France and died quietly in 1815 close to the village where he had been born.

AFTER MESMER IN FRANCE

Following the departure of Mesmer from France, not all of his associates ceased their interest and work with animal magnetism. Arguably the most noted of these was the Marquis A.M.J. de Puységur. In the late 1700s and early 1800s, he established a laboratory in which he conducted experiments on animal magnetism. He was a man of benevolence who not only treated but also fed the sick who flocked to him. As a result of his experiments, Puységur concluded that it was not necessary to induce the mesmeric convulsions of the crisis. He also noted that his subjects displayed behavior that resembled sleep walking, and therefore Puységur renamed the phenomenon *artificial somnambulism.* He observed that somnambulists would often speak spontaneously of matters that were of concern to them, following which they would report feeling relief (Puységur 1784). This observation was the beginning of the later emergence of catharsis and free association as psychotherapeutic techniques in the work of Sigmund Freud.

Puységur applied his method of induced somnambulism to a variety of medical problems. He treated more than 300 persons, some of whom suffered from severe chronic illness. There were numerous cases of fever, hernia in a child, urinary retention, "sickness in the whole body," functional paralyses, "entrails not performing any of their functions," headaches, "nerves due to a fear," epileptoid seizures and deafness, among other problems (Puységur 1784). It is apparent from his description of these medical problems that today many would be diagnosed as emotional in origin and thereby more responsive to psychologically oriented techniques of treatment. In that sense, his work can be considered as a forerunner of modern psychotherapy.

Puységur himself was convinced of the significance of psychological factors in using his therapeutic method. This was expressed by his motto, which was "believe and will." He later expanded this to a firm belief in one's power and full confidence in using it. By such conclusions, Puységur parted with the theory of animal magnetism of Mesmer and began, without realizing it, to develop the constructs upon which modern psychotherapy and behavioral medicine are based. Thus, the work of Puységur is a bridge between Mesmer, with his mechanistic and physical theory of a universal fluid, and those later hypnotists who rejected physicial explanations in favor of psychological understanding.

Puységur "magnetized" trees in the countryside so that when he was away local citizens could gather around these "magnetized" trees, touch them, and obtain reported therapeutic relief. A later observer, Francois-Joseph Noizet, made the insightful observation that "to me it is obvious that the effect of the tree was nonexistent and that which occurred in its shade was entirely the result of the confidence that was placed in its magnetic virtues" (Noizet 1854). Noizet also emphasized the importance in the treatment process of suggestions made by the therapist, the facilitation of positive anticipation and outlook within the patient, and the establishment of mutual feelings of trust between the therapist and the patient. Important implications for the practice of medicine were derived from these early 19th century conclusions (e.g., bedside manner and the confidence that the patient has in the physician are important elements in the treatment process).

Also in France, in the early 1800s, Jose Custudio de Faria proposed a theory that no special fluid, as maintained by Mesmer, was transmitted by the magnetizer. Instead, Faria suggested that it was the patient himself or herself who generated what he termed *lucid sleep.* Furthermore, he believed that lucid sleep explained why there were individual differences in the response of patients to the magnetic instructions for treatment (Faria, 1819). Another contribution by Faria was that he introduced a new trance induction technique in which the patient was asked to fix his or her gaze on a particular point in their environment, such as the physician's raised hand. This technique was then accompanied by loudly given commands for the patient to sleep. While in the state of lucid sleep, the patient was then given therapeutic suggestions for positive changes in the presenting symptoms. These developments were the forerunners of what came to be known, later that century, as posthypnotic suggestions. Such suggestions continue, today, to be potent means of facilitating positive therapeutic change through clinical hypnosis.

Alexandre Bertrand agreed with Faria that the underlying causes of therapeutic somnambulistic behavior were the result of the patient's own imagination (i.e., mental forces) (Bertrand 1826). These were important views that were later enlarged upon and made a part of the successful methods of treatment by the Nancy school of hypnosis, and they form the basis of modern hypnotic therapy.

It remained, however, for another Frenchman to revive the course of magnetic treatment in France following the decline after Mesmer. Joseph Philippe Francois Deleuze authored an important textbook (Deleuze 1810/1837) and a number of other works. The textbook, *Instruction Pratique sur le Magnétisme Animal,* was widely known throughout France and its possessions, and it was translated into several other languages, notably English. Deleuze's text was one of the important influences in the early history of mesmerism in the United States.

There was another important development in the early 1800s, this time in the area of nomenclature. During those early years, one of the important theories of mesmerism was that it was a variation of nocturnal sleep. Etienne Felix d'Henin de Cuvillers, a contributor to early developments in the field of animal magnetism (Gravitz 1993b), did not accept the fluid theory of classic animal magnetism as proposed by Mesmer but instead considered that mental forces were responsible for the origin of many medical disorders, the so-called magnetic diseases. Further, he proposed that the therapeutic benefits of animal magnetism also had a mental basis. In these views, Cuvillers was many decades in advance of the developments in dynamic psychology and psychiatry that began to evolve in the late 1800s. He proposed, described, and used a system of magnetic nomenclature based on the "hypn-" prefix, referring for example to "hypnologie" and related terms. He did not claim to have originated this vocabulary, noting that the term had earlier been listed in other French publications; however, the terminology beginning with the "hypn-" prefix used by Cuvillers and his predecessors did not enter into wide use after their publication in the early 1800s, likely because there was no strong advocacy for such use. On the other hand, as will be noted, James Braid, many years later in England, actively utilized that vocabulary in his writings, and Braid's medical colleagues soon adopted the more scientifically acceptable term of *hypnotism.* Although the term hypnotism was derived from the Greek word for sleep, this theory is a misnomer, and many years later, this explanation was finally discarded by scientific researchers.

In the early 1800s, mesmerism was utilized for a variety of medical problems. One of the most important of these applications was the use of the modality as a benign anesthetic agent in patients undergoing surgery for a variety of conditions. At that time, surgery, if it was even undertaken at all, resulted in the death of more than half the patients who suffered through it (Gravitz 1988a). The application of hypnosis as surgical anesthesia was first used in France and later in the United States and England. The first documented use for such purposes took place on April 12, 1829, 14 years after the death of Mesmer.

Jules Cloquet, a Parisian surgeon, reported that he had performed a mastectomy on a 69-year-old woman. That case was presented before the Section Surgery of the French Academy of Medicine. (Even this early date may not have been the first case, however, as there are other undocumented reports that much earlier another physician, N. Dubois, had also performed a mastectomy, in 1797, with mesmerism as the anesthetic agent.) Then, in 1829 Jules Charpignon described the use of the method as a surgical anesthetic in the influential *Gazette des Hopitaux* (Bernheim 1889). Jean-Victor Oudet, another Parisian physician, extracted a tooth from a mesmerized patient in 1836 with the patient displaying no apparent reaction of discomfort or pain. A decade later, Loysel, a physician in the city of Cherbourg, amputated a leg and extirpated a gland (Podmore 1909), using mesmerism. Another example of developments in those days occurred in 1847 when a tumor was painlessly removed from the jaw of a man (Bernheim 1889).

DEVELOPMENTS IN ENGLAND

News of the new technique of animal magnestism was brought to England in 1788 by a French practitioner, J. B. de Mainauduc. He arrived in England to present a series of lectures on the method, and soon others, too, presented public demonstrations of mesmeric phenomena throughout England. Also, textbooks that described the theory and methodology began to be published. In addition to the English language translation of Deleuze's textbook, noted previously, Richard Chevinix, who had studied with Faria, published a number of scientific articles on animal magnetism that created much comment in the British medical community. As a result, a number of English physicians became interested in mesmerism and began to practice it. One of the leaders of this group was John Elliotson, a dedicated and caring physician and an important medical educator

and innovator of medical practice aids. It was he who introduced the stethoscope to England. For daring to do so, incidentally, Elliotson was criticized by a number of conservative medical figures. He became interested in animal magnetism and invited a noted French mesmerist, Jules Denis du Potet de Sennevoy (1838), to come to London in 1837 to present a series of lectures and demonstrations. Du Potet was well known for his work with mesmerism in Paris, and his theories stressed the importance of mental influence, or "the soul," in treatment (du Potet de Sennevoy 1838). Elliotson's interest was heightened by his work with du Potet de Sennevoy, and the former began to treat his own patients in England in the 1830s. Elliotson's work in surgery became known even in the far-off United States (Elliotson 1843).

The British medical establishment, though, was antagonistic to his efforts, and he was consequently unable to publish his work on animal magnetism in the traditional journals of the day because of that opposition. Therefore, in 1843 Elliotson established a new journal that he called *The Zoist,* which soon became the most important English language mesmeric periodical of its time. His harsh critics in the medical hierarchy, however, eventually provoked him so that he resigned his academic honors and hospital appointments in 1849. With that development, and the consequent professional demise of Elliotson, mesmerism in England soon became discredited as a legitimate area of medical practice. Interestingly, the same had previously occurred to Mesmer, but as in those earlier times, animal magnetism in England survived. It did so principally through the work of James Braid and several others.

James Braid

Braid was a surgeon in Manchester who was introduced to mesmerism in 1841 by a noted Swiss magnetizer, Charles Lafontaine. Lafontaine came to Manchester to present a number of public lectures and demonstrations of somnambulism. Braid, who originally was a skeptic of mesmerism, initially came to scoff at Lafontaine's presentations, but he was soon impressed by what he observed. Braid then began his own experiments with the magnetic treatment of his own patients (Braid 1843).

At first, Braid proposed the theory that the effects of animal magnetism were the result of fatigued eye muscles, which he believed in turn led to a physiologically based variant of natural sleep. That explanation was neither novel nor new by then, as reflected in the derivation of the term hypnotism by the French in the early 1800s. Braid later coined the term *neurypnology* in 1843 (Braid 1843), which he then replaced by the word hypnotism. Athough Braid is frequently given credit for originating that nomenclature, the credit was not due him; the term was earlier used by the French (Gravitz 1997a). In any event, the word hypnotism, shortened several decades later to hypnosis, was sufficiently popularized by Braid and his colleagues so that it has remained the preferred term. (In certain countries, the field is sometimes referred to as *sophrology,* which is also a derivation of a term for sleep; in most of the world, today's preferred term is hypnosis.)

Another important contribution by Braid was that he influenced the traditionally cautious British medical community to accept his new physiology-based theory of hypnotism principally because it was based upon accepted anatomical and physiological processes. In addition, he rejected the traditional concept of an invisible magnetic fluid and the use of mesmeric passes, which thereby facilitated the acceptance of the field. Braid, furthermore, emphasized the significance of subjective elements in the patient and in the relationship between the patient and the therapist. He was a strong supporter of the view that the mind and the body influenced each other; eventually, he came to believe that the fundamental mechanism in hypnotism was both psychological as well as physiological in nature, and he proposed that hypnotic phenomena were the result of mental concentration on a fixed idea. Thus, Braid's contributions included that he gave his considerable prestige as a surgeon and physician in support of a new and at times controversial therapy. He also popularized a new nomenclature for the old "mesmerism," which made it more acceptable, and he proposed an explanation for hypnotism based on a frame of reference familiar to his medical colleagues.

James Esdaile

A contemporary of Elliotson and Braid was James Esdaile, a Scottish surgeon working in India. Esdaile was familiar not only with the work being done with hypnotism in England but also with the altered states utilized for therapeutic purposes by the local Indian physicians. Esdaile performed several thousand surgical procedures using hypnotism as the anesthetic agent (Esdaile 1846). That number included over 300 major operations, and his mortality rate was about 5% compared with about 50% in surgery elsewhere; because of this dramatic decrease, the work of Esdaile received wide publicity in Europe and America. His reports encouraged the use of the method by other members of the medical community, and they also served to generate considerable interest in the public at large. But soon after his work was published in the early 1840s, the arrival of chemical anesthetic agents diminished the use of hypnotism in surgery. Even though it was undoubtedly successful in

its purpose, hypnotism still was unacceptable to important segments of the medical community. The chemical agents required little training, were more reliable, and perhaps most of all they were part of the medical mainstream that was based in those days upon mechanistic formulations of diagnosis and treatment.

THE LATE 1800s

There was a published report in 1846 that hypnosis was successfully used in Boston, Massachusetts, to put into remission the palpable medically diagnosed breast tumor of a female patient. Several similar cases were contemporaneously published in Elliotson's journal, *The Zoist,* and there are a number of modern reports as well. Among the possible explanations considered in reviewing these accounts is that hypnosis in some people, in an unidentified way, can enhance the body's immune system so that it acts more effectively against the disease process. In modern times, such reports have been subjected to scientific scrutiny, and it does appear evident that hypnosis can in some instances beneficially impact bodily defense mechanisms (Gravitz 1985a).

By the third quarter of the 19th century, the field had begun to decline once again. In addition to the chemical anesthetics that began to be used, another reason for the decline was that the reputation of the field was negatively impacted by fringe practitioners who were outright charlatans, stage entertainers, spiritualists, and other similarly unqualified persons. In the United States in particular, the field was infiltrated by unqualified persons, and there were some hypnotists who unfortunately blended the method with occult beliefs like phrenology, telepathy, clairvoyance, and so on. There is a lesson in this historical development for those practicing clinical hypnosis in our modern times: The professional and scientific community must constantly be aware of and counter the attempts of unqualified persons to infiltrate the field. These days many such persons tend to identify themselves as "lay hypnotists" (Gravitz 1997b). On numerous occasions, the history of medicine has shown that when science and respectable practice are left open to unqualified elements, then respectability and the field itself will inevitably decline (Gravitz 1985b).

DEVELOPMENTS IN AMERICA

Opposition to hypnotism in the United States was not as strong as that in England. News of Mesmer's work had been brought to the attention of no less a figure than George Washington by the noted Marquis de Lafayette in 1784; however, neither Washington nor any other prominent Americans at the time were interested in animal magnetism.

In the early 1820s, Charles Caldwell of Kentucky developed a version of mesmerism, and nearly 20 years later he wrote a book on the subject that reflected the influence of Elliotson, whom Caldwell had met while on a trip to England. In 1829, Jospeh du Commun, an immigrant from France, lectured on hypnosis in 1829 to large audiences in New York City (du Commun 1829). In 1835, Oliver published a physiology textbook that contained the earliest American account in print of the European uses of mesmerism as surgical anesthesia. The work of Charles Poyen, another Frenchman who resided in the United States in the late 1830s, introduced many others to hypnotism, including the noted physicians Amariah Brigham and William L. Stone. (Brigham was a prominent founder of American psychiatry who practiced hypnotism.) Poyen published numerous articles in the *Boston Medical and Surgical Journal* (now named the *New England Journal of Medicine*). In 1837, an American translation of Deleuze's influential textbook also was an important reference source at the time (Gravitz 1993a).

Against the background of these developments, the first recorded use of hypnosis as surgical anesthesia in the United States occurred in Boston in June 1836, which was 2 years before its initial application in England. Benjamin West, who was affiliated with Harvard University, reported the case of an adolescent girl whose decayed molar was painlessly extracted. This dramatic account was an encouragement to others to use hypnotism as anesthesia, and numerous other reports of such applications soon followed (Gravitz 1988a). In the 1840s, professional societies and scientific journals devoted to hypnotism began to organize in the United States. These organizations occurred in various locales, especially in the South and New England. The Medical College of Georgia was a center of hypnotism applied as anesthesia, and New Orleans was an important research and practice center because of its strong French influence. In fact, reports of the Magnetic Society of New Orleans were published by a Paris-based journal.

The United States was also the location for the first applications of hypnotism in treating smoking cessation and dietary management. This occurred in 1847 when a Massachusetts physician, J. W. Robbins, successfully used hypnotic suggestions combined with aversive suggestion with two different subjects. The techniques he used closely resembled those of today (Gravitz 1988b). Such applications anticipated the uses of hypnosis, begun in the mid 20th century, for the modification of noxious habits.

LATER DEVELOPMENTS

Although the use of hypnotism in medicine was dormant in both the United States and Europe from the late 1840s until some 30 years later, renewed interest in the method surfaced in France with the publication in French of Braid's work. His book served to influence a generation of serious French theorists and practitioners, most notably Charles Richet, a Nobel Laureate in physiology. Richet's experimentation with the modality led his colleague, Jean Martin Charcot, to utilize hypnotism himself in 1878. Charcot, who was the most noted and influential neurologist at this time, was a world renowned teacher and researcher and the medical director of a large hospital for the neurologically and mentally disordered in Paris. Theoretically, he conceptualized hypnotism to be somatically determined, and he was a neo-mesmeric fluidist who believed that magnets, auditory stimulation, tactile pressure, and certain metals could induce a trance state. He also held that hypnotism was a pathological condition of physiological and anatomical origins virtually synonymous with hysteria. He and his associates published many contributions in support of his theories, although other investigators did not concur with his views. In the French city of Nancy, a rural physician named August Ambroise Liebeault became familiar with Braid's teachings through the work of Richet and Braid. Liebeault offered his patients the choice of traditional care at full fee or hypnotic treatment at no charge. It was no surprise that the number of those who opted for hypnotism was large, especially because the method proved to be effective in many instances. Liebeault proposed that hypnotism was a mental state similar to natural sleep with the principal difference that hypnosis was produced by suggestion. He also emphasized that the patient–doctor relationship was important in the induction of the trance state (Gravitz 1993a). He emphasized the interpersonal aspects of hypnotic treatment, a point of view that has continued into modern times. Although initially his work was met with benign neglect by many of his colleagues, Liebeault's views became more acceptable when he successfully treated a severely sciatic patient who had not been helped by traditional medical treatments. That case was referred to him by a professor at the University of Nancy Medical School, Hippolyte Bernheim. Bernheim wrote a number of important books, many of which were translated into other languages, and from the beginning he theorized that the key to hypnotism was suggestion (Bernheim 1889). Although the Paris School and the Nancy School were bitter intellectual opponents, and there ensued a struggle of philosophy about hypnotism that lasted several years, eventually the Nancy adherents prevailed, and their theories have shaped professional scientific views on hypnotism to the modern day.

Students throughout Europe and elsewhere came to Paris to study neurology and psychopathology with Charcot. Among them, beginning in October 1885, was a young Viennese physician, Sigmund Freud, who came to Paris for a brief stay of 4 months intending to study neurology and neuropathology. However, as a result of his exposure to Charcot's influential views on mental disorder and hypnotism, Freud changed his career field to psychopathology (in modern terms, *psychiatry*). Freud already was somewhat familar with hypnosis; he had been interested in the field since his medical school days. He and his medical colleague and friend, Josef Breuer, had often discussed the latter's puzzling hypnosis patient, who became known in the scientific literature as the famous case of "Anna O" (Breuer and Freud 1895/1957). Freud's subsequent development of psychoanalytic theory was based initially and importantly on the hypnotically based relationship dynamics (transference) of the Anna O case and other cases. Whereas Freud went on to become a significant figure in the development of the larger field of psychoanalysis and psychoanalytic psychotherapy, he has been a relatively minor force in the larger history of hypnotism. His clinical techniques were limited to direct verbal commands for remission of symptoms, and his theoretical position was that hypnotism was essentially an eroticized-dependant relationship.

In 1896, however, Freud abandoned the use of hypnosis for several reasons, which included his own emotional reactions to his personal experiences with hypnotic patients, as well as to Breuer's traumatic reaction to the Anna O case. Furthermore, Freud rejected hypnotism at a time when his own prestige was rising because of the rapid growth and influence of his evolving psychoanalytic theories. When Freud adopted a negative stand and stopped using hypnosis, other professionals quickly followed his lead and also abandoned the study and use of hypnosis.

Fortunately, because of the successful application of hypnosis to numerous medical and psychological disorders, a number of practitioners continued to apply the technique to their own work. In the United States such practitioners included Morton Prince, Boris Sidis, and John Duncan Quackenbos. In other countries, best known practitioners included Ivan Pavlov (Russia); Pierre Janet and Alfred Binet (France); C. Lloyd Tuckey, Ralph Henry Vincent, and R. W. Felkin (England); and Oskar Vogt, Rudolf Heidenhain, and Albert Moll (Germany). Until the outbreak of the first World War, however, hypnosis and its therapeutic applications were in a period of decline, largely because of Freud's announcement of his "abandonment." During those war years, though, there was a brief revival of the use of hypnosis in trenchline surgical anesthesia and for the psychological treatment of "shell shock." (Today, shell shock has become known as *post-traumatic stress disorder.*)

After the war, although once again hypnosis fell into disrepute, the theories and methods of the Nancy School, based on the psychology of suggestion, remained viable, and continue to influence us even in the present day. The work of Janet in France and Prince in the United States became the basis for our present-day understanding of such psychological phenomena as dissociative disorders and hysteria-based psychosomatic problems.

In the 1920s, two important contributors came forward in the United States. Clark L. Hull was a university professor of psychology who designed a series of laboratory experiments to test some of the underlying and then unresolved questions about hypnosis (Hull 1933). His work served to generate interest in the method among colleagues in the academic community. One of Hull's students was the physician Milton H. Erickson. Although the two initially were collaborators, they eventually parted because Erickson disagreed with his professor's theoretical emphasis on the primary role of the hypnotist and the research-based need for a standardized induction procedure. Erickson himself emphasized the individual subject's own complex and dynamic inner processes, and he developed an approach that was naturalistic, permissive, and indirect (Rossi 1980).

Hull moved away from hypnosis into a distinguished career in other areas of psychology, notably learning theory. Erickson went on to become a prolific and innovative contributor to hypnotic treatment and is perhaps the best known American practitioner in the 20th century and an important influence in other countries as well.

In conceptualizing a psychological link between the mind and the body, Ernest Rossi has recently commented on the unifying role of hypnosis and hypnotic-like phenomena in both the biology and the treatment of a large variety of psychobiological disorders (Rossi 1993). He assembled extensive evidence from the evolving fields of molecular genetics, neurobiology, psychoneuroimmunology (see Chapter 4), and neuroendocrinology, together with new concepts of hypnosis.

SUMMARY

Modern-day applications of clinical hypnosis in medicine and related fields have their historical origins dating back decades and even centuries. These therapeutic applications are considered in detail throughout this textbook. In more recent decades, practitioners have used forensic hypnosis for the retrieval and refreshment of memories from witnesses to, and victims of, crime (Brown 1997). This use has important legal consequences and also has raised research issues regarding hypnosis and the psychology of memory and forgetting.

Currently, hypnosis is on the crest of a wave of interest in application that has increased significantly since the 1930s. Scientific research is voluminous, and modern techniques are pointing the way for increased effective utilization of hypnosis in a variety of clinical and other settings.

REFERENCES

Bernheim H: Suggestive therapeutics: A treatise on the nature and uses of hypnotism (translated from the 2nd French edition). New York, Putnam, 1889

Bertrand AJF: Du magnétisme animal en France. Paris, Ballière, 1826

Braid J: Neurypnology, or the rationale of nervous sleep considered in relation with animal magnetism. London, Churchill Livingstone, 1843

Breuer J, Freud S: Studies in hysteria (translated from the German edition). New York, Basic Books, 1895/1957

Brown D, Scheflin AW, Hammond DC: Memory, trauma treatment, and the law. New York, Norton, 1997

Deleuze JPF: Practical instruction in animal magnetism (translated from the French edition). Providence, Cranston, 1810/1837

Diethelm O: The medical teaching of demonology in the 17th and 18th centuries. J Hist Behav Sci 6:3–15, 1970

du Commun J: Three lectures on animal magnetism. New York, Desnous, 1829

du Potet de Sennevoy JD: An introduction to the study of animal magnetism. London, Sanders and Otley, 1838

Ellenberger H: The discovery of the unconscious. New York, Basic Books, 1970

Elliotson J: Numerous cases of surgical operations without pain in the mesmeric state. London, Baillière, 1843

Esdaile J: Mesmerism in India, and its practical applications in surgery and medicine. London, Longmans, Brown, Green, and Longmans, 1846

Eslon CD: Observations sur le deux rapports de MM. les commissaires nommés par Sa Majeste pour l'examen du magnétisme animal. Paris, Clousier, 1784

Faria JC: De la cause du sommeil lucide. Paris, Horiat, 1819

Forster TIM: Observations on the casual and periodic influence of peculiar states of the atmosphere on human health and diseases, particularly insanity, ed 2. London, The Pamphleteer, 1819

Franklin B: Report of Benjamin Franklin and other commissioners charged by the King of France with the investigation of the animal magnetism as practiced at Paris (original work published in 1784). Philadelphia, Perkins, 1837

Gravitz MA: An 1846 report of tumor remission associated with hypnosis. Am J Clin Hypn 28:16–19, 1985a

Gravitz MA: Early theories of hypnosis: A clinical perspective. *In* Lynn SJ, Rhue JW (eds): Theories of Hypnosis: Current Models and Perspectives. New York, Guilford, 1993a, pp 19–42

Gravitz MA: Early uses of hypnosis as surgical anesthesia. Am J Clin Hypn 30:201–208, 1988a

Gravitz MA: Early uses of hypnosis in smoking cessation and dietary management: A historical note. Am J Clin Hypn 31:68–69, 1988b

Gravitz MA: Etienne Felix d'Hènin de Cuvillers: A founder of hypnosis. Am J Clin Hypn 36:7–11, 1993

Gravitz MA: First uses of "hypnotism" nomenclature: Clarifying the historical record. Hypnos: Swedish Journal of Clinical Hypnosis 24:42–46, 1997a

Gravitz MA: First use of self-hypnosis: Mesmer mesmerizes Mesmer. Am J Clin Hypn 37:49–52, 1994

Gravitz MA: Lay hypnotists and professional psychologists. Presented at the Annual Meeting of the American Psychological Association. Chicago, Illinois, 1997b

Gravitz MA: Scientific responsibility and hypnosis. Am J Clin Hypn 28:90–92, 1985b

Hull CL: Hypnosis and suggestibility. New York, Appleton-Century-Crofts, 1933

de Jussieu AL: Rapport de l'un des commissaires chargés par le Roi de l'examen du magnétisme animal. Paris, Veuve Herissant, 1784

Laver AR: Miracles no wonder! The mesmeric phenomena and organic cures of Valentine Greatrakes. J Hist Med Allied Sci 33:35–46, 1978

Maxwell W: De medicina magnetica. Frankfurt, Zubrodt, 1679

Mead R: De imperio solis ac lunae in corpora humana et morbis inde oriundis. London, Raphaelis Smith, 1704

Mesmer FA: Dissertatio physico-medica de planetarum influxu. Vienna, Ghelen, 1766

Mesmer FA: Mémoire sur la découverte du magnétisme animal. Paris and Geneva, Didiot, 1779

Mesmer FA: Précis historique des faits relatifs au magnétisme animal jusques en Avril 1781. London, 1781

Noizet FJ: Mémoire sur le somnambulisme et le magnétisme animal. Paris, Plon, 1854

O'Doherty B: The strange case of Mademoiselle P. New York, Pantheon, 1992

Pattie FA: Mesmer and animal magnetism. Hamilton, NY, Edmonston, 1994

Podmore F: Mesmerism and Christian Science. London, Methuen, 1909

Puységur AMJ: Mémoires pour servir a l'histoire et a l'establissement du magnétisme animal. Paris, Dentu, 1784

Rossi EL: The Collected Papers of Milton H. Erickson, vol 1–4. New York, Irvington, 1980

Rossi EL: The psychobiology of mind-body healing. New York, Norton, 1993

Vincent RH: The elements of hypnotism. London, Kegan Paul, Trench, and Trubner, 1893

4

Contemporary Context: Psychoneuroimmunology

Karen N. Olness

INTRODUCTION

Psychoneuroimmunology is a term coined by Dr. Robert Ader in the late seventies. The textbook *Psychoneuroimmunology*, published in 1981, actually contained no specific definition of psychoneuroimmunology. In this edition, Dr. Ader wrote the following:

There is a growing awareness of an intimate and relatively unexplored relationship between the immune system and the central nervous system, and an analysis of this relationship might reveal much about the operation of the immune system—and about the brain.

Other people provided definitions, usually those that implied the existence of intentional immunomodulation by humans, something that was not yet proved. The majority of material of Ader's first and second editions of *Psychoneuroimmunology* (Ader 1981) is devoted to animal experiments; however, in the second edition, he became a little bolder in reflecting on a definition:

There is now abundant data documenting neuroanatomical, neuroendocrine, and neurochemical links to the immune system. . . . The existence of bidirectional pathways of communication between nervous and immune systems provides an experimental foundation for the observation of behavioral and stress-induced influences on immune function and, conversely, the effects of immune processes on behavior.

(Ader 1991)

CONDITIONING OF IMMUNOSUPPRESSION AND IMMUNOENHANCEMENT

A serendipitous discovery in mice led Ader into psychoneuroimmunology research: Linking a taste stimulus to an immunosuppressive drug, cyclophosphamide, led to, after relatively few pairings, conditioning the physiological effects of that drug, including not only nausea but also immunosuppression. There have been scores of studies that confirm his initial observation. Immunoenhancement has also been conditioned in animals (MacQueen 1989).

During the past decade a number of human studies have demonstrated the conditioning of immune responses. A study from Germany (Buske-Kirschbaum 1992) demonstrated the conditioned release of natural killer cell (NK) activity in 24 university students. A neutral sherbet was paired four times with a subcutaneous injection of 0.2 mg of epinephrine. Subsequently, the conditioned subjects showed significantly increased NK cell activity after re-exposure to the sherbet. A control group in which the sherbet was paired with subcutaneous saline showed no similar increases in NK cell activity. A study in women receiving cyclic chemotherapy for ovarian cancer found that they not only demonstrated conditioned nausea but also conditioned cellular immune responses (Bovbjerg 1990).

Intrinsic Immune Status Impacts on Animal Behavior

Several studies have shown that animals develop a preference for flavors (CS) that have been paired with drugs associated with recovery from naturally occurring or experimentally induced illness. In Ader's studies, the mice with autoimmune disease failed to show the aversion to the CS that healthy mice manifest (Ader 1991). In further experiments with cyclophosphamide-laced chocolate milk (CY), healthy animals showed a dose-related decrease in consumption. However, lupus-prone mice with symptoms of autoimmune disease drank more CY, enough to reduce their elevated autoantibody titers. Ader concluded that this behavior of animals provides evidence that the nervous system acts on information from the immune system in a manner that is in the best interests of animal survival.

Stress and the Mind/Body Connection

The body's network of immune defenses is intertwined with the nervous and endocrine systems. There are direct physical links and also molecular links via interleukins, neurotransmitters, and hormones. Immune regulators such as interleukins can stimulate nerves to transmit signals rapidly to the brain. The perception of distress by the brain can also activate immune messengers to trigger physiological changes. For example, the sight of something frightening might stimulate production of

corticotropin-releasing factor (CRF) by the hypothalamus of the brain, leading to release of corticosteroids and, in turn, to reduction of inflammatory responses. This reaction could ultimately lead to decreased ability to fight infections, as has been demonstrated by studies of stressed medical students at Ohio State (Kiecolt-Glaser 1984). On the other hand, a depressed hypothalamic pituitary adrenal axis may make some individuals susceptible to allergies or to autoimmune disease.

More recently, Glaser et al have reported that 48 medical students were inoculated with a series of hepatitis B vaccine to coincide with the third day of a 3-day examination series. Students who reported greater social support and lower anxiety and stress demonstrated a higher antibody response to the vaccine and a more vigorous T-cell response to hepatitis B surface antigen at the end of the third inoculation (Glaser 1996).

A meta-analytic study on the effects of stress and relaxation on the in vitro immune response in man reviewed 24 stress studies and 10 relaxation studies (Van Rood 1993). The weakness of the meta-analysis was that it assumed parity among interventions that were, in fact, very different. Some of the studies included in the "relaxation" group asked subjects to focus on changing specific immune parameters; other studies simply asked subjects to relax. The two requests were very different. Relaxation alone and intention alone, without relaxation, have both been associated with changes in laboratory measures of immune responses (Hall 1996). Some of the studies in the meta-analysis included imagery with relaxation. Investigators concluded from the stress study results that observed changes in interleukin-2 (IL-2) receptor expression on lymphocytes and antibody titers against Epstein-Barr virus were consistent for the direction of change and globally significant. Observed changes in percentage of NK cells, salivary immunoglobulin A (IgA) concentration, and antibody titers against herpes simplex virus HSV) were inconsistent and not significant. Analysis of results from the relaxation studies indicated that the observed changes in secretory IgA concentrations were consistent for direction of change and significant, but results for white blood cell counts were consistent but not significant.

Many studies have examined immune responses in depressed individuals. A recent study evaluated immune differences in children with and without depression (Bartlett 1995). Eighteen children who met the criteria for unipolar minor depressive disorder were compared with 18 healthy age-and gender-matched controls. None of the depressed children had ever been on medications for their illness. Each child was seen on one occasion for psychopathological assessments and for blood draws. Total white blood cell and differential counts, T cell, B cell, monocyte, NK, CD4+, and CD8+ cells were measured. Mitogen-induced lymphocyte stimulation was performed, and NK cell activity was assessed. Bartlett et al found lowered NK activity but increased response to ConA (lymphocyte stimulation) in the depressed children. This finding was comparable to those of similar studies with depressed adults (Irwin 1990; Evans 1992).

The measurement of immune measures is complex. For example, only about 5% of neutrophils are circulating at any given time. Measurement of numbers of neutrophils from blood may be a poor measure of what is really going on in the entire organism. Many factors such as nutrition and sleep may impact on immune measures. Perhaps researchers in the next century will laugh about the efforts some of us made in this century to demonstrate that immune measures were affected by relaxation or stress.

Cohen has noted that there is substantial evidence for the plausibility of psychosocial influences on infectious upper respiratory disease in humans and for a role of psychological stress in determining susceptibility for few infectious agents (Cohen 1995). Cohen emphasizes that we still know very little about mechanisms.

The direction or magnitude of the effects of conditioning or "stress" in modulating immune responses of humans depends on the following factors:

1. Host factors such as age, sex, genes, or intrinsic immune status.
2. Quality and quantity of behavioral interventions.
3. Amount and type of relaxation practice, if required.
4. Quality and quantity of antigenic stimulation or exposure to infectious agents.
5. Temporal relationship between behavioral and antigenic stimulation.
6. Nature of the immune response and method of measuring it.
7. Other unknown factors.

Is There Evidence for Intentional Immunomodulation by Humans? What Role Does Hypnosis Play?

The short answer to the first question is a yes, but most reported studies are essentially laboratory studies in normal humans. Clinical implications from laboratory studies are not clear (Halley 1991). There are over 30 reported studies in the English language. Some of the earliest research efforts were made more than 35 years ago by Black in England and Good in Minnesota (Black 1963; Good 1991). Black worked with 28 subjects, each of whom had daily hypnosis practice for 12 days and was then asked to suppress his Mantoux reaction. The majority of subjects were successful. Good's study included three subjects, each of whom had one hypnotherapy session and was encouraged to inhibit delayed cutaneous hypersensitivity response. Each was successful. Black trained a second group of 18 selected adults (Black 1963). Two thirds demonstrated inhibition of immediate hypersensitivity responses.

In 1970 Beahrs et al published an account of a study with five "extremely well experienced, highly hypnotizable" subjects who attempted to suppress the delayed hypersensitivity response; however, there were no changes. In a well publicized study, Smith worked with one experienced meditator who was able to inhibit her response to the varicella-zoster antigen and could replicate this 9 months later (Smith 1985). In 1989, Smith published another study involving 28 "experienced meditators" and demonstrated that this group was successful in both enhancing and suppressing the Prausnitz-Küstner (i.e., delayed cutaneous hypersensitivity) reaction.

Locke et al recently studied 24 college students, selected for their high hypnotizability and ability to change skin temperature with hypnotic suggestions (Locke 1994). Students were assigned randomly to undergo a predetermined sequence of four different experimental conditions with each condition including varicella-zoster (VZ) skin testing: 1) hypnosis with suggestions to enhance the delayed-type hypersensitivity (DTH) response to VZ antigen; 2) hypnosis with suggestions to suppress the DTH response; 3) hypnosis with suggestions for relaxation only; and 4) skin testing without hypnosis. They found no significant effects on the area of the DTH response. Limitations of the study included use of a standardized script and induction technique, hypnotic suggestions given *after* injection of the antigen, and the assumption that high hypnotizability and skin temperature changes were predictors for success. The study found a few individuals who achieved changes in the suggested directions. Such individuals should be studied carefully to guide experimental methods in future studies of intentional immunomodulation.

Kiecolt-Glaser et al conducted an intervention study with the previously mentioned medical students who were randomly assigned to a hypnotic/relaxation group that met in the interval between baseline and examination blood draws (Kiecolt-Glaser 1986). There were no significant differences between the groups who learned the hypnosis/relaxation and those who did not. The number of times of practice by students ranged from 5 to 50. Subsequent regression analyses found that frequency of practice was a significant predictor of the percentage of T helper cells in the examination sample but did not predict either the percentage of suppressor cells or NK cell activity. In a sample of 45 geriatric residents from four retirement homes, Kiecolt-Glaser et al found that those randomly assigned to a relaxation training group showed statistically significant enhancement in NK cell activity and in control of latent HSV-1 virus. (Kiecolt-Glaser 1985). Again, there was no evidence for clinical changes as a result of the relaxation practice in either the medical student or geriatric groups.

Zachariae et al measured effects of relaxation and guided imagery on cellular immune function. Ten healthy subjects were given two sessions of training, one involving general relaxation with a music background and the second involving a procedure to imagine different cells of their immune systems and elimination of an intruding virus. Results found significant differences in NK cell function and no changes in numbers of major mononuclear leukocyte subsets (Zachariae 1990).

A few studies have been done with HIV-1 infected individuals. These have not documented significant clinical changes as a result of meditation or self-hypnosis. A weakness in all of these studies is that group analysis does not recognize important individual differences that need to be considered and that may explain results.

REVIEW OF CHILD STUDIES IN PSYCHONEUROIMMUNOLOGY

The first study related to children was done at the University of Rochester in 1962 (Meyer 1962). This study examined the clinical manifestation of Group A streptococcal infection in children and found that environmental stress was associated with increased clinical streptococcal infections.

The first study to examine the possibility that children might intentionally modulate a humoral immune response was done in Minnesota in 1986 (Olness 1989). The specific aims of the study were to determine if children who learned self-hypnosis would be able to increase salivary IgA and if laboratory values varied according to whether or not children gave themselves specific, directive suggestions. Fifty-seven children were randomized to an attention control group, a group that did self-hypnosis alone, and a group that did self-hypnosis with specific suggestions to increase salivary IgA. Prior to the experiments, children watched a videotape made to teach youngsters about the immune system. The 19 children in the group who did self-hypnosis with suggestions demonstrated a significant increase in salivary IgA.

Subsequently, Dr. Hewson-Bower of Australia replicated the above study and extended the work into a clinical application (Hewson-Bower 1996). The purpose of her clinical work was to determine if children who learned self-hypnosis and stress reduction methods would have fewer colds and flu symptoms than a matched control group. Her results indicated that children who participated in training sessions over a 14-week period were healthier during that period than those in the control group. Their improved clinical status was associated with higher levels of salivary IgA than in the control group.

We did several preliminary studies to investigate the possibility that children might intentionally immuno-modulate white cell function. These studies began in 1977. Although early results were encouraging, the validity of the laboratory tests was in question. Interpretation of results was also confounded by the evidence that most children found the need for blood drawing to be frightening. Therefore, we continued this work with adolescents.

We designed controlled studies involving normal adolescents who were randomized to experimental or control groups. Those in the experimental groups were taught a self-hypnosis strategy associated with suggestions to "increase the stickiness of white cells" (i.e., increase neutrophil adherence). There were two experimental groups named B and C. Group B received no relaxation training prior to the experimental sessions. Group C received four relaxation training sessions 2 weeks prior to the experimental days. Subjects in the control groups (A) were coached to "rest" during the experiments. During experiments, pulse and peripheral temperature were monitored. Following the initial experiment, participants were asked to practice the intervention daily (either self-hypnosis or "resting") for 2 weeks; then they returned for a repeat of the first experiment. Heparin locks were placed in the arms of each experimental subject at the beginning of the intervention. These were analyzed for neutrophil adherence measures (Hall 1992). The control group demonstrated no major changes in neutrophil adherence during either experimental session. The untrained experimental group (B) had decreases in neutrophil adherence during both experimental sessions. The experimental group with prior training experience had increases in neutrophil adherence.

Although practice of self-hypnosis was associated with success in increasing neutrophil adherence, the most successful subjects did not demonstrate physiological evidence of relaxation (Hall 1993). This result suggests that some cognitive effort is associated with intentional changes in neutrophil adherence. The control group, who simply rested, did demonstrate physiological evidence of relaxation.

In a subsequent study, we evaluated the possibility of bidirectional changes in neutrophil adherence. Fourteen subjects were assigned randomly to one of three conditions. Two experimental groups were trained to use relaxation and imagery to either increase or decrease neutrophil adherence in four training sessions over a 2-week period. A control group had the same number of resting sessions without training in relaxation and imagery. Subsequently, all subjects had blood samples collected before and after 30 minutes of self-hypnosis or resting practice. Both experimental groups showed decreases in neutrophil adherence. The control resting group had slight increases in neutrophil adherence. These results suggest that alterations in neutrophil adherence do not follow simply as a result of actively imagining selective bidirectional changes. Active imaging may result in decreases in adherence regardless of the type of imagery. Resting practice may lead to increased neutrophil adherence. Much more research is needed in this area (Hall 1996).

Warts

There are numerous clinical reports about warts remitting in association with nonpharmacological treatment involving some type of relaxation and suggestion (Noll 1994). We designed a consortium study involving seven institutions to study the effects of nonpharmacological intervention on juvenile warts. Children were randomized to either topical or a self-hypnosis treatment group. Each child viewed a videotape about warts, made expressly for this study. Photos of warts were taken when the child entered the study and at subsequent visits for review of self-hypnosis or to participate as an attention control. The logistics of this study were enormously complex, and the study ultimately took more than twice the anticipated time. Seventy-eight children completed the study. There was a diminution of warts in both the pharmacological and the nonpharmacological treatment groups. In these and similar studies there remains uncertainty about what may be predictors for which children are most likely to respond to nonpharmacological interventions.

Juvenile Migraine and Mast Cell Responses

The pathogenesis of juvenile migraine remains unclear. There is evidence in adult migraineurs that mast cell function may be disturbed. It has been known for some time that self-hypnosis tranining in children is an effective and practical strategy to prevent migraine episodes. We investigated whether or not there is evidence of increased reactivity in mast cells of children who have migraines and whether or not self-hypnosis in these children may impact mast cell function (Olness 1996). Thirty-two juvenile migraineurs were randomized to either self-hypnosis training or to a control group. Prior

to intervention they collected 24-hour urine samples. These collections were repeated during a migraine episode and again at 4, 12, and 24 weeks after beginning either self-hypnosis or participation in the control group. Fourteen children in each group completed the study. Although group analysis did not detect significant changes in mast cell function as reflected in urine tryptase measures, the individual children who were successful in reducing migraine frequency also tended to have reduced urine tryptase. At 12 weeks we offered self-hypnosis training to children in the control group who had completed the first part of the study. Two children who began the training shortly after 12 weeks had decreases in urine tryptase at the 24-week sampling. Results suggest that the mechanism by which juvenile migraineurs successfully use self-hypnosis is via stabilization of mast cells.

STRESSORS AND INTRINSIC DIFFERENCES IN BIOLOGICAL REACTIVITY

Boyce et al began a study in 1989 to assess immunologic changes that might occur at kindergarten entry (Boyce et al 1993). Their study protocols focused on individual differences that might mediate responses to stress. Twenty 5-year-old children were enrolled, and blood for immune measures was drawn 1 week before they began kindergarten and again 2 weeks later. At enrollment mothers completed a variety of psychometric instruments including problem behaviors, stressful life events, child temperament, and family environment. During the 12-week follow-up period, the incidence, severity, and duration of respiratory illnesses were assessed from parent interviews every 2 weeks. At 6 weeks, the Loma Prieta earthquake struck; therefore, data assessment was divided into two periods, before and after the earthquake. Six weeks following the earthquake the child behavior checklist was readministered along with a Child Earthquake Experience Checklist, and a Parent Earthquake Impact Scale.

For the three immune measures—the helper:suppressor ratio, pokeweed mitogenesis, and antibody responses to Penumovax—there was broad variability in change scores. This variability was also true for respiratory illness incidence. Upregulation of either helper:suppressor ratio or pokeweed mitogenesis was associated with increased respiratory illness incidence following the earthquake. Change in behavior problems was significantly related to scores from the Parent Impact Scale and inversely associated with pokeweed mitogenesis (i.e., high earthquake-related parental distress and low immune reactivity was predictive of an increase in parent-reported problem behaviors). With low parental distress neither highly nor minimally reactive children experienced a marked change in respiratory illness incidence. By contrast, under conditions of high parental distress, highly reactive children showed a marked increase in illness, whereas minimally reactive children showed a marked decrease.

Boyce believes that the health effects of psychologically stressful events are best predicted by an interaction between the intensity of environmental stressors and the biological reactivity of the individual host. Only a subset of children within any given population are truly at risk under conditions of environmental stress and adversity.

FUTURE RESEARCH RELATED TO HYPNOSIS AND INTENTIONAL IMMUNOMODULATION

The ideal system for the study of immunomodulation does not yet exist. To move toward a clinical intervention that is practical, research would benefit from a biofeedback system capable of providing minute-to-minute evidence of immune changes. For example, if a sensor could be placed over a blood vessel near the skin surface that was able to interpret movements or function of white cells passing by, it would be possible for experimental subjects to recognize whether or not changes in their mental processes affected the white cells. Another variable that has not yet been addressed is that only 5% of polymorphonuclear white cells are in the circulation at any time. The function of those not in the circulation is undoubtedly different from the function of those lying in other areas of the body.

With respect to humoral immunomodulation, research would be more meaningful if there were techniques for monitoring the amount of various immunoglobulins in saliva or tears on a minute-to-minute basis. Development of such techniques seems possible at this time but will require a collaboration among creative biomedical engineers, knowledgeable in tiny sensors, and skilled computer scientists.

In general, researchers in this area need more information about better surrogate markers for immune function. In our recent migraine work, we have examined mast cell products in the urine. Although these tests are practical because they are noninvasive, they give no information about the origin of the mast cell products.

Future research into clinical applications of hypnosis must begin to account for individual differences that predict responsivity, success, or failure—for both adults and children. Research review committees, often not knowledgeable about hypnotherapy, too often demand identical protocols for all participants in a study, which reduces the likelihood of success by individuals. Training in hypnosis must be tailored to individual preferences, imagery skills, communication styles, attentional skills, fears, and likelihood of practice at home. There is little point in developing elegant immune function biofeedback systems if we continue to proceed without more knowledge about individual differences that affect outcomes.

FUNDING ISSUES AND COLLABORATIONS

About a decade ago the National Institutes of Health funded a group of training fellowships in the area of psychoneuroimmunology. As a result, research in this area has burgeoned, most of it being done in animal laboratories. However, most people working in this area find that obtaining funding is difficult. The types of laboratory tests required are very expensive, and studies often take long periods of time. Most groups find that they cannot sustain research for long periods without finding other ways to support themselves.

RESOURCES

The Psychoneuroimmunology Society was founded by Robert Ader and colleagues in 1992. It supports the journal *Brain, Behavior, and Immunity* and sponsors a yearly conference. Membership is by nomination. For further information contact the PNIRS Administrative Office by phone at (217) 244-3156 or via e-mail at esampson@staff.uiuc.edu.

The Biobehavioral Research Consortium was organized in 1985 by pediatricians and psychologists from eight institutions. This group has written several protocols related to hypnosis and has completed one study, the complex multi-institutional controlled study of hypnosis for warts. The most recent meeting of this group was in February 1997. Several protocols have been planned, but, like all of these studies, progress is slow because of funding difficulties.

The International Society for Neuroimmunomodulation supports the journal *Neuroimmunomodulation.* For further information, contact Dr. James M. Lipton, University of Texas Southwestern Medical Center, Department of Physiology, Dallas, Texas 75235-8873. (Phone: (214) 648-3630; Fax (214) 648-7933.)

SUMMARY

A great deal of progress has been made in the science of psychoneuroimmunology during the past 20 years. There is documentation that both immunoenhancement and immunosuppression can be conditioned in animals, that stressors impact immune responses, and that intentional immunomodulation by humans is possible. We believe that humans may be inadvertently conditioning their own immune systems with either positive or negative outcomes. The exciting work of Hewson-Bower has taken these ideas into the clinical arena. Hypnosis may turn out to be an important facilitator of intentional immunomodulation, but more research is needed. We need more information about predictors of success or failure when interventions are used to impact the human immune system via either conditioning or intentional means.

REFERENCES

Ader R: Psychoneuroimmunology. New York, Academic Press, 1981

Ader R, Felten DL, Cohen N: Psychoneuroimmunology, 2nd ed. New York, Academic Press, 1991

Bartlett JA, Schleifer SJ, Demetrikopoulos MK, et al: Immune differences in children with and without depression. Biol Psychiatry 38:771–774, 1995.

Beahrs JO, Harris DR, Hilgard ER: Failure to alter skin inflammation by hypnotic suggestion in five subjects with normal skin reactivity. Psychosom Med 32(6):627–631, 1970

Black S: Inhibition of immediate-type hypersensitivity response by direct suggestion under hypnosis. BMJ 1:925–929, 1963a

Black S, Humphrey JH, Niven JS: Inhibition of Mantoux reaction by direction suggestion under hypnosis. BMJ 1:1649–1652, 1963

Bovbjerg DH, Redd WH, Meirer LA, et al: Anticipatory immune suppression and nausea in women receiving cyclic chemotherapy for ovarian cancer. J Consult Clin Psychol 38:153–157, 1990

Boyce WT, Chesterman EA, Martin N, et al: Immunologic changes occurring at kindergarten entry predict respiratory illnesses after the Loma Prieta earthquake. J Dev Behav Pediatr 14:296–303, 1993

Buske-Kirschbaum A, Kirschbaum C, Stierle H, et al: Conditioned increase of natural killer cell activity in humans. Psychosom Med 54:123–132, 1992

Cohen S: Psychological stress and susceptibility to upper respiratory infections. Am J Respir Crit Care Med 152:553–558, 1995

Evans D, Folds JD, Petittio JM, et al: Circulating natural killer cell phenotypes in men and women with major depression. Arch Gen Psychiatry 49:388–395, 1992

Felt B, Hall H, Coury D, et al: A prospective comparison of self-hypnosis and topical treatment in the management of juvenile warts. Am J Clin Hypnosis, in press, 1998

Glaser R, Kiecolt-Glaser JK, Malarkey WB, et al: The effect of stress on viral vaccine responses [abstract]. Proceedings of the Congress of the International Society for Neuroimmunomodulation 56:13–15, 1996

Good RA: Interactions of the body's major networks: Foreword in Ader R (ed): Psychoneuroimmunology. New York, Academic Press, 1991

Hall HR, Minnes L, Tosi M, et al: The psychophysiology of voluntary immunomodulation. Int J Neurosci 69:221–234, 1993

Hall HR, Minnes L, Tosi M, et al: Voluntary modulation of neutrophil adhesiveness using a cyberphysiologic strategy. Int J Neurosci 63:287–297, 1992

Hall HR, Papas A, Tosi M, et al: Directional changes in neutrophil adherence following resting versus active imagery. Int J Neurosci, 85:185–194, 1996

Halley FM: Self-regulation of the immune system through biobehavioral strategies. Biofeedback and Self Regulation 16:55–74, 1991

Hewson-Bower B, Drummond PD: Secretory immunoglobulin A increases during relaxation in children with and without recurrent upper respiratory tract infections. J Dev Behav Pediatr 17:311–316, 1996

Irwin M, Patterson T, Smith TL, et al: Reduction of immune function in life stress and depression. Biol Psychiatry 27:22–30, 1990

Kiecolt-Glaser JK, Glaser R, Strain EC, et al: Modulation of cellular immunity in medical students. J Behav Med 9:5–21, 1986

Kiecolt-Glaser JK, Glaser R, Williger O, et al: Psychosocial enhancement of immunocompetence in a geriatric population. Health Psychol 4:25–41, 1985

Locke SE, Ransil BJ, Zachariae R, et al: Effect of hypnotic suggestion on the delayed-type hypersensitivity response. JAMA 272:47–52, 1994

MacQueen GM, Marshall J, Perdue M, et al: Pavlovian conditioning of rat mucosal mast cell to secrete rat mast cell protease II. Science 243:83–85, 1989

Meyer R, Haggerty R: Streptococcal infections in families: Factors altering individual susceptibility. J Pediatr 29:539–549, 1962

Noll RB: Hypnotherapy for warts in children and adolescents. J Dev Behav Pediatr 15:170–173, 1994

Olness K, Culbert T, Uden D: Self-regulation of salivary immunoglobulin A by children. Pediatrics 83:66–71, 1989

Olness K, Hall H, Schymidt W, et al: Mast cell activation in juvenile migraineurs [abstract]. Pediatr Res 39:20A, 1996

Pennisi E: Tracing molecules that make the brain-body connection. Science 275:930–931, 1997

Smith GR, McKenzie JM, Marmer DJ, et al: Psychologic modulation of the human immune response to varicella zoster. Arch Intern Med 145:2110–2112, 1985

VanRood YR, Bogaards M, Goulmy E, et al: The effects of stress and relaxation on the in vitro immune response in man: A meta-analytic study. J Behav Med 16:163–181, 1993

Zachariae R, Kristensen JS, Hokland P, et al: Effect of psychological intervention in the form of relaxation and guided imagery on cellular immune function in normal health subjects. Psychother Psychosom 54:32–39, 1990

part two

Hypnosis and the Medical Specialty

Hypnotic Preparation in Anesthesia and Surgery

Rodger Kessler
Thomas Whalen

INTRODUCTION

There are more than 23 million surgical procedures performed in the United States each year (Davis 1987). Although there has been a dramatic increase in outpatient surgeries, almost 50% continue to be inpatient procedures (American Medical Association 1993). Increasingly, providing the best clinical care to surgery patients in the least amount of time is a key requisite of surgical care. Over the last years we have been assisting that process by preparing patients hypnotically and psychologically for surgery. Our experience agrees with the 30 years of research that suggests that outcomes are improved and costs reduced when patients are prepared.

In some areas of surgery and technology the level of surgical and anesthetic skills has improved outcomes to the extent that no further improvement in postoperative return of function, as defined by discharge, is expected (e.g., laparoscopic cholecystectomy). In every other aspect of functioning, the rate of postoperative recovery is determined by the individual's response to the surgical intervention (Kessler 1993; Dane 1993; Mumford 1982). This chapter discusses physiologic and psychologic dimensions that influence each other and the course of surgery and postsurgical recovery. We then elaborate on specific hypnotic and psychological intervention strategies and present two case studies. We conclude with observations about the future of this work.

THE ENDOCRINE AND METABOLIC RESPONSE TO STRESS

Anesthesia and surgery generate a complicated set of stress-producing stimuli. Selye has defined stress as a generalized nonspecific set of responses to protect the organism from harm (Selye 1976). Thus stress can be defined as any demand, exogenous or endogenous, that is *perceived* as a threat to homeostasis. The response that it engenders is the individual's attempt to either maintain the original internal homeostasis or to arrive at a new place of balance. The type and degree of response are dependent upon the individual's perception (which always has an affective component) of the magnitude of the demand and the availability of personal resources (Goldstein 1987; Bandura 1985).

The stress response is easily appreciated in the following scenario. TW is walking in the woods and comes upon a brown bear. As the bear growls, TW is filled with fear. His pulse and blood pressure go up; his skin turns cold and his hair is on end, and without thinking, he is running faster than he has ever run in his life. This reaction exemplifies what we know as the classical stress response, the fight-or-flight response, a physiologic response through the psychological pathway of fear. The fight-or-flight response is mediated by the sympathetic nervous system. Now consider this. It is the next day, a beautiful April day in the north woods. TW walks down to the pond, which is filled with the run-off of melting snow. He decides to jump in. The moment he hits the water, his breathing stops and he can hear his heart beat at an extremely low rate. He cannot move his arms or legs and with no panic he thinks, "I might die here." This physiologic response is yet another classical stress response, the diving reflex, mediated via the parasympathetic nervous system. Most literature (see upcoming information on Bohus) equates stress response with predominant sympathetic response. We ask you to reframe your thinking to allow other possibilities.

The stress response is a complex neuroendocrine affector–effector response that is elicited by a large number of exogenous and endogenous stimuli, including but not limited to surgical stimulation, fear, anxiety, physical trauma, pain, fever, hypothermia, malnutrition, infection, or exogenous drugs. The putative benefit of this response is to mobilize energy and substrate to either avoid injury or to repair injury. This stress response has been most extensively studied in two systems, the hypothalamo-pituitary-adrenocortical and the hypothalamo-sympatho-adrenomedullary, but also involves other neuropeptide and tissue cytokine systems such as insulin, glucagon, vasopressin, angiotensin-renin-aldosterone, growth hormone, testosterone, interleukins, tumor necrosis factor, and so forth. The evolutionary development of this system presumed that the source of all energy and substrate would of necessity be endogenous and of course did not anticipate the availability of exogenous supports routinely available in the practice of modern allopathic medicine. The initial endocrine response to surgical stimulation is an increase in tissue catabolism due to an increase in levels of adrenocorticotropic hormone (ACTH), cortisol, antidiuretic hormone (ADH), growth hormone (GH), catecholamines (epi norepi), renin, angiotensin, aldosterone, glucagon, interleukin (IL 1-8), and a simultaneous decrease in insulin and testosterone.

Elective Surgery and Hypothalamo-Pituitary-Adrenocortical Axis

Plasma ACTH and cortisol levels show a rapid (20–30 minutes) rise to levels two to five times baseline following skin incision and remaining at this level for at least 24 hours (Lush 1972; Scott 1973). The magnitude of the response correlates well with the intensity of the surgical stimulation. The levels of ACTH are greater than the amount required to produce maximal cortisol release. Thoren showed that the usual adrenocortical-pituitary negative feedback loop is not intact, with levels of both hormones elevated above baseline (Thoren 1974). The administration of exogenous corticosteroid does not abolish the postsurgical elevated cortisol-ACTH response. Elevated levels of cortisol and ACTH persist for 3 to 6 days (Johnston 1964); if there are intervening complications, levels are elevated for longer periods.

In total abdominal hysterectomy (TAH), the increase in plasma cortisol can be blocked by adequate epidural or spinal anesthesia but only if the blockade is maintained from S5-T4 (Kehlet 1979; Enqvist 1977). However, Bromage demonstrated that in upper abdominal and thoracic surgery there was no inhibition of the adrenocortical response even in the face of complete analgesia with epidural anesthesia as high as C6 (Bromage 1971). These findings suggest that both autonomic fibers (which follow both intra- and extra-spinal pathways) and somatic afferent nerve fibers are involved in initiating the response. It should also be noted that the inhibition of the adrenocortical response only persists as long as the neural blockade is maintained. High-dose opiate anesthesia (e.g., fentanyl 75 μg/kg) for coronary artery bypass grafting (CABG) surgery has been shown to prevent the increase in cortisol until the patient goes on bypass circulation, at which time there is a profound neuroendocrine response (Stanley 1979). The site of action of high-dose opiates is the hypothalamo-pituitary axis, blocking the release of corticotropin-releasing factor (CRF). Other anesthetic agents do not block the adrenocortical response, except for etomidate, which directly interferes with adrenocortical enzyme activity, temporarily blocking cortisol synthesis without interfering with ACTH levels.

The effect of increased levels of cortisol is to produce a catabolic state. There is hyperglycemia from increased gluconeogenesis and tissue resistance to insulin. There is tissue protein breakdown, especially muscle breakdown, to provide amino acids for the synthesis of acute-phase reactants (as well as gluconeogenesis), which are important in repairing tissue damage. There is increased lipolysis, retention of water and sodium, and increased urinary excretion of potassium. Teleologically these effects would be important to maintain homeostasis in the face of injury; however, continued over time, this response will weaken the individual's reserves. Much of postsurgical care is aimed at supporting the individual to minimize these effects and promote quicker long-term healing. Kehlet and Kehlet and Schulze have shown, however, that the administration of exogenous cortisol plus substrate (glucose, amino acids, fat) plus fluids fails to prevent the changes in cortisol, gluconeogenesis, and tissue protein breakdown that follows surgery (Kehlet 1984; Kehlet 1986).

Elective Surgery and Hypothalamo-Sympatho-Adrenomedullary Axis

Data are inconsistent on the adrenomedullary response to surgical stimulation. Pelvic surgery has been shown to increase levels of plasma epinephrine but not norepinephrine (Nistrup 1978). Both epinephrine and norepinephrine levels are elevated in upper abdominal surgery (Halter 1977). In both of these situations, the greatest elevation in catecholamine levels occurred at the end of anesthesia. The confounding influences of the type, dose, and duration of the anesthetic no doubt contribute to the variability in observations. Each anesthetic agent has its own spectrum of excitatory or depressant effects upon the sympathetic nervous system and may be reflected in varying levels of circulating catecholamines. Other factors of influence include patient individual responses (age, diet, exercise, etc.), depth of anesthesia, fluid or blood volume status, temperature, and presence or absence of neural blockade.

The adrenal medulla and its principal messengers, epinephrine and norepinephrine, are best known for their role in the fight-or-flight response. The hallmarks of this response include increased heart rate, increased cardiac output, increased respiratory rate, and internal shunting of blood flow (more to muscle, heart, and lungs and less to skin and gut), pupillary dilatation, increased auditory acuity, generalized cerebrocortical arousal, analgesia (mediated by catecholamines and endogenous opioids), hyperglycemia, lipolysis, and tissue (muscle) protein catabolism. Although this response is exquisitely developed to protect the individual from injury from an external threat, it may be counterproductive to the recovering surgery patient. Consider the patient with coronary artery disease who has just had bowel surgery: The fight-or-flight response will increase heart rate, pos-

sibly causing myocardial ischemia, and will attempt to decrease blood flow to the gut, possibly causing ischemia at the surgical site.

Neuroendocrine Stress Response to Pain

Sherrington defined pain as the psychic adjunct to an imperative protective reflex (Sherrington 1906). Thus pain includes not only reflex motor responses (to avoid the source of the pain stimulus) but also a perceived unpleasantness that gives pain an affective dimension. The application of a given stimulus, whether damaging to tissue or not, is not a necessary or sufficient condition to produce pain. The aphorism "One person's pleasure is another person's pain" proves true. As well, it should be appreciated that pain may be classified in many ways: imminent superficial/deep pain (related to immediate tissue damage), neuropathic pain (related to morphofunctional CNS changes after the damaging stimulus is no longer present (Fields 1987), psychogenic pain (not related to a prior damaging stimulus), and existential pain (as felt in endogenous depression) (Agnati 1991).

It is beyond the scope of this chapter to review in depth the neuroanatomical correlates of pain. There is general agreement that pain signals are received by both site-specific wired transmission and nonspecific volume transmission (Agnati 1991) in the thalamus and hypothalamus. Next, pain signals are projected to the somatosensory cortex (areas SI and SII of the parietal lobe) for appreciation of the stimulus modality/location/intensity (e.g., burn/hand/30% amplitude) and to the frontal cortex and limbic structures where the affective component of the response is located (comfort/distress; attention/disattention).

The neuroendocrine response to the perception of pain has been studied mainly in the two systems we have discussed previously: the hypothalamo-pituitary-adrenocortical axis and the hypothalamo-sympatho-adrenomedullary axis. Corticotropin releasing factor (CRF) may be the initiating agent for both systems (Dunn 1990), which could account for the integrated response seen throughout systems. Activation of the stress response is not an all-or-none phenomenon but is reflective of the pain modality, its intensity, its location, magnitude of perceived threat versus perceived personal control (Bandura 1985; Davis 1987), prestimulus psychological state (Bandura 1985; Weiss 1970), level of attention/disattention (Bowers 1968; Houston 1972), and other factors.

Various physical and psychic stressors can induce hypalgesia, known as *stress-induced analgesia* (Zieglgansberger 1986). This hypalgesia is mediated by both opioid and nonopioid mechanisms. Catecholamines modulate pain at the peripheral and spinal levels. In addition, the stress response elicits release of opioids from the pituitary (endorphins, dynorphins) and the adrenal medulla (enkephalins), which have peripheral, spinal, and supraspinal effects to decrease pain.

Neuroendocrine Stress Response to Anxiety

Psychological and social stimuli are potent activators of the stress response (Mason 1968; DeWied 1982). Once again, the major effectors studied are the hypothalamo-pituitary-adrenocortical axis (HPA) and the hypothalamo-sympatho-adrenomedullary axis (HSA). Likewise, the end-organ results are the same as those described previously. Research suggests that there are distinctive neuroendocrine responses that are preferred by the pre-existing coping behavioral style. There is also evidence indicating that the kind of control (active/avoidance versus passive/denial) used in coping with a given stress determines whether an adrenomedullary catecholamine response (favoring active control) or an adrenocortical corticosterone response (favoring passive control) is preferred (Bohus 1982). Clinically, this distinction may be operative in the differences between a patient who reads everything he can about a surgery or anesthetic agent (active control) and a patient who tries not to think about what is going to happen, leaving it all in the hands of his doctor (passive control).

Specific dominance of one axis response over the other may determine the resulting affective/behavioral response to a stressor. Animals that are behaviorally active show predominantly sympathetic responsivity to stress (high cardiac, blood pressure, epinephrine, norepinephrine, and corticosterone reactivity to stress), whereas passive animals show predominantly parasympathetic responsivity to stress (Fokkema 1985). Some suggest that the amygdala is the locus of control of the active adrenomedullary response, and the hippocampus-septum is the locus of control of the passive adrenocortical response (Henry 1977).

EFFECT OF HYPNOSIS ON STRESS RESPONSE

Studies have demonstrated variable responses of catecholamines and cortisol to hypnotic intervention (Barber 1984; Goldstein 1987). In a study that dramatically demonstrated the inherent variability associated with hypnotic interventions, Sturgis showed that heart rate, blood pressure, galvanic skin response, and electromyogram responses varied dramatically depending upon the task required of the hypnotic suggestion; for example, heart rate increased with suggestion of arm rigidity/levitation, whereas heart rate decreased with suggestion of deep relaxation (Sturgis 1990). The hypothesis can be made that very different neuroendocrine responses would be measured coincidental with these different suggestions. Another study demonstrated that as subjects face a series of tasks that induced increasing levels of anxiety, catecholamine levels increase (Bandura 1985). Subjects were then taught relaxation strategies to master the anxiety associated with certain tasks. As anxiety ratings fell, catecholamine levels fell to baseline. In the middle of some tasks, it was suggested to subjects that they had lost the ability to master the task, and anxiety and catecholamine levels were found to be even greater than had been seen previously.

The variability seen in HPA and HSA responses to hypnotic intervention is both interesting and encouraging. Rather than bemoaning the lack of "a consistent biochemical response" we can recognize that the *individual's* preferred style of biochemical response was assisted in producing a more rapid and favorable outcome.

The effect of hypnotic suggestion on evoked potentials has been found to be more consistent. Somatosensory- (Spiegel 1989), auditory- (Crawford 1994), and olfactory- (Barbasz 1983) evoked potentials have all been shown to have increased amplitudes following hypnotic suggestions of heightened awareness of the stimulus and decreased amplitudes with suggestions of diminished awareness of the stimulus. Crawford also reported that increased theta electroencephalogram activity during hypnosis corresponded with increased levels of focused attention. Previously, it has been demonstrated that the source of EEG theta activity is deep frontolimbic areas (Michel 1992), which also happens to be the area of origin of response of HPA and HSA axes.

Arendt-Nielsen et al have developed an argon laser model for experimental pain that has been used to measure effects of hypnosis on somatosensory-evoked potentials. Threshold measurements are made to determine the intensity of laser energy at which subjects can first feel any sensation as well as the intensity that elicits the sensation of pain. Hypnotic suggestions of hyperesthesia decreased the threshold of sensory perception by 47% and the threshold of pain by 48%. Conversely, suggestions of analgesia produced increased thresholds of 316% and 190%, respectively (Arendt-Nielson 1990). Irrespective of the biochemical changes that might occur, the electrophysiological response (a measure of the final common pathway) demonstrates consistently favorable responses to hypnosis.

THE PSYCHOLOGY OF CRITICAL EVENTS: MULTIPLE CONTRIBUTORS TO THE STRESS

Psychologically, surgery is a critical event. Prior, during, and after the surgical process, emotional and cognitive reactions generate autonomic arousal. This arousal is a stress activator that is an additional pathway to generating the sequelae previously reviewed. We view surgery and anesthesia as psychologically critical and stress-generating events that are affected by physician–patient interaction, hospital environment, and procedures, current medical and life events, and the individual patient differences that affect their response. Hypnosis focuses on assessing the varieties of patient experiences in each of these dimensions. It generates interventions that target rapid physician–patient relationship development. It helps to overcome obstacles such as developing trust, difficulty talking about a problem, views of medical problems as being independent from psychological issues, and an inability to see solutions to problems.

It should not be surprising that physician–patient relationship is a key factor in compliance with medical advice and in patient openness about medical concerns (Kessler 1996). It is also clear that since this factor began to be investigated by Egbert et al in 1963, such relationship factors contributed to patient readiness, tolerance of and recovery from anesthesia and surgery. Some patients feel best prepared for surgery when they feel they have an active partnership with their surgeon and anesthesiologist. Others feel more comfortable having little active involvement and are most comforted knowing they are in the capable hands of the "expert" anesthesiologist and surgeon. Simple direct questioning about patient preference can establish an important tone for this brief but critical relationship as well as give the physician clues about the types of preparation strategies that can be most helpful. Physician flexibility in responding to patient preference will enhance the relationship and enhance treatment compliance.

It is particularly important to emphasize active relationship development when one considers the hospital environment. Hospitals and operating rooms must function as organized processors of people. Except in acute situations, the hospitalization process is primarily institution and physician driven, and the patient is expected to adapt to hospital, operating room, and physician expectation. This process is frequently isolating and sometimes dehumanizing for patients. Thus the relationship between surgeon, anesthesiologist, and patient and the adaptive skills and strategies patients can learn as part of that relationship strongly influence the patient's response to surgery (Blacher 1987b).

For some patients, life events are not a significant part of their surgical process or recovery; for others, their life events seriously influence the surgical process. A surgeon colleague of ours referred a woman for presurgical preparation for a colostomy closure. He had operated on the woman before and described the experience as "a disaster." He reported that she had come to the hospital for the surgery with an entourage of people, one of whom she insisted had to be in the operating room during the procedure. Prior to surgery she also insisted on calling someone from the operating room. Even though the procedure was technically routine, the surgeon said it was one of the most difficult surgeries he had done because of the psychological, emotional, and behavioral sequelae. Prior to the colostomy closure we did a two-visit preparation. The suggestions focused on a successful, stable procedure that went smoothly. Greater detail of the strategies employed is discussed later in this chapter in a case study. The postoperative course progressed without the sequelae of the first. The patient left the hospital functioning well, 2 days earlier than the surgeon's initial prediction.

INDIVIDUAL PATIENT DIFFERENCES

The hypnosis literature has primarily discussed individual differences with reference to differences in hypnotic susceptibility and the nature of response to hypnosis. However, variation in contextual factors and individual patient characteristics can significantly alter a participant's motivation and response to the surgical experience. Specifically, there are three individual differences of which physicians need to be aware: coping style, prior medical and surgical experiences, and hypnotic ability.

Implications of Coping Strategies

It is frequently agreed that helping patients generate and use coping strategies appears to be the most effective set of intervention strategies in presurgical preparation (Salmon 1994). Patients characterized by avoidance or denial frequently have less positive surgical results (Rogers 1986). It has been shown that patients characterized by avoidance may experience more pain and anxiety if given increased information presurgically (Andrew 1970; Cohen 1973) or gain no benefit from presurgical information provision (Wilson 1981), whereas coping sensitizers increase their rate of surgical recovery with specific information (DeLong R, unpublished data 1970). Taenzer et al have demonstrated that more extroverted patients who are given standard care use more analgesics postsurgically (Taenzer 1986).

Van Dalfsen and Syrjala have suggested that whatever characteristic coping style is used, a patient's sense of self efficacy and confidence in using a coping skill is critical (Van Dalfsen 1990). This need for self efficacy and confidence in being able to cope suggests that in developing a psychological or hypnotic intervention, characteristic coping style must be assessed to shape interventions that patients will believe in and use to influence their medical and surgical behavior (Cohen 1973; Dane 1993). Some evidence suggests that when interventions are tailored to individual patient's coping style, the benefit of the intervention is enhanced (Miller 1988; Mumford 1982).

Previous Medical Surgical Experiences

When a patient comes to surgery, his own prior negative experiences with medical and surgical procedures (or those of his family members) sometimes profoundly influence his function (Blacher 1987a; Kessler 1996). It is often the role of presurgical assessment and hypnotic treatment to identify whether historic medical and surgical events are influencing current patient functioning and, if so, pursue resolution of that conflict. At times the connection may be subconscious. At other times the connection between current and historic events may be obvious to the patient but still significantly interfere.

A 42-year-old woman was scheduled to have a fibroid removed. She was in good health but was panicked by her upcoming surgery. When she was seen, even walking into the hospital was extremely difficult and panic-generating. She related that her father had come to the hospital 5 years before in the terminal stages of lung cancer. She was with him through the hospitalization and at the time of death when he apparently was gasping for breath as he expired. The patient had a vision of his passing in that terrible way any time she thought of hospitals or her uncoming surgery. In this case, brief hypnotic intervention helped her dissociate her father's passing from her own experience, and she went on to have an uneventful surgery.

Hypnotic Ability

A number of studies have recently suggested that hypnotic ability may be associated with the efficacy of presurgical and intrasurgical interventions and influence surgical recovery and psychophysiologic change (Disbrow 1993; Greenleaf 1992; Rapkin 1991; Rondi 1993). Disbrow et al found that suggestion shortened the time to first flatus (60 versus 100 hours), which is an accurate measure of recovery from ileus; time to first flatus had

a nearly significant negative correlation with hypnotic ability; which means the higher the measured hypnotic ability, the shorter the time to the return of bowel function. Rondi et al (Rondi 1993) found that patients with high measured hypnotic ability used significantly less patient-controlled analgesia–delivered morphine than persons with low-measured hypnotic ability, regardless of whether they received intraoperative suggestion or not. In a study evaluating the effects of different preoperative preparation strategies, Greenleaf et al found that measured hypnotic ability was a predictor of surgical recovery independent of experimental condition (Greenleaf 1992). Lastly, in a study of 36 head and neck cancer surgery patients, Rapkin et al found that patients with higher measured hypnotic ability had fewer surgical complications and significantly less blood loss during surgery (Rapkin 1991).

Individual patient differences can psychologically impact presurgical functioning and postsurgical outcome. The isolation of the surgical/hospital experience and current or historical coping style and hypnotizability interact to generate formidable psychological consequences that can negatively influence surgical outcomes.

DEVELOPMENT OF THE PRESURGICAL INTERVENTION HYPOTHESIS

Because of concerns about the physical, biochemical, and psychological stress of surgery and anesthesia and their potential negative consequences, a considerable amount of literature has developed identifying potential stressors and evaluating interventions designed to influence these concerns and effect surgical outcomes. Since Egbert initially evaluated the utility of a support visit the night prior to surgery more than 30 years ago, over 200 citations have evaluated a variety of psychological interventions in anesthesiology and surgery (Kessler 1996). The four major review papers that summarized these 30 years of diverse literature and findings suggest that such interventions consistently provide psychological and economic benefit (Blankfield 1991; Rogers 1986; Johnston 1993; Mumford 1982). In addition, two recent studies continue to support the position that a variety of hypnotic and nonhypnotic interventions both improve dimensions of surgical and postsurgical functioning and demonstrate dramatic cost savings (Disbrow 1993; Rapkin 1991).

A number of authors have found that overall postoperative recovery and functioning is only partially related to a patient's physical state and significantly related to a variety of psychological factors (Kessler 1993; Kessler

1996; Mumford 1982; Blankfield 1991; Kinsmen 1977; Volicier 1977). Such observations have generated the hypothesis that influencing a patient's presurgical beliefs, attitude, and behaviors should influence the course of recovery from surgery, both emotionally and physically. As noted previously, perhaps the best known early effort in this direction was that of Egbert et al, who found that brief procedural information or a supportive visit from an anesthesiologist the night before surgery was related to rapid recovery (Egbert 1963). Since then, other interventions have been used to alter psychological functioning. Information about the steps of procedures, how a patient will physically feel during and after surgery, and sensory experiences have been used with some success (Van Dalfsen 1990; Johnson 1978). Suggestions for shunting blood at the surgical site for rapid resolution of gastrointestinal (GI) ileus and to influence wound healing have been used as strategies prior to surgery (Johnston 1980; Evans 1990).

Effectiveness of Interventions

In the last 16 years, four meta-analyses of the effects of presurgical psychological intervention (including hypnosis) on postoperative psychophysiological recovery have been published. Mumford et al performed a statistical meta-analysis of 34 controlled outcome studies and concluded that (1) surgical patients who were given preoperative information, psychological support, or hypnosis preoperatively recovered more rapidly, physically, and felt better psychologically than those patients receiving ordinary care; and (2) patients receiving psychological intervention had a 2.4 day shorter hospital stay (Mumford 1982).

A review by Rogers and Reich of surgical and obstetrical procedures came to similar conclusions (Rogers 1986). Blankfield then reviewed 18 studies utilizing hypnosis, suggestion, or relaxation to prepare patients for surgery and found that 16 studies credited the intervention with improved psychological or physical postoperative function. Two studies showed no benefit. Blankfield's review showed the following results:

- Seven studies demonstrated shortened hospital stay
- Seven studies demonstrated less narcotic use
- Five studies demonstrated less postoperative pain
- Six studies demonstrated less postoperative anxiety
- Two studies demonstrated less blood loss
- Three studies demonstrated earlier return of GI function (Blankenfield 1991).

It should be noted that not all studies targeted or followed the same outcome variables. For instance, few studies specifically looked at blood loss or return of GI function as outcome variables. In the two studies he

reviewed that failed to show improved outcomes, those patients *did not* have a poorer outcome than controls.

Finally, a review by Johnston and Vogele came to the conclusion that there is substantial agreement that psychological preparation for surgery is beneficial for patients (Johnston 1993). Now we examine the contribution of hypnosis to the improved outcomes found in these reviews.

Hypnosis has been used as a preparation strategy in such procedures as laparotomies, thyroidectomies, mastectomies, cholecystectomies, colectomies, and cardiac and orthopedic surgeries (Evans 1990). Specifically, hypnosis has had multiple uses in reducing anxiety so that use of procedural and sensory information could be effective. It has also diminished the intrusions of worries about surgery or previous surgical experiences (Rogers 1986; Enqvist 1991); reduced premedications and chemoanesthesia (Ridgeway 1982), diminished postoperative pain medication use, reduced units of blood needed postoperatively (Fredericks 1978), and reduced the length of postoperative hospitalization (Salmon 1986). Intervention formats have included taped and face-to-face interventions that were sometimes standardized and sometimes tailored to the identified needs of the patient (Johnston 1993; Fredericks 1978; Hart 1980; Syrjala, Cummings and Donaldson, 1992; Sapirstein 1992).

A significant decrease in perioperative blood loss was found following both preoperative hypnosis (Bennett 1986; Enqvist 1991) and a taped intraoperative protocol (Hart 1980). In a study of radical head and neck surgery patients (Rapkin 1991), average blood loss was 904 mg for high hypnotizables and 2056 mg for low hypnotizables. A significant decrease in required narcotic pain medication has been shown for general surgery (Doberneck 1959; Egbert 1964), oral surgery (Enqvist 1997), radiographic angiographic procedures (Lang 1996), and coronary angioplasty (Weinstein 1997). In the angioplasty setting, patients were able to tolerate significantly longer balloon inflation times (usually leading to greater pain) while requiring less narcotics.

Earlier return of normal gastrointestinal function has been demonstrated with both preoperative suggestions (Disbrow 1993) and with audio taped suggestions for rapid resolution of ileus played for the patient while under general anesthesia (Evans 1988). Significant decreases in the length of hospital stays have been shown with both preoperative hypnosis (Disbrow 1993; Rapkin 1991; Egbert 1964; Bonilla 1961) and with taped suggestions under general anesthesia (Pearson 1961; Evans 1988).

As noted, the literature suggests that hypnotic and psychological preparation for surgical procedures not only impacts physiologic parameters but also decreases the costs of care. In May 1993, Disbrow et al reported in the *Western Journal of Medicine* that in a study of patients undergoing intra-abdominal surgery, the preparation group had a 1.5-day more rapid return of intestinal motility and a 1.6-day shorter time to discharge than the control group, with a cost savings of $1200 per surgery (Disbrow 1993). Also, Rapkin et al compared the use of hypnotic preparation with the usual preparation for head and neck cancer surgery. In their study, hypnotic preparations were associated with fewer complications and postoperative stays 5 days shorter, with an average reduction in cost of $6725 per hospitalization (Rapkin 1991). It must also be recognized that there are small numbers of reported studies that have shown no benefit for either preoperative hypnosis (Surman 1974; Greenleaf 1992) or intraoperative suggestions (Abramson 1966).

There is emerging support for the position that perioperative tailored interventions are superior to standardized interventions. Enqvist has demonstrated that use of preoperative hypnosis had a greater effect in controlling the amount of blood loss than did therapeutic suggestion during surgery (Enqvist 1991; Enqvist 1995). Also, Syrjala et al found individualized hypnosis to be superior to information alone in association with coping strategies for pain reduction in bone marrow transplants (Syrjala 1992).

Hypnosis is such an appealing intervention that it may seem intuitive to want to use it with a broad variety of patients. Be reminded that individual variation in hypnotic ability or hypnotic susceptibility varies. Hilgard established that 15% to 20% of the population is highly susceptible, 15% to 20% of the population has very limited susceptibility, and the remaining population falls somewhere in the middle. An earlier review suggests that hypnotic ability may influence both surgical recovery and the efficacy of presurgical interventions; given the limited time available for hypnotic interventions with surgical patients, some sense of hypnotic susceptibility may predict the rapidity of patient involvement in hypnosis and whether to use hypnosis as the primary preparation intervention or whether to consider a different psychological preparation strategy. For a more thorough discussion of this issue see Kessler and Dane, 1996.

HYPNOTIC AND PSYCHOLOGICAL INTERVENTION STRATEGIES

Earlier in the chapter we discussed our view of hypnosis as part of a set of psychological strategies in response to the critical event of anesthesia and surgery. To understand the utility of hypnotic intervention strategies, it is important to understand the range of strategies that can be used within and outside of hypnosis. We discuss strategies for preoperative preparation (prior to arrival for surgery) and then discuss strategies for use in and around the operating room environment.

The initial focus of preparatory strategies was the provision of information about what a patient would feel during and after a procedure, information about how long a procedure and recovery would take, and information about what would happen during anesthesia and surgery. Research has concluded that the usefulness of providing information as a primary preparation strategy is limited (Salmon 1994). It was observed earlier that *patients who cope best by knowing more benefit from information provision as part of their preparation (Kessler 1996), but patients who avoid information will function poorly when it is provided* (Cohen 1973; Wilson 1981). For example, if after being told that surgery is imminent a patient has asked questions about diagnosis, procedure, recovery, or other similar issues, ask him if all of his questions have been answered or if additional information is required. Conversely, if presented with the same scenario about an upcoming surgery a patient asks very little and has minimal external response, take more time with the patient, express confidence in the physicians involved in the care, help your patient to understand what is important to their care, and provide no more information than is necessary.

Over the last number of years there has been support for the position that cognitive coping strategies are a key component in successful presurgical preparation (Salmon 1994; Kessler 1996; Kessler 1997). Patients are taught ways of responding to specific situations that will occur during anesthesia and surgery, strategies to accomplish difficult activities that enhance recovery, and general strategies to respond to unanticipated events. An example is teaching a patient to deepen relaxation while riding in the car coming to the hospital. This strategy is a general one for responding to increased anxiety. Rehearsing the steps to recovering successfully, including each of the stages up to, through, and after the procedure, would be taught to a patient who needs to preserve a sense of control.

For many patients we have discovered that the key to successful preparation is a patient's perceived self control, whether through active or passive strategies. We attempt to provide skills that allow the patients to control how they are presenting and conducting themselves during anesthesia and surgery. For example, preparation strategies can be rehearsed just prior to surgery. Just being able to play an audio tape of music or suggestions for rapid recovery even under general anesthesia can enhance perceived control. This sense of increased effectiveness or self-efficacy has been long studied by

Bandura, with consistent findings of positive relationships between improved self-efficacy and clinical outcome.

Hypnosis can create rapid patient involvement and a rapid relationship development between physician and patient. Hypnosis can also quickly generate useful physiologic changes such as temperature, respiration, muscle tension, and pain in the patient. These changes are important to the process and are a direct feedback to the patient about his ability to change his physical response. Hypnosis allows patients to identify cognitive and emotional factors influencing an upcoming procedure and targets the direction of preparatory intervention. Hypnosis is a procedure that allows access to cognitive emotional and physiologic parameters at the same time, helping patients to understand and experience the relationship between mind and body. This multi-sensorial access allows a patient to experience the situation in a greater variety of ways, providing broader sets of possibilities. Use of "hypnotic" as opposed to "nonhypnotic" strategies enhances effectiveness. Kirsch et al have demonstrated that beliefs and expectancies are powerful predictors of patient response. They have shown that if one gives the same cognitive behavioral treatments to two different groups of patients, including relaxation training, by labeling one treatment hypnosis one creates significantly better outcomes than the other treatment that was not labeled hypnosis (Kirsch 1995).

This result suggests that we have the ability to influence the patient's experience in a variety of senses. We can help create certain beliefs, attitudes, ways of viewing and doing things to amplify the most favorable outcomes. Among the sensations that are part of a patient's life experiences related to upcoming surgery are thinking, coping, remembering, believing, feeling, autonomic arousal, and sensory experience. For example, a patient may think that surgery is going to be difficult because of past memories of surgical difficulty, hyperarousal, and pain when exposed to any medical procedure involving insertion of needles. This patient needs (1) assistance to change this perception (thoughts) of surgery as a difficult experience, (2) to separate the memory and feelings of prior experience from the present situation, and (3) to learn control of autonomic reactivity in the presence of a stressor, such as a needle. Another patient may have a coping need for information, fears the unknown of the future, and is physically tense and hyperanxious about an upcoming surgery. This patient needs (1) information, (2) a sense of active partnership with the physician, (3) training in relaxation and diaphragmatic breathing, and (4) rehearsal of moving through the steps before, during, and after the surgery leading to a successful outcome. Parenthetically, switching the strategies for these patients could produce negative consequences and perhaps negative complications and outcomes of both the preparation and the surgery.

STRATEGIES FOR MEDIATING THE EFFECT OF THE OPERATING ROOM ENVIRONMENT AND PROCEDURES IN THE SURGICAL PROCESS

The surgical experience begins with the preoperative anesthesia visit and extends through the period of convalescence. Pennebaker has shown that anxiety as measured by the Spielberger State Trait Anxiety Inventory (STAI) is elevated 2 to 4 days preoperatively (this represented the earliest testing of subjects, so it is likely that anxiety levels are increased for an even longer preoperative period) and remains elevated for at least 2 weeks postoperatively (Pennebaker 1977). At the time of the preoperative visit, medical, anesthesia, and nursing-related questions should be answered. Also during this period, ideally 2 to 7 days preoperatively, appropriate psychological support should be initiated. The psychological support may include a focused one-on-one session or taped suggestions, as well as routine supportive suggestions that should be embedded within the medical/anesthesia/nursing assessment process. The approach of the caregiver to the patient, especially with regard to language and images, should be tailored to support the individual's coping response to surgery. Avoiders should not be given more information than they want. When a patient states that "it's all in the hands of my doctors and I trust them," this is a very clear message that the patient will not be helped by a lot of detailed information. For avoiders, it is far more appropriate to support their belief that everything is being handled well by their doctors; suggestions that encourage nonconscious healing may be helpful as in the following example. "As you are given any information, you can choose to pay attention to as much or as little as you wish and you know that your body is doing everything that is necessary to ensure a quick recovery without your having to even think about it."

Patients who are clear that they need answers to their questions to feel ready for surgery should be given as much information as they desire, while keying this information into the recovery process. A physician can easily ask such patients if they feel that all of their questions have been answered and supply any other information that is needed. For example:

Postoperatively, you may experience some discomfort, especially in the area of your incision. The discomfort is actually a sign that the healing process is progressing; the chemicals that are released at the site of the incision that promote healing are also the chemicals that cause the sensation of pain. By taking several deep breaths and then gently exercising the muscles, you will be helping the healing process. In addition, you will always be able to receive as much pain medicine as you need (especially if patient-controlled analgesia is used) to control the discomfort.

Often language used by operating room personnel such as anesthesiologists, surgeons, and nurses communicate to patients how they *will* feel, such as "you will be given medication for your pain" or "you won't be able to move your legs when you awake." At no time should patients be told what they *will* feel; rather, information should be framed to enhance broad, positive possibility, such as the following statements:

- Some people experience nausea after surgery but you . . .
- You may experience some discomfort postoperatively, but you may be surprised at just how comfortable you can feel . . .
- If you feel distress that needs assistance, medicine will be available . . .
- As your body heals and readjusts from surgery and anesthesia, your legs will slowly regain their regular movement.

Allow patients to experience their own recovery without the overlay of the caregivers' positive or negative impressions. Similarly, we feel that it is unwise to tell patients that they will not experience something, such as pain. If the person does experience pain, he may then assume that something is very wrong and expect and influence negative consequences.

If the patient has had a one-on-one preoperative preparation, strategies for dealing with the operative and the recovery periods will be developed. These may include hypnosis/suggestion, guided imagery, relaxation, and cognitive restructuring. We recommend that a written plan of the strategies be conveyed to the anesthesiologist, surgeon, and nurses involved in the person's care.

When the patient arrives for surgery, the admitting nurses can continue care of the person by keying into the developed preoperative strategy. If no specific preoperative strategy was developed, the nurse can use permissive suggestions that allow the patient to be more in control of his experience or experience events in a new way. For example, when starting an intravenous drip, the following suggestions foster patient control:

I'm going to clean your skin with some alcohol, and you might be surprised to find that the coolness is already beginning to numb your skin, the way that ice on a bruise sometimes makes it feel better. Now I'm going to give you some local anesthetic (or numbing medicine). One of the

extra benefits of the local is that it often dilates the blood vessels in the area, making it easier to start your IV . . . so, if you feel a pin prick now or any discomfort as I inject the numbing medicine, I want you to tell me. That's good; everything's going just fine (no matter what the response).

This same type of approach can be easily adapted to more invasive procedures in the preoperative area (central lines, arterial lines, epidural catheters, peripheral nerve blocks, etc.) as well as in the operating room. In addition, while in the preoperative area, the patient should be given as much control over the environment as is consistent with the well-being and privacy of the other patients in the preoperative area: allowing the presence of family or friends, listening to music or taped suggestions, controlling the ambient temperature, lying/sitting/walking, or involving other nonallopathic health support people.

All operating room personnel should understand that each surgical patient is in a highly suggestible and potentially vulnerable period. Unnecessary traffic, loud noises, and loud talking should be discouraged because the patient may easily misinterpret these sounds. Psychological preparation is not meant to replace chemoanesthesia. Occasionally, certain patients will specifically try to minimize their chemoanesthesia. The anesthesiologist should always use whichever anesthetic regimen he feels is safest for the patient. There is no need to avoid using benzodiazepines out of concern that an amnestic response will interfere with the psychological preparation. If a specific hypnotic strategy has been developed, the anesthesiologist should use agreed-upon suggestions at significant times: during induction, prior to incision/surgical start time, during periods of intense stimulation, after diseased organs are removed, during emergence, after extubation, and upon arrival in the recovery room.

If the patient wishes to listen to tapes, even under general anesthesia, the anesthesiologist should assist throughout the operation. If no specific strategy has been developed preoperatively, the anesthesiologist is free to use his or her own imagination to develop a strategy. Most anesthesiologists find that a core strategy is easily adaptable to most patients. Here is a brief example of a strategy that you should feel free to modify:

I'm giving you some medicine now that may begin to make you feel relaxed and comfortable so that as you take your next deep breath in and then out (keying the pace to the patient's respiratory cycle) you may be pleasantly surprised to find that you are beginning to feel more relaxed and more comfortable. If you would, with your next deep breath in and then out, I'd like you to picture a place, it can be a real place or an imaginary place, where you feel completely safe and very comfortable, so that as you breathe in and then out you are in a place that is safe for your body to begin to heal. . . .

A script like this can be easily completed during the time it takes to induce a general anesthetic and is invariably well received by the patient. The biggest obstacle to talking with patients in this manner usually comes from the anesthetist's fear of saying something wrong or from fear of sounding foolish in front of other staff. With a little practice, anyone can develop an effective script. Stage fright disappears with time, and the realization develops that, far from being critical, other operating room staff will actually be more appreciative of efforts to help the patient in every way possible.

It is now well recognized that awareness under anesthesia occurs (Mainzer 1979; Blacher 1984; Guerra 1980). For our purposes, it should be assumed that all patients have some degree of awareness under anesthesia. Rather than being a problem, awareness can be viewed as an opportunity. As noted previously (Pearson 1961; Hart 1980; Evans 1988), taped suggestions given

---

Case study 5–1

A.H. is a 39-year-old woman. Five months prior to the present admission she had been admitted with an accidental gun shot wound to the abdomen. At emergency exploratory laparotomy, she was found to have a perforated proximal sigmoid colon. A partial sigmoid colectomy was performed with creation of a colostomy and Hartmann's pouch. She had a prolonged (greater than 3 weeks) postoperative course, which was characterized by prolonged ileus, prolonged use of higher than usual narcotics, supplemental doses of benzodiazepines for anxiety, and frequent demands for nursing attention despite an uncomplicated (by standards of normal wound healing, absence of fever or other signs of infection, normal fluid and electrolyte balance, normal urination) recovery in other respects. The nursing staff viewed her as a difficult patient with exaggerated complaints and "drug-seeking behavior."

Four months after her initial surgery, she was scheduled for elective sigmoid reanastomosis and colostomy take-down. Her surgeon, noting that she remained very anxious at her interval check-ups, was anticipating a very stormy admission. In the 2 weeks prior to her scheduled surgery, she was seen twice by R.K.

During the initial contact, A.H. was extremely anxious, nervous, and scared. She clearly recognized the need for preoperative assistance and was eager to avoid the sequelae of the first surgery. There continued to be high levels of interpersonal stress in her life and she was in regular psychotherapeutic treatment. She knew Dr. Kessler "did hypnosis" and was interested, but prior attempts at "relaxation stuff" had been unsuccessful. Assessment revealed a mixed coping style, considerable negative medical and surgical experience, and modest hypnotic ability. Three goals were identified: (1) separating the previous surgery from the upcoming surgery; (2) generating strategies for effective psychological handling of the surgery and recovery; and (3) targeting a psychophysiological focus on rapid return of ileus, minimal blood loss, and rapid postoperative recovery. The remainder of the first session was spent learning and practicing physical self-regulation (diaphragmatic breathing and muscular relaxation) and developing a safe dissociated imagery to enable the patient to organize how she wanted to feel during the surgery. Practice between sessions was assigned. At the time

of the second appointment, A.H. was visibly more calm and relaxed. She had a clear mental attitude of taking charge of her responses to the procedure. She easily engaged in the relaxed dissociative imagery, altering her respiration, generating muscle relaxation, closing her eyes, and smiling for the next 30 minutes; she was able to emotionally and psychologically stay in the present as she watched the sequelae of the prior surgery fade into the distance. The remainder of the session included reinforcement of the previous suggestions and future rehearsal of a successful operation and recovery. After the second session I summarized the strategies to T.W. who would follow the case as anesthesiologist.

When seen in the preoperative holding area on the morning of surgery, she was calm and relaxed, much to the surprise of her surgeon. Reiteration of suggestions for relaxation, early return of normal bowel function, minimal postoperative discomfort, and redirection of blood flow to minimize operative blood loss were made by T.W. in the preoperative area as well as in the operating room during induction and at various times during the procedure. In the operating room, she had an epidural catheter placed for postoperative analgesia and a general anesthetic. The procedure lasted approximately 3 hours and was uncomplicated. Blood loss, estimated independently by the surgeon and two experienced operating room nurses as less than 300 ml, was felt by the surgeon to be unusually low for the amount of adhesions he encountered.

On the first postoperative day, she was walking in her room with minimal complaints. On the second postoperative day, she asked to have her epidural removed, and her nasogastric (NG) tube was clamped. On the third postoperative day, the NG was discontinued, and she began taking liquids. On the fourth day, T.W. witnessed the following event: A second surgeon who had assisted with the second surgery and who had been involved with several difficult days of cross-coverage during the first hospitalization was once again cross-covering; while standing at the nursing station, he looked up to see A.H. walking comfortably in the hall; in surprise, he called out to her "Hey! You are not supposed to be walking around." A.H. smiled and went on her way. She was discharged on the fifth hospital day, and her recovery as an outpatient proceeded well.

under general anesthesia can sometimes have beneficial effects on recovery. If technical difficulties are experienced by the surgeon, such as greater than expected oozing blood loss or difficulties with exposure, specific suggestions can be given to decrease blood flow to the oozing sites or to relax in such a way to allow better exposure (Bennett 1986; Enqvist 1991). It costs nothing, and it works. Sometimes, inappropriate comments are made either advertently ("There's tumors everywhere; this patient isn't going to live long") or inadvertently ("Oh no, I dropped it" after dropping a clamp, which can be interpreted many ways by a sedated/anesthetised patient).

The anesthesiologist can intervene through such techniques as rephrasing, explaining, or redirecting the patient's attention. An example of rephrasing might be, "so the surgery can remove those tumors and help you recover as best you are able." An example of explaining might be "so we will remove that clamp and replace it. It caused no problem and your surgery is continuing to proceed." An example of redirection might be "as the surgeons continue with their work, you can just focus on that pleasant comfortable place where you can rest pleasantly and comfortably."

The process can and should continue in the recovery room and then on the hospital ward. Caregivers in these areas can aid the recovery process by employing the following practices:

- Encouraging the strategy previously developed by the patient.
- Using language that allows the patient to have his or her own experience, while framing the experience so that it can be viewed in a context of rapid, safe, comfortable healing.
- Honoring the individual's coping style on the sensitizer–avoider continuum.
- Allowing the patient as much control (visitors, noise, temperature, medications) as possible.

These efforts to improve recovery require no new technology and little if any extra time by caregivers. The potential benefits include fewer transfusions, less pain and fewer pain medication requests, earlier return of bowel function, less nausea and vomiting and fewer requests for anti-emetics, less anxiety and less need for anxiolytics, quicker recovery, and earlier discharge from hospital. These benefits only require increased awareness by caregivers and the support for patients to more

---

Case study 5–2

N.W. is a 35-year-old woman who was scheduled for elective open Nissen fundoplication for symptoms of severe reflux. She was seen once by R.K. 48 hours before surgery. She had no specific concerns about the upcoming procedure, was actively using her own strategies to relax and prepare, and wanted the best surgical outcomes. N.W. was assessed to have no significant negative medical surgical history, was a coping sensitizer who did well with much information, and she was assessed to have substantial hypnotic skill. As part of our conversation a light hypnotic involvement was generated by asking her what it would be like to just allow herself to be very comfortable, very relaxed, breathing easily and comfortably, and noticing her mind and body working together to find a place from which to continue her preparation. Imagery was developed for time distortion by asking her to imagine as she goes into the operating room, visualizing herself lying on a special beach for hours feeling the warmth of the sun and sand and the cool of the breeze. When the procedure is finished, she should become alert and find herself in the recovery room ready to continue her healing. Because of her sensitizing coping style and the demands of the postoperative recovery, we also rehearsed her recovery after surgery both in the hospital and at home, which included deep breathing soon after she went to her hospital room, with an ensuing discomfort being a signal of healing. Suggestions for rapid appropriate healing were also given.

Little blood loss was anticipated with this proce-

dure, so no suggestions for redirecting blood flow were developed. In the operating room, she had an epidural catheter placed for postoperative analgesia, and general anesthesia was induced. The suggestions developed preoperatively were reinforced in the preoperative holding area, during induction, and at various times throughout the procedure. It happened that the attending surgeon was the same surgeon who had attended A.H. As he made his way down through skin, muscle, and fascia he jokingly commented to T.W., "She is really oozing a lot. I thought these people weren't supposed to bleed." T.W. asked him to wait a moment, leaned over to N.W.'s ear and told her that she could safely direct her blood flow away from the operative site so that her surgeon could work more effectively and that at the end of the procedure, she could return the blood flow to the operative site to promote healing. And with that, the oozing stopped.

Early on the second postoperative day, the epidural inadvertently came out when the tape loosened. N.W. was in quite a bit of discomfort when seen by T.W. that day. After discussing several options, including placing a second epidural catheter, it was elected by N.W. to try a hypnotic approach. A glove anesthesia was induced that N.W. then placed over the operative wound with dramatic improvement in her level of comfort. The remainder of her postoperative course was complicated by a urinary tract infection that delayed her discharge, but all other facets of her recovery were unremarkable.

consistently use the skills that many patients already possess.

SUMMARY

This is a very complex area of intervention and investigation. There are multiple possible environmental stressors, multiple neural pathways, and multiple neuroendocrine transmitters. In surgical studies, there are multiple endogenous variables (patient anatomy and physical status, disease process) and multiple exogenous variables (surgical technique and skill, anesthetic technique and skill, postoperative supportive measures). There are an infinite number of prior experiences that the individual brings to the affective component of the response to surgery. This last set of variables impacts not only the individual's perception of and response to the stressor (e.g., surgery) but also the individual's perception of and response to the images used in hypnotic/relaxation/cognitive techniques. An image of flying like a bird will elicit different responses from a jet pilot than from an agoraphobic.

Our usual scientific model of inquiry is a Cartesian map-making model that presumes that all independent variables, except the dependent variable being studied, are held constant while an experimental intervention is employed. The effect upon the dependent variable is then measured, and conclusions are drawn. We propose that this is not likely to occur in a setting with so many clearly interdependent variables. We feel that it is wise to heed Heisenberg's Uncertainty Principle, which has two basic tenets:

- In any multi-variable system, the moment an observer focuses on any single variable, he loses sight and control of other variables.

- The mere act of observing a variable changes that variable.

Developed within the field of quantum physics, these tenets appear applicable to this field of scientific inquiry. In spite of these inherent difficulties, the hypnotic interventions that have been clinically investigated have shown consistently impressive improvement in the outcomes: less blood loss, sooner return of normal bowel function, less postoperative pain, and shorter length of stay.

We conclude that (1) The things that you say and do with surgical patients change both the situation of the surgery and patient response; (2) the process of the surgery and its outcome are a product of anesthetic and surgical procedures *and* patient response to their history, the context of their experiences, and their encounters with and responses to you, all of which affect the biochemic and physiologic response to surgery; and (3) you can tailor, even very briefly, the perioperative experience to enhance surgical outcomes and return to functioning.

It may be that our clinical outcomes are positive as judged by generally accepted standards and the biochemical or electrochemical results are confusing, contradictory, or not readily explainable. It may be that just as our use of these techniques in anesthesia and surgery is in its early stage of development, so too the scientific methods used to evaluate these interventions are still to be understood more fully.

It is our contention that future investigations and interventions take into account the variables that we have discussed as important influences upon outcome: coping style, prior medical/surgical experiences, hypnotic ability, and the variables that the caregiver brings to this experience. It is our hypothesis that hypnotic interventions tailored to these variables will improve upon the impressive results so far and will produce the best possible results for our patients.

REFERENCES

Abramson M, Greenfield I, Heron WT: Response to, or perception of, auditory stimuli under deep surgical anesthesia. Am J Obstet Gynecol 96:584–585, 1966

Agnati FL, Tiengo M, Ferraguti F, et al: Pain, analgesia, and stress: An integrated view. Clin J Pain 7(1):23–37, 1991

American Medical Association: Socioeconomic characteristics of medical practice. Annual Report, American Medical Association, Chicago, 1993

Andrew JM: Recovery from surgery, with and without preparatory instruction, for three coping styles. J Pers Soc Psychol 15:223–226, 1970

Arendt-Nielsen L, Zacharie R, Bjerring P: Quantitative evaluation of hypnotically suggested hyperesthesia and analgesia by painful laser stimulation. Pain 42:243–251, 1990

Bandura A: Self-efficacy: Toward an unifying theory of behavior change. Psychol Rev 84:191–215, 1977

Bandura A, Reese L, Adams NE: Microanalysis of action and fear arousal as a function of differential levels of perceived self-efficacy. J Pers Soc Psychol 43:5–21, 1982

Bandura A, Taybor CB, Williams SL et al: Catecholamine secretion as a function of perceived coping self-efficacy. J Consult Clin Psychol 53:406–414, 1985

Barabasz AF, Lonsdale C: Effects of hypnosis on P300 olfactory evoked potential amplitudes. J Abnorm Psychol 92:520–523, 1983

Barber TX: Changing "unchangeable" bodily processes by hypnotic suggestion. *In* Sheikh M (ed): Imagery and Healing. New York, Baywood Publishing, 1984

Bennett HL, Benson DR, Kuiken DA: Preoperative instructions for decreased bleeding during spine surgery. Anesthesiology 65:A245, 1986

Blacher R: Brief psychotherapeutic intervention for the surgical patient. *In* Blacher R (ed): The Psychological Experience of Surgery. New York, John Wiley, 1987a, pp 207–220

Blacher R: General surgery and anesthesia: The emotional experience. *In* Blacher R (ed): The Psychological Experience of Surgery. New York, John Wiley, 1987b, pp 1–25

Blacher RS: Awareness during surgery [editorial]. Anesthesiology 61:1–2, 1984

Blankfield RP: Suggestion, relaxation, and hypnosis as adjuncts in the care of surgery patients: A review of the literature. Am J Clin Hypn 33:172–187, 1991

Bohus B, DeKloet ER, Veldhuis HD: Adrenal steroids and behavioral adaptation: Relationship to brain corticoid receptors. In Ganten D and Pfaff D (eds): Adrenal Actions on Brain: Current Topics in Neuroendocrinology, vol. 2, Berlin, Springer-Verlag, 1982, pp 107–148

Bohus B, Benus RF, Fokkema OS, et al: Neuroendocrine states and behavioral and physiological stress responses. Prog Brain Res 72:57–70.

Bonilla KB, Quigley WF, Bowers WF: Experiences with hypnosis on a surgical service. Mil Med 126:364–370, 1961

Bowers KS: Pain, anxiety and perceived control. Consult Clin Psychol 32:596–602, 1968

Bromage PR, Shibata HR, Willoughby HW: Influence of prolonged epidural blockage on blood sugar and cortisol responses to operations upon the upper part of the abdomen and thorax. Surgery, Gynecology and Obstetrics 132:1051–1056, 1971

Cohen F, Lazarus R: Active coping processes, coping dispositions and recovery from surgery. Psychosom Med 35:375–387, 1973

Crawford HJ: Brain dynamics and hypnosis: Attentional and disattentional processes. Int J Clin Exp Hypn 42:204–232, 1994

Dane J, Kessler R: Pain management in the critically ill and acutely injured. A matrix model for psychological assessment and treatment of acute pain. In Hamill R, Rowlingson J (eds): Handbook of Critical Care Pain Management. New York, McGraw-Hill, 1993, pp 53–82

Davis H, Porter JW, Livingstone J, et al: Pituitary-adrenal activities and leverpress shock escape behavior. Physiol Psychol 5:280–284, 1977

Davis J: The major ambulatory care center and how it developed. Surg Clin North Am 67(4):671–692, 1987

DeWied D, Jolles J: Neuropeptides derived from pro-opiocortin: Behavioral, physiological and neurochemical effects. Physol Rev 62:976–1059, 1982

Disbrow EA, Bennett HL, Owings JT: Effect of preoperative suggestion on postoperative gastrointestinal motility. West J Med 158:488–492, 1993

Doberneck RC, Griffin WO, Papermaster AA, et al: Hypnosis as an adjunct to surgical therapy. Surgery 46:299–304, 1959

Dunn A, Berridge C: Is corticotropin-releasing factor a mediator of stress response? In Koot G (ed): A Decade of Neuropeptides. Annals of New York Academy of Sciences. New York, New York Academy of Sciences, 1990, pp 183–191

Egbert L, Battit G, Turndorf H: The value of the preoperative visit by the anesthetist: A study of doctor–patient rapport. JAMA 185:553–555, 1963

Egbert LD, Battit GE, Welch CE, et al: Reduction of postoperative pain by encouragement and instruction to patients: A study of doctor–patient rapport. New Engl J Med 270:825–827, 1964

Enqvist A, Brandt MR, Fernandes A, et al: The blocking effect of epidural analgesia on the adrenocortical & hyperglycaemic responses to surgery. Acta Anaesthesiol Scand 21:330–335, 1977

Enqvist B: Preoperative hypnotherapy and preoperative suggestions in general anesthesia: Somatic responses in maxillo-facial surgery. Hypnosis 28:72–77, 1991

Enqvist B, Fischer K: Preoperative hypnotic techniques reduce consumption of analgesics after surgical removal of third mandibular molars. Int J Clin Exp Hypn 45:102–108, 1997

Enqvist B, von Konow L, Bystedt H: Pre- and perioperative suggestion in maxillofacial surgery: Effects on blood loss and recovery. Int J Clin Exp Hypn 18:97–105, 1995

Evans B, Stanley R: Psychological interventions for coping with surgery: A review of hypnotic techniques. Australian Journal of Clinical and Experimental Hypnosis 18(2):97–105, 1990

Evans BJ, Stanley RO: Hypnoanaesthesia and hypnotic techniques with surgical patients. Australian Journal of Clinical and Experimental Hypnosis 19:31–39, 1991

Evans C, Richardson PH: Improved recovery and reduced postopera-
tive stay after therapeutic suggestions during general anesthesia. Lancet 2:491–498, 1988

Fields H: Pain. New York, McGraw-Hill 1987

Fokkema DS, Koolhaas JM: Acute and conditioned blood pressure changes in relation to social and psychosocial stimuli in rats. Physiol Behav 34:33–38, 1985

Fredericks I: Teaching of hypnosis in the overall approach to the surgical patient. Am J Clin Hypn 20:175–183, 1978

Goldstein S, Halbreich U: Hormones and stress. In Nemeroff C, Loosen P (eds): Handbook of Clinical Psychoneuroendocrinology. New York, John Wiley and Sons, 1987, pp 460–469

Greenleaf M, Fisher S, Miaskowski C, et al: Hypnotizability and recovery from cardiac surgery. Am J Clin Hypn 35:119–128, 1992

Guerra F: Awareness under anesthesia. In Guerra F, Aldrete A (eds): Emotional and Psychological Responses to Anesthesia and Surgery. New York, Grune & Stratton 1980, pp 1–8

Halter JB, Pflug AE, Porte D Jr: Mechanisms of plasma catecholamine increases during surgical stress in man. J Clin Endocrinol Metab 45:936–944, 1977

Hart RR: The influence of a taped hypnotic induction treatment procedure on the recovery of CABG surgery patients. Int J Clin Exp Hypn 28:324–331, 1980

Henry JP, Stephens P: Stress, Health and the Social Environment: A Sociobiological Approach to Medicine. New York, Springer, 1977

Hilgard J: Sequelae to hypnosis. Int J Clin Exp Hypn 22:281–298, 1974

Houston BK: Control over stress, locus of control and response to stress. J Pers Soc Psychol 21:249–255, 1972

Johnson JE, Fuller SS, Endress MP, et al: Altering patients' responses to surgery: An extension and replication. Research Nursing Health 1:111–121, 1978

Johnson M, Carpenter L: Relationship between pre-operative anxiety and post-operative state. Psychol Med 110:361–367, 1980

Johnston IDA: Endocrine aspects of the metabolic response to surgical operation. Ann R Coll Surg Engl 35:270–286, 1964

Johnston M, Vogele C: Benefits of psychological preparation for surgery: A meta-analysis. Ann Behav Med 15:245–256, 1993

Kehlet H: The stress reponse to anaesthesia and surgery: Release mechanisms and modifying factors. Clinical Anaesthesia 2:315–323, 1984

Kehlet H, Brandt MR, Hanson AP, et al: Effect of epidural analgesia on metabolic profiles during and after surgery. Br J Surg 66:543–546, 1979

Kehlet H, Schulze S: Modification of the general response to injury—pharmacological and clinical aspects. In Little RA, Frayn KN (eds): The Scientific Basis of Care of the Critically Ill. Manchester, Manchester University Press, 1986

Kessler R: Psychological and hypnotic interventions in anesthesiology and surgery: A hopeful and cautious analysis. Presented at the Scientific Meeting of The Society for Clinical and Experimental Hypnosis. Chicago, 1993

Kessler R, Dane J: Psychological and hypnotic preparation for anesthesia and surgery: An individual differences perspective. Int J Clin Exp Hypn 44(3):189–207, 1996

Kessler R: The consequences of individual differences in preparation for surgery and invasive medical procedures. Hypnos December xxiv:181–192, 1997

Kinsmen R, Dahlem N, Spector S: Observations on subjective symptomatology, coping behavior, and medical decisions in asthma. Psychosom Med 39:102–119, 1977

Kirsch I, Montgomery G, Sapirstein G: Hypnosis as an adjunct to behavioral cognitive psychotherapy: A meta-analysis. J Consult Clin Psychol 63:214–220, 1995

Lang EV, Joyce JS, Spiegel D, et al: Self-hypnotic relaxation during interventional radiological procedures: Effects on pain perception and intravenous drug use. Int J Clin Exp Hypn 44:106–119, 1996

Lush D, Thorpen JN, Richardson DJ, et al: The effect of epidural analgesia on the adrenocortical response to surgery. British Journal of Anaesthesia 44:1169–1172, 1972

Mainzer J: Awareness, muscle relaxants and balanced anesthesia. Canadian Anaesthesia Society Journal 26:386–393, 1979

Mason JW: A review of psychoneuroendocrine research on the pituitary–adrenal cortical system. Psychosom Med 30:576–607, 1968

Michel CM, Lehmann D, Henggeler B, et al: Localization of the sources of EEG delta. Theta, alpha and beta frequency bands using the FFT di[pole] approximation. Electroencephalogr Clin Neurophysiol 82:38–44, 1992

Miller SM: The interacting effects of coping styles and situational variables in gynecologic settings: Implications for research and treatment. J Psychosom Obstet Gynaecol 9:23–24, 1988

Mumford E, Schlesinger HJ, Glass GV: The effects of psychological intervention on recovery from surgery and heart attacks: An analysis of the literature. Am J Public Health 72:141–151, 1982

Pearson RE: Response to suggestions given under general anesthesia. Am J Clin Hypn 4:106–114, 1961

Pennebaker JW, Burnam MA, Schaeffer MA, et al: Lack of control as a determinant of perceived physical symptoms. J Pers Soc Psycho 35:167–174, 1977

Rapkin DA, Straubing M, Holroyd JC: Guided imagery, hypnosis and recovery from head and neck cancer surgery: An exploratory study. Int J Clin Exp Hypn 39:215–226, 1991

Ridgeway V, Matthews A: Psychological preparation for surgery: A comparison of methods. British Journal of Clinical Psychology 21(4):271–280, 1982

Rodin J: Aging and health: Effects of the sense of control. Science 211:1271–1276, 1986

Rogers M, Reich P: Psychological intervention with surgical patients: Evaluation outcome. Adv Psychosom Med 15:25–50, 1986

Rondi G, Bowers K, Buckley D, et al: Postoperative impact of information presented during general anesthesia. *In* Sobel P, Bonke B, Winograd E (eds): Memory and Awareness in Anesthesia. New Jersey, Prentice Hall 1993, pp 187–195

Salmon P: Psychological factors in surgical recovery. *In* Gibson HB (ed): Pain and Anesthesia. London, Chapman and Hall, 1994, pp 229–258

Salmon P, Evans R, Humphrey D: Anxiety and endocrine changes in surgical patients. British Journal of Clinical Psychology 25(2):135–141, 1986

Sapirstein G, Montgomery G, Kirsch I: Hypnosis as an adjunct to cognitive behavioral theory. *In* Rhue J, Lynn S, Kirsch I (eds): A Handbook of Clinical Hypnosis. Washington, DC, American Psychological Association, 1992, pp 151–172

Scott H: Hypnoanalgesia for major surgery—A psychodynamic process. Am J Clin Hypn 16:84–90, 1978

Selye H: The stress of life. New York, McGraw-Hill, 1976

Sherrington CS: The integrative action of the nervous system. New Haven, Yale University Press, 1906

Spiegel D, Bierre P, Rootenburg J: Hypnotic alteration of somatosensory perception. Am J Psychiatry 146:749, 1989

Stanley TH, Berman L, Green O, et al: Fentanyl-oxgyen anesthesia in coronary artery surgery: Plasma catecholamine and cortisol response. Anaesthesiology 51:S139, 1979

Sturgis LM, Coe WC: Physiological responsiveness during hypnosis. Int J Clin Exp Hypn 38:196–207, 1990

Surman OS, Hackett TP, Silverberg EL, et al: Usefulness of psychiatric intervention in patients undergoing cardiac surgery. Arch Gen Psychiatry 30:830–835, 1974

Syrjala K, Cummings D, Donaldson G: Hypnosis or cognitive behavioral training for the reduction of pain and nausea during cancer treatment. Pain 48:137–148, 1992

Taenzer P, Melzack R, Jeans ME: Influence of psychological factors on postoperative pain, mood, and analgesic requirements. Pain 24:331–342, 1986

Thoren L: General metabolic response to trauma including pain influence. Acta Anaesthesiol Scand 18(suppl):55:9–14, 1974

Van Dalfsen P, Syrjala K: Psychological strategies in acute pain management. *In* Hoyt J (ed): Pain Management in the ICU. Critical Care Clin 6(2):421–432, 1990

Volicier B, Burns M: Pre-existing correlates of hospital stress. Nursing Research 26:408–415, 1977

Weinstein EJ, Au PK: Use of hypnosis before and during angioplasty. Am J Clin Hypn 34:29–37, 1991

Weiss JM: Somatic effects of predictable and unpredictable shock. Psychosom Med 32:397–408, 1970

Wilson J: Behavioral preparation for surgery: Benefit or harm? J Behav Med 4(1):79–102, 1981

Zieglgansberger W: Central control of nociception. *In* Mountcastle VB, et al (eds): Handbook of Physiology. Bethesda, American Physiological Society, 1986, pp 581–645

6

Hypnosis in the Emergency Room

Dabney Ewin

TRANCE–EQUIVALENT STATES

One of the common definitions of hypnosis or trance is that it is a state that occurs when there is a central focus of attention with surrounding areas of inhibition. In acute trauma, most individuals will focus on the injury and ignore their surroundings and arrive in the Emergency Room in a "trance–equivalent" state. This state is either good or ominous because there is increased susceptibility to suggestion, both good and bad. In addition, the Law of Pessimistic Interpretation says that if a suggestion can be interpreted either optimistically or pessimistically, a *frightened* person will interpret it pessimistically. Because many equivocal phrases can be heard in the Emergency Room—"uh oh," "this is it," "get some oxygen," "we're out of blood," or "that's not sterile"—the patient can easily assume those statements are predicting a negative outcome.

Even before the patient arrives in the Emergency Room, the trance–equivalent state is apparent. We can assume that most patients carried by an ambulance are frightened and in trance. Unintentional comments can be pessimistically interpreted, and emergency medical technicians (EMT) should be taught to remain aware of this danger. In one case, a Navy plane commander was accompanying a crewman in the ambulance following a painful fall from the plane to the tarmac. The ambulance came to a stop because an 18-wheel rig was making a turn ahead of them, and his trailer was obviously going to hit the street lamp post. The EMT, intent on this drama, said "He's not going to make it!" The commander realized that his crewman on the stretcher could not see what was going on and put a hand on his shoulder and said, "Joe, he's not talking about you." A few words of explanation at the right time can be very reassuring.

Only one controlled study has been done with EMTs. M. Eric Wright at the University of Kansas trained one set of EMTs in suggestion theory and matched them against a naive crew (Wright 1990). After 6 months, he compared the outcomes of patients brought to the ER by the two crews. Patients brought by the trained crew had significantly lower mortality, shorter hospital stays, and more discharges from the ER (i.e., fewer hospital admissions) than those brought by the naive crew.

If a patient is not traumatized when he arrives at the ER he might soon become so during the admission process. In my hospital if a patient needs surgery, the release he or she must sign says, "I understand that I may die, be paralyzed, lose use of a limb, or be permanently scarred." The alert physician will pick up on this and find a way to protect the patient by interpreting the sounds of the ER, and by pointing out to the surgical patient that the law requires that we get every patient to sign a general release that includes all the worst possibilities, even though we intend to protect against any of these things happening.

There is controversy about getting informed consent for the use of hypnosis. I agree with Bierman that this is not necessary in emergencies, and is probably counterproductive (Bierman 1989).

EMOTIONAL TONE

Sir William Osler, often referred to as the "Father of Medicine" in the United States, titled his farewell address to the graduating students at Johns Hopkins, *AEQUANIMITAS* (Osler 1904). He communicated that the most important single attribute of the physician, aside from knowledge, is equanimity (imperturbability). The physician sets the emotional tone in the Emergency Room, and this tone is rapidly communicated to the patient. No matter how chaotic the situation, the quiet confidence of a calm and empathetic physician can direct the patient's focus toward trust and put the chaos into the surrounding areas of inhibition. Rudyard Kipling wrote, "If you can keep your head, when all about you are losing theirs and blaming it on you, If you can trust yourself when all men doubt you, but make allowance for their doubting too . . . Yours is the world, and everything that's in it. . . ."

Never hesitate to call for help if it's needed, but when the ultimate responsibility is yours, then even when you feel uncertain you should keep your head and trust yourself for the sake of your patient. Don't be fooled into thinking that a nonresponsive patient is unaware of you or your actions. Special care with loose talk is needed around an unconscious patient. Just because the verbal left brain is shut down does not mean that the survival-oriented nonverbal right brain is inactive. Often, following recovery from a concussion, a patient who

is amnesic in the waking state can go into trance and repeat almost verbatim things that were said while he or she was unconscious. I have an audiotape of a hypnotic age regression of a boy who was hit by a car and was unconscious for 3 months. He reports several things that were clearly never told to him after regaining consciousness, such as the fact that the ER nurse knew who his father was and was especially kind to him. In seeking to validate this, I found that that nurse had moved out of town shorly after the accident and never made further contact. She was gone by the time the patient regained consciousness. When reviewing the case with the father, it was a detail he overlooked until he was asked if he had recognized anyone in the ER.

The maxim is that one should never say anything around an unconscious patient that you would not say if you knew the patient to be awake.

ANALGESIA

Anesthesia is not feeling anything, while analgesia is simply not feeling pain. Analgesia is easy to induce in light trance, and generally suffices for most ER procedures. Anesthesia requires more time and deep trance and is generally unnecessary.

DISLOCATED SHOULDER

These patients experience excruciating pain with any motion, and you can make the diagnosis from 100 feet away. The patient walks in with an attitude of great concern, firmly holding the elbow of the affected arm with the other hand to prevent any motion, and seeking immediate help. Knowing that the longer a joint is dislocated, the more likely there will be permanent nerve or vascular injury, this diagnosis gets some priority in triage.

The hypnosis is easy and consists of simply inserting oneself into the patient's spontaneous trance and relieving him or her of the responsibility for pain control. I say, "I'm Dr. Ewin. I can help you. Will you do what I say?" When I get a "yes" to that question, it is as good as any formal hypnotic induction I can do because the patient has agreed to set aside critical testing and unconditionally follow my instructions. If the answer is "no" (which is rare), then conventional care is indicated. A radiograph should be taken because there are occasional complicated fracture-dislocations that require reduction in the operating room, even though nearly all are simple anterior dislocations.

First, with the patient in the sitting position I apply a Velcro sling and swath so the patient can feel safe letting go of the elbow. Then I tell him or her to lie down and relax and "let your thoughts and feelings go to your laughing place, leaving your shoulder and arm here for us to x-ray." This may sound a little silly to us in the waking state, but with the shoulder immobilized and finally feeling safe after being very frightened, it is easy for the patient to respond to this simple suggestion for dissociation and the comfort it brings. When the radiograph shows a simple anterior dislocation, I deepen the trance, enhance the imagery, and ask for an ideomotor signal to confirm that the dissociation has occurred. Then *I gently abduct the arm about 30 degrees, take off my shoe and put my foot in the axilla and firmly pull on the arm* while suggesting relaxation of the shoulder. As the deltoid muscle relaxes, the arm stretches out about an inch, and when it stops stretching I simply externally rotate it while my nurse puts some pressure on the head of the humerus, popping it back through the hole in the capsule. Then the patient can come fully alert and sit up to reapply the sling and swath. It is important to stress the necessity of maintaining immobilization for several weeks while the tear in the capsule heals; failure to heal it results in recurring dislocations on reaching overhead so that a surgical closure may be required.

LACERATIONS

Light trance is very helpful in calming a frightened patient who is bleeding from a laceration. It works best as an adjunct to local anesthesia. Equanimity here is imperative. I hold a sterile pressure dressing on the wound to control bleeding while I take a short history of what happened. Then I get the patient to lie down and I say, "Close your eyes for a few moments and relax, and let me examine this part." I examine for injury to deeper structures, particularly nerves and tendons. Lidocaine is an excellent topical anesthetic, and I first drop some into the open wound, then infiltrate some into the skin on both sides through the anesthetized tissue. At this point it is easy for my nurse to clean the wound under running water and I proceed with the repair in the waking state with the wound now adequately anesthetized.

Splinters and other foreign bodies in the palm of the hand present a special problem. Exploration must be done in a completely dry field so the foreign body can be seen without damaging any of the many arteries, nerves, and tendons in the palm. A tourniquet on the

forearm inflated to 300 mm Hg will dry the field but causes considerable ischemic pain after 5 to 10 minutes in the waking state. *In trance, tourniquet time can be extended to 20 to 30 minutes rather easily.* This extra time allows for more meticulous exploration.

ATRIAL FIBRILLATION

Bierman reports a case of paroxysmal atrial fibrillation with conversion to normal sinus rhythm in an 84-year-old man (Bierman 1989). As the cardiologist arrived, the patient aroused spontaneously and reported, "I did it; I went back there and did just what the doctor said to do."

COLLES' FRACTURE

A fall on the outstretched hand is the precursor of the common Colles' fracture. The distal radius is broken transversely and displaced dorsally, producing the classic "silver fork" deformity. Anatomical reduction can usually be accomplished by first hyperextending the wrist, then aligning the dorsal edge of the fragment with the dorsal edge of the distal radius and snapping the wrist into full flexion and ulnar deviation to pull the radial styloid to its full length. This procedure is quite painful and cannot be accomplished without some form of anesthesia. In addition, the hyperextension is resisted by spasm in the powerful flexor muscles of the forearm.

It is easy to combine local anesthesia with hypnosis for relaxation and anxiety. To assure sterility, I use 5 mL or 2% lidocaine from a previously unopened vial and inject it into the hematoma at the fracture site. While this is diffusing and the pain is rapidly diminishing, I talk to the patient about letting "the whole forearm and wrist go limp and floppy so it will be very easy for us to slip it back into its *normal* position." With that thought accepted, I proceed to the same induction I use for dislocated shoulder and have the patient go to his laughing place leaving the arm with me. I find the manipulation and reduction much easier than with local anesthesia alone.

ASTHMA

Asthma has become an increasingly dangerous disorder in terms of both morbidity and mortality. Increasingly potent medicines are not lowering the mortality rate but are producing serious side effects in some people. Few things are more frightening than being unable to breathe. In an acute episode the patient may be so focused on the next breath that he mentally places the whole ER and the physician in the "surrounding areas of inhibition" mentioned in our earlier definition of trance.

When you cannot get the patient's conscious attention, it is necessary to insert yourself into his trance by having a sham asthma attack too and take over control. Face and hold the patient by the shoulders, breathing in synchronous rhythm and effort, and say something he can only agree with, like "hard to breathe?" If he says "yes" you simply repeat "yes," and whatever else he says. This is a feedback induction that works particularly well with children. At some point the patient realizes he is not in this alone and looks up to make eye contact. That is when you take control and start giving simple, short suggestions: "enough air" . . . "blow it out" (asthmatics hoard air) . . . "breathe easy" . . . and so on. As you do this you pace your own breathing just a little slower and easier than the patient. In less than 5 minutes, most patients will not be filled with panic and will be able to cooperate with your treatment plan. Some will require very little medication, and most will respond to it well. In a life-threatening situation, medication and resuscitation must be given immediately, but this technique can still be useful as secondary support.

CHEST PAIN

When a patient comes to the ER complaining of chest pain, it is a given that he fears it is a heart attack. There is such a thing as being frightened to death. In the 1993 Northridge earthquake, 15 uninjured people died of heart attacks within an hour of the shock (Leor 1996). In the ER, the patient is hypervigilant for disaster. Just starting oxygen can be interpreted as a bad omen unless the nurse says something like "we routinely give oxygen while we're discovering the cause of chest pain." Anything reassuring that sounds honest is calming. Immediately after taking the pulse, say something. If the pulse is regular, say "That's a good, regular pulse." If it's irregular, say something like "That's a good strong pulse (pause) with some extrasystoles like we see sometimes when a person is under stress." The patient probably doesn't know what extrasystoles are, but he's just found out that they come with stress, and the logic is that he needs to be calm and turn off all the stress he can.

BURNS

Thermal burns are remarkably responsive to early hypnosis. Anyone who has ever had a sunburn knows that when you leave the sun, you're not in much trouble. It's after 10 or 12 hours that the blisters and fever occur. This is the "normal" progression of a burn from first to second degree, and it also occurs from second to third degree. This progression is an inflammatory process and is apparently the body's attempt to reject the injured tissue.

In a good hypnotic subject, the *suggestion* that a hot object is being placed on the skin will produce a blister (Ullman 1947), even though there is no thermal stimulus. By the same token, a *suggestion* that the skin is "cool and comfortable" given in the first 2 hours after the burn will prevent the usual progression of the burn. In addition, burn pain is attenuated by early hypnosis because pain is part of inflammation (calor, dolor, rubor, and tumor), and the inflammatory response has been aborted by perceiving the involved area as "cool and comfortable."

With burns of less than 15% of body surface that can be treated on an outpatient basis, a single hypnosis session will suffice and help the patient all the way through to healing. For patients who must be admitted to a burn unit, multiple reinforcement sessions are usually needed. Patterson et al have done controlled studies on a Burn Unit showing that the patients in the most severe pain are the most responsive to hypnotic pain palliation, whereas those with the least pain were less responsive to hypnosis but could be adequately treated with opioids (Patterson 1995)

The acutely burned patient is often a stranger to the physician, and the first communication is an introduction. I immediately insert a hypnotic suggestion, couched in the form of a question:

Doctor: "I'm Dr. Smith, and I'll be taking care of you [pause]. Do you know how to treat this kind of burn?"

Comment: This question brings to the patient's attention the fact that he does not know how to care for his burn, and so must trust the medical team. Precise wording is important because if you ask "Do you know *anything* about treating burns?" he may think he knows something and tell you about butter, Solarcaine, and so forth. That latter response avoids recognizing the dependence, which is what you are after.

Patient: "No."

Comment: The standard reply. In the rare instance of a physician or nurse who actually does know about burns, you simply use that knowledge to say "Then you already know that you need to turn your treatment over to us, and we will take good care of you."

Doctor: "That's all right, because we know how to take care of this, and you've already done the most important thing, which was to get to the hospital quickly. You're safe now, and if you will do what I say, you can have a comfortable rest in the hospital while your body is healing. Will you do what I say?"

Comment: This exchange lets the patient know that he is on the team and he has already done his biggest job. It includes a prehypnotic suggestion that he is safe and can be comfortable if he makes a commitment. Now he can safely lay aside his fight-or-flight response (he's already *flown* to the hospital). The fight-or-flight response mobilizes adrenal hormones that interfere with normal immunity and metabolism.

Patient: "Yes," or "I'll try."

Comment: With his affirmative answer, he has made a hypnotic contract that is as good as any trance.

Doctor: "The first thing I want you to do is turn the care of this burn completely over to us, so you don't have to worry about it at all. The second thing is for you to realize that your own thoughts will make a great deal of difference in your healing. Have you ever seen a person blush red or blanch white with fear?"

Comment: Frightened patients tend to constantly analyze each sensation and new symptom to report to the doctor. By turning his care over to *us* (the whole team), he is freed of this responsibility and worry. Next, his attention is diverted to something he has not thought of before.

Patient: "Yes."

Comment: Even dark-skinned patients are aware of this phenomenon in light-skinned people.

Doctor: "Well, you know that nothing has happened but a thought or an idea, and all of the little blood vessels in the face have opened up and turned red or clamped down and blanched. Your thoughts are going to affect the blood supply to your skin, and that affects healing, and you can start right now. You need to have happy, relaxing, enjoyable thoughts to free up all your healing energy. Brer Rabbit said, 'Everybody's got a laughing place,' and when I tell you to go to your laughing place, I mean for you to imagine that you are in a safe, peaceful place, enjoying yourself, totally free of responsibility, just goofing off. What would you choose for a laughing place?"

Comment: The patient needs something he perceives as useful to occupy his mind. The laughing place may be the beach, television, fishing, golfing, needlepoint, playing dolls, and so on. The "laughing place" becomes the key phrase that can be used for subsequent rapid induction for dressing changes or any other type of medical maintenance. I simply say, "Go to your laughing place."

Patient: "Go to the beach . . . or. . . ."

Comment: It helps to know what the laughing place is and to record it. Later, it may be necessary to enhance it with specific visual imagery.

Doctor: "Let's get you relaxed and go to your laughing place right now, while we take care of the burn. Get comfortable and roll your eyeballs up as though you are looking at the top of your forehead and take a deep, deep, deep breath. And as you take in that breath, gradually close your eyelids. And as you let the breath out, let your eyes relax and let every nerve and fiber in your body go [slow and cadenced] loose, and limp, and lazy, as if your limbs are like lumps of lead. Then just let your mind go off to your laughing place and enjoy . . . [visual imagery of laughing place]."

Comment: This easy induction usually produces a profound trance almost immediately.

Such a short bit of conversation does not ordinarily delay the usual emergency care. Most often, when the burned patient arrives in the Emergency Room an analgesic is given, blood is drawn, intraveneous drips are started, and cool water applications are put in place. These procedures can go on while the conversation takes place. A towel dipped in ice water produces immediate relief of the burning pain that occurs right after a fresh burn. Because frostbite is as bad an injury as a burn, the patient should not be packed in ice; ice water towels are very helpful. In fact, Chapman et al showed that applying ice water to a burn holds the release of inflammatory enzymes in check for several hours, so there is ample time to call for the assistance of a qualified hypnotist if the primary physician is not skilled in the techniques of hypnosis (Chapman et al. 1959).

Doctor: "Now while you are off at your laughing place, I want you to also notice that *all of the involved areas* are cool and comfortable. Notice how cool and comfortable they actually are, and when you can really feel this, you'll let me know because this finger (touch an index finger) will slowly rise to signal that *all of the involved areas* are cool and comfortable."

Comment: By this time the patient has iced towels on and the analgesic is taking effect, so that he actually is cool and (relatively) comfortable.

It is much easier hypnotically to continue a sensation that is already present than it is to imagine its opposite. The suggestion "cool and comfortable" is anti-inflammatory, and if he accepts it he cannot be hot and painful. From now on, the words *involved* or *injured* are substituted whenever possible for the word burn, because patients use the term *burning* to describe their pain. Do not specify a particular area such as hand or neck because although these areas may do well, some area you omitted may do poorly. I had one case (Ewin 1986) where I specified the hand and forearm that went into boiling oil, and neglected some oil that had splattered onto the shoulder. The hand and forearm stayed second degree and healed in 2 weeks. The shoulder area that I had considered inconsequential went on to third degree and required a skin graft.

Doctor: (After obtaining ideomotor signal) "Now let your inner mind lock in on that sensation of being cool and comfortable, and you can keep it that way during your entire stay in the hospital. You can enjoy going to your laughing place as often as you like, and you'll be able to ignore all of the bothersome things we may have to do, and *anything negative* that is said by anybody."

Comment: I just leave the patient in trance, go ahead

with his initial care, and get him moved to the Burn Unit. Often, he will drop off to sleep.

Doctor: "Go to your laughing place."

Comment: On subsequent days, this is all the signal the patient usually needs to drop into a hypnoidal state and tolerate bedside procedures, physical therapy, or the like.

Joseph Dane has produced an excellent videotape of a terrified and difficult burn patient quietly accepting whirlpool and debridement of both legs in hypnosis, then walking back to the ward (standing on his own two feet) for the first time. It is available from the video library of the American Society of Clinical Hypnosis.

REFERENCES

Bierman SF: Hypnosis in the emergency department. Am J Emerg Med 7:238–242, 1989
Chapman LF, Goodell H, Wolff HG: Changes in tissue vulnerability induced during hypnotic suggestion. J Psychosom Res 4:99–105, 1959
Ewin DM: Emergency room hypnosis for the burned patient. Am J Clin Hypn 26:9–15, 1986
Leor J, Poole K, Kloner RA: Sudden cardiac death triggered by an earthquake. New Engl J Med 334:413–419, 1996

Osler W: Aequanimitas with Other Addresses, ed 3. New York, Blakiston, 1953
Patterson DR, Goldberg ML, Ehde DM: Hypnosis in the treatment of patients with severe burns. Am J Clin Hypn 38:200–212, 1996
Ullman M: Herpes simplex and second degree burn induced under hypnosis. Am J Psychiatry 103:828–830, 1947
Wright ME: Suggestions for use of spontaneous trances in emergency situations. *In* Hammond CD (ed): Handbook of Hypnotic Suggestions and Metaphors. New York, W.W. Norton, 1990, pp 234–236

7

Hypnosis in Obstetrics and Gynecology

Larry Goldman

INTRODUCTION

Hypnosis can be a valuable tool throughout the entire course of pregnancy and into the postpartum period, from controlling hyperemesis gravidarum (excessive nausea and vomiting of early pregnancy) to the prevention and control of postpartum depression. The pregnant patient can learn techniques that will reduce her chances of cesarean section and lower the risk of premature delivery. Hypnosis can control blood pressure also.

Obstetric and gynecologic patients can use hypnotic techniques for a wide variety of uses. Hypnosis is an incredibly powerful tool for treating mind/body problems, and these patients present us with myriad problems and situations that intertwine psychological and physiological aspects so thoroughly that to adequately treat the body we must also attend to the mind. The uses of hypnosis in obstetrics and gynecology are limited only by your imagination and creativity. I hope that this chapter stimulates you to incorporate some of these techniques into your practice.

HYPNOSIS IN OBSTETRICS

Our obstetric patients remind us that pregnancy and delivery are normal physiological processes. Pregnancy is not an illness and delivery need not be a surgical event. Women have demanded the right to be included in the decision-making process—the process that determines how they will experience their labor and delivery. Hypnosis during pregnancy and delivery helps the woman accomplish her personal goal, established along with her obstetrician, of just how she will manage her labor and delivery. When the obstetric patient learns to use hypnosis she gains greater control over whatever challenges her pregnancy presents. Through the use of hypnosis the pregnant patient becomes a valuable ally to her obstetrician because they work as a close-knit team throughout the pregnancy, greatly improving the odds for a successful atraumatic outcome. The delivery becomes a shared endeavor between the mother, father, and physician that reduces the stresses of pregnancy, delivery, and the postpartum period for all concerned, including baby.

Controlling Nausea and Vomiting

Nausea and vomiting can make the first 3 months or more of pregnancy a nightmare for many women. The dehydration and acidemia, resulting from the patient's inability to hold down even water, pose a substantial health risk to both mother and child. Over the years, many remedies have been tried with varied levels of success. A plethora of medication has been used, the most notorious of which was thalidomide. The catastrophic birth defects and resulting lawsuits caused most drug companies to abandon product distribution and research in this area. Bendectin, the last remaining medication primarily indicated for nausea and vomiting of pregnancy, was removed from the market after multiple unsubstantiated lawsuits were filed alleging teratogenic effects. Hypnosis offers an effective, rapid, and safe method to control this problem. A very important factor is that the patient herself learns to control her own problem; this is a good start to the team approach to obstetric care.

Various techniques have been described detailing successful methods for controlling hyperemesis (Fuchs 1967; Fuchs 1980; Crasilneck 1985; Goldman 1990). Most deal with regaining control of the digestive tract through relaxation and positive reinforcement. Suggestions focus on control of both the physiological (hormonal and intestinal motility changes) and psychological (stresses from multiple sources) components of the problem. Hypnosis is used as both a therapeutic and diagnostic tool. Before formulating a treatment approach, it is imperative to ascertain the possible causes of the problem.

Ideomotor questioning can rapidly uncover hidden agendas that may need to be dealt with before therapy can be effective. Patients may be consciously unaware of psychological stressors. Stress may originate from family, friends, previous negative experiences, or from the patient herself. There may be a considerable amount of secondary gain obtained through the persistence and severity of the nausea and vomiting. In some cases hyperemesis is a learned response (e.g., "My mother and sister both vomited throughout their pregnancies and they had healthy babies").

There are situations in which the unconscious requires nausea and vomiting as reassurance that everything is okay. This scenario is common in women with a previous history of miscarriage, who mistakenly believe that the more you vomit the healthier the baby. An effective question for uncovering this line of thinking using ideomotor questioning under hypnosis would be, "Is there any reason why you might not wish to stop vomiting?" If the yes finger comes up, successful treatment will be impossible without further elucidating this reason.

The physiological portion of this problem is solved by teaching the patient self-hypnotic techniques that she can use to regain control over her alimentary tract. One of the easiest and most effective techniques is to first teach her how to make her nausea worse. Once she has accomplished this, the suggestion is then given, "If you can make it worse, then you can make it better." This suggestion seems quite logical to the unconscious mind, especially when it is in the hypnotic state. While under hypnosis, patients may also be given positive suggestions about the importance of good nutrition for development of a healthy, normal baby. Rapid self-hypnosis induction

---

Case study 7–1

I was asked to see a patient (S.R.) in consultation by one of my obstetric colleagues. This 19-year-old primigravida was seven weeks into her pregnancy. She had been hospitalized for the second time because of hyperemesis and dehydration. Her vomiting had been unresponsive to conventional therapy with intraveneous fluids, Tigan suppositories, and so forth.

S.R. appeared quite cheerful for someone in her condition. She seemed to actually enjoy her hospital stay. She readily consented to the use of hypnosis and was an excellent hypnotic subject. After rapidly entering a moderate depth trance, ideomotor questioning revealed the source of her problem. Her mother-in-law did not approve of her marriage, and S.R. felt that her vomiting in some way punished her mother-in-law. Every time the patient had contact with this lady, whether it be in person or by phone, S.R. would become violently ill and vomit.

Reframing was carried out under hypnosis. (During reframing a patient changes the way in which she views her problem and its solution.) The patient was given the suggestion that she could punish her mother-in-law far more effectively if she were able to appear happy and healthy whenever they had contact. It was suggested to S.R. that smiling at her mother-in-law would aggravate her much more than would vomiting. S.R. was discharged the following morning and had an uneventful course the rest of her pregnancy.

Hypnotic Suggestions for Control
of Hyperemesis

The normal peristaltic motion of your bowel and esophagus move food down into the stomach, then into and through the intestine, for absorption of nutrients. The unconscious mind controls the direction of peristalsis and the path food is supposed to take. The unconscious mind also knows how important nutrition is to the proper growth and development of your baby.

The unconscious mind also knows there are many times when the vomiting center of the brain needs to be stimulated (i.e., in case of food poisoning or intestinal flu), and it does this automatically. But during a normal physiological state, like pregnancy, it knows that this center should be suppressed, because vomiting and nausea are counterproductive to good nutrition. The unconscious mind knows nutrition is vital to a normal pregnancy outcome.

There may be times during the pregnancy when the conscious mind feels there is a need for nausea, but these times will be short-lived, lasting 30 seconds or less, and will not interfere with your ability to eat, digest, and absorb your meals in a normal, profitable fashion, assuring you and your baby proper nutrition throughout the pregnancy.

Your unconscious mind knows that your pregnancy is a normal, physical state and *does not* and *will not* have any need for vomiting.

Your unconscious mind knows that good nutrition is essential to the normal progress of your pregnancy and will work to assure you of this.

Now, I would like you to picture, very clearly, your favorite food, prepared as you like it. And see yourself with this food in a relaxed atmosphere, where you feel comfortable, safe, and secure. When you can vividly see and smell the food, please signal me.

Now, begin to eat your favorite food. I wonder how good it tastes, and how easily it goes down into your relaxed stomach and does not cause any nausea or urge to vomit.

Feel how satisfying it feels to eat and digest your favorite meal and know that you are giving vital nutrition to your normally developing infant—nutrition that cannot be obtained through intravenous feeding.

Now, at your own rate, finish your meal, and see how there is no sign of nausea or vomiting. Once you have finished your meal, please signal me.

Now, I would like you to begin to become more awake and aware, feeling very confident in your ability to eat and digest meals without any significant nausea and no vomiting, knowing that your unconscious mind will not allow you to vomit, because vomiting deprives both you and your baby of needed nutrition.

As you return to the awake, aware state, you will look forward to eating and enjoying your meals.

---

techniques can be useful in stressful situation to allow the patient to relax quickly and prevent the onset of nausea. Patients are also allowed to retain a small amount of nausea each day if they feel this is necessary to assure a healthy pregnancy.

Once the patient has learned to deal with her stressors and understands the physiology of her problem, she is then able to control her problem and enjoy her pregnancy.

In the majority of less severe cases of nausea and vomiting formal trance induction is not necessary. Waking hypnotic suggestions can be quite effective if properly presented. Anchoring a positive suggestion to an important landmark of the pregnancy can make the suggestion very therapeutic. For patients who are still vomiting at 10 weeks into the pregnancy, my favorite suggestion is, "I have found that once we can hear the baby's heartbeat, nausea and vomiting disappear within a week in most of my patients." Following this statement the patient is taken to an exam room where in 90% of the cases we can hear the baby's heartbeat for the first time. The excitement of the moment combined with the previously implanted suggestion usually results in a rapid cessation of the problem within a few days. Waking hypnosis by any other name would be called rapport!

Prevention of Premature Labor

Premature delivery is one of the leading causes of fetal loss in the United States and is the major contributor to the exorbitant costs of neonatal intensive care. Newton et al showed that pregnancies resulting in premature labor were far more common in pregnancies complicated by high levels of psychosocial stress (Newton 1979). Omer has shown that hypnosis combined with conventional pharmacological therapy can significantly prolong the duration of pregnancies threatened by premature labor (Omer 1987). Omer found that the addition of hypnotic techniques to standard therapeutic regimens prolonged pregnancies an average of 18% over those treated with conventional therapy alone.

Hypnosis improves treatment in several ways. First, patients learn to control the psychosocial stress that may be a precipitating factor in the onset of premature contractions. Second, patients can be taught to use hypnosis to become more vigilant. By recognizing their contractions earlier, they are able to initiate pharmacological therapy sooner, at a more effective point in the labor process. Third, the relaxation effect of hypnosis not only helps the patient tolerate the side effects of the pharmacological agent (usually Betamimetic drugs that cause nervousness and irritability) but also may serve to relax

---

Case study 7–2

L.P., a 31-year-old gravida 5, para 0222 (two live preemies, two spontaneous abortions) with a history of progressively earlier deliveries was initially seen at 6 weeks into her latest pregnancy. She considered termination of the pregnancy because of her well-founded fear of having another, even more severely premature infant. She had used pharmacological agents and bedrest with her last pregnancy with little success, delivering a 2 pound, 12 ounce little girl at 28 weeks' gestation. L.P. was anxious and depressed. Hypnosis was discussed and the patient opted to give it a try.

She was enrolled in our regular prenatal hypnosis class but at a much earlier stage in her pregnancy. Most of our patients do not begin class until their 28th week; L.P. began at 16 weeks. Four weeks later, she was already experiencing significant contractions and uterine irritability. Although others in the class received suggestions for comfortable, controlled childbirth, L.P. was given suggestions for uterine relaxation and heightened awareness of premature uterine contractions. The importance of having a full-term infant who wouldn't require tubes and other costly special care was also stressed while she was in trance. Being in class with patients who were excited, happy, confident, and close to term also served as an incentive to her. She was given oral tocolytics to be used on an as necessary (PRN) basis only.

The patient was able to continue all normal activities with the exception of sexual activity. Self hypnosis and tocolytics were used whenever she felt it was indicated. At 41 weeks' gestation, she arrived at the hospital, and with a great deal of pride and comfort delivered an 8 pound male infant without complication. Two years later, she returned and delivered another term male infant weighing 7 pounds, ¼ ounce.

---

chronic hypertension with exacerbation secondary to pregnancy. More commonly, however, it is a primary occurrence caused by the pregnancy. Treatment regimens depend on the severity of the disease and the stage of pregnancy. Hypnosis has been shown to be an effective adjunct to any of the more conventional modes of treatment (e.g., bedrest, pharmacological agents, or delivery). In an article in Lancet, Little et al described the effective use of hypnosis alone and hypnosis with biofeedback in the treatment of pregnancy-induced hypertension (PIH) (Little 1984). Groups containing hypnosis-trained patients require half the number of hospitalizations as the controls. Hypnotic groups also had significantly lower systolic and diastolic blood pressures than controls.

Many factors that influence the onset and degree of PIH are well understood, but the exact cause is still unknown. Stress and varying levels of renin, angiotensin, and other renal and adrenal substances all play a part in the disease. Hypnosis can be used to control stress levels and also directly reverse the vasoconstrictive effect of the disease process. Reduction of stress levels, through hypnosis and rest, reduces catecholamine levels that may be responsible for elevating blood pressure. The patient may also be taught to use hypnosis to dilate blood vessels, directly reducing peripheral resistance and decreasing mean arterial blood pressure.

In my own experience, early hospitalization is avoided. Patients are able to keep their blood pressures at a safe level using rest, hydration, and hypnosis, which

---

the smooth muscle of the uterus itself. Using imagery and projection techniques, hypnosis can also be used to increase the patient's motivation to continue her pregnancy to term. The extra attention and social support given to patients during their hypnosis training may also contribute to the reduction in prematurity rates.

Getting patients into hypnosis training early and making control of the problem a shared responsibility helps prevent premature labor. I recommend hypnosis training to all of our mothers who are at increased risk for premature births, especially those with twins.

Pregnancy-Induced Hypertension

Hypertension can present during pregnancy in many different ways. It can be a continuation of an ongoing

---

Case study 7–3

A 28-year-old gravida 2, para 1001 with one previously uncomplicated delivery developed an elevated blood pressure at 35 weeks into her pregnancy. Blood pressures varied between 132/88 mm Hg and 170/96 mm Hg during the 5 weeks prior to delivery.

The patient had already received hypnosis training in our hypnosis-prepared childbirth classes. Two extra hypnosis sessions were required to teach the patient methods to help control blood pressure while increasing circulation to the baby. The patient was also given suggestions, while in trance, that would enable her to be more alert to signs or symptoms of worsening disease (e.g., headache, vision changes, increasing edema, or decreasing fetal movement).

Delivery was accomplished at 40 weeks' gestation. The patient spontaneously delivered a 6 pound, 11 ounce female infant with excellent Apgar scores. Mom's diastolic pressure during labor and delivery never exceeded 94. No medications were required.

allows them to remain home until delivery of a mature baby can be accomplished.

It should be stressed that hypnosis is only one of many therapeutic and diagnostic regimens required to assure a safe, healthy delivery for mom and baby. The physician must be careful to follow all standards of care when dealing with this serious and potentially life-threatening complication of pregnancy. Hypnosis is an aid to, not a replacement for, good medical care.

Labor and Delivery

Of all the uses for hypnosis during pregnancy, labor and delivery is the premier occasion. The improvements made in the birth experience through the use of hypnosis, at times, appear to be miraculous. Although exact training methods vary greatly, the ultimate effect has been uniformly excellent. Some physicians emphasize only relaxation and pain control, whereas others include education about the birthing process and actually teach patients to control the entire delivery and recovery experience. My classes are focused on the latter.

The "Hypnoreflexogenous Technique" developed by Roig-Garcia and brought to this country by William Werner is the model from which I have developed my childbirth preparation course (Roig-Garcia 1961; Werner 1963). The premise expounded by both men is that labor is a normal physiological process, and that no normal physiological, within-the-body process causes pain. It is a basic simple fact. Unfortunately, without the use of hypnosis most patients are unable to accept this idea.

Roig-Garcia, Werner, and many others before them, including Grantley Dick-Read, believe that pain with labor is a learned response (Read 1953). Young women are programmed from early childhood to expect painful childbirth. It fact, in some ethnic cultures it is unacceptable not to have pain with childbirth. "If you don't suffer enough you won't appreciate what you have" is the attitude. Peer pressure, television, movies, magazines, and even the Bible teach women to expect pain. "To the woman he said, 'I will greatly increase your pains in childbearing; with pain you will give birth to children' " (Genesis 3:16). Women are bombarded from all directions with negative expectations about labor. Friends and relatives are quick to describe their worst labor experiences. Sometimes it seems that each person must top the other with horror stories.

The goal in our hypnosis classes is not painless childbirth but to empower the patient to experience labor the way she wishes and to always be in control. Hypnosis returns control of the problem to the patient. Once she has control, she can ignore negative suggestions from

friends, family, and even medical staff members. "Hi, Mrs. Jones. How often are your *labor pains*?" is a negative statement frequently heard on admission to the hospital.

In 1953, Grantley Dick-Read, the father of the Lamaze movement in the United States, wrote the book called *Childbirth Without Fear* (Read 1953). In this book, Read theorized that the pain of childbirth resulted from a reverberating triad of fear, tension, and pain. He believed that fear caused tension; tension caused pain; and pain caused more fear. Read proposed that fear was produced by possession of bad information or a lack of correct information. He believed that the most effective way to control fear was through proper education of patients.

During our 12-week course, we attempt to do exactly what Read proposed. Our goal is to educate the patients and their partners. We discuss, in great detail, every facet of the labor, delivery, and recovery process. This discussion is done both in the waking and hypnotic states. It is our hope that this thorough education will eliminate the fear component and reduce the possibility of pain during labor. Along with the naturally sedating effect of hypnosis, this education process significantly reduces the tension that drives the pain arm of the triad.

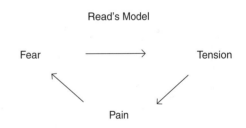

Read's Model

Our patients begin their training between 28 and 30 weeks into their pregnancy. If a patient is high risk for premature labor or hypertension, she will start earlier, usually around 20 weeks' gestation. Classes are done in a group setting, with no more than 6 couples in a group, and meet every 2 weeks. This format gives the couples plenty of time to practice between classes. Fathers of the babies are required to attend classes. We stress that this is a joint effort. Fathers are taught to be hypnotechnicians for their wives. It is an absolute necessity to have support from the fathers if hypnotic techniques are to be successful. Their support helps the mothers ignore negative suggestions from those who don't believe in hypnosis and from those who have had negative birth experiences.

During the first session, the couples learn the basics of hypnosis. We discuss and dismiss the myths and false information most people have learned about hypnosis. At this first meeting both partners are invited to experience trance states and relaxation. This experience gives the husbands a better idea of what their wives are experiencing when they are practicing at home. During this initial class, patients view a video of one of our previous hypnosis moms having her baby. This film helps to give the group confidence that this "hypnosis stuff" really works.

In the second class, patients and their partners view a video that teaches them the physiology and anatomy of childbirth. This is the beginning of the education process that will eventually alleviate the fear component. In trance (moms only) the suggestion is given, "You can look forward to each contraction because each contraction brings you closer to the delivery of your baby." The contraction of the uterus is equated to the contraction of other muscles in the body such as the heart. Patients are reminded that under normal circumstances the heart causes no pain when it contracts because, just like the uterus in labor, this is a normal physiological process. Therefore, if there is no pain when the heart works there should be no pain when the uterus contracts doing its work. During this second class, fathers learn basic hypnotic induction and deepening techniques that they can practice with their partners at home. We start with progressive relaxation and some imagery.

Contrary to Lamaze training in which patients learn techniques to divert attention away from contractions, we teach patients to focus on their contractions. They are taught that most hypnotic inductions go from a state of tension to one of relaxation. Their contractions (tension) can serve as a cue to the unconscious mind to begin the relaxation process. The contraction causes a reflex relaxation response, hence the name *Hypnoreflexogenous Technique*.

During the third class a couple who recently delivered using hypnosis address the class. This visit helps to motivate the class as well as legitimize the theories they are learning. Both mom and dad are encouraged to discuss their birthing experience. During this class couples also learn more rapid induction techniques, such as Chiasson's technique (Chiasson 1984). In this way they can spend less time with induction and more time on suggestions. Music as an induction and deepening technique is also introduced during this session. Following this introduction, couples are taught the basics of self-hypnosis—Garver's modified six-step approach (Garver 1990).

At each of these first three classes, demonstrations of hypnotic phenomena are done on different classmates. These demonstrations serve as trance ratification for

the expectant couple and again helps to motivate them to practice at home. We emphasize that practice is the key to success, and it will take a great deal of practice to change their expectations and eradicate the negative conditioning they have been exposed to throughout most of their lives. We remind them that all learning occurs through repetition. The more they practice, the more they will be able to control.

The fourth class is a tour of the areas of the hospital they will be in during their labor. I am the tour guide for this field trip. During the tour we discuss everything that might occur when they are in labor. The couples are instructed to focus on and remember as many physical details about the hospital as possible. These images will serve as a background for the rehearsals they will conduct under hypnosis during the next 4 weeks before delivery. Visiting the hospital removes one of the new mother's biggest fears, the fear of the unknown.

The fifth class begins with the same video seen in the second class, which enables the couples to incorporate the hospital tour and the anatomy and physiology of delivery into their labor and delivery rehearsal imagery. More rapid induction techniques are added, including eye roll techniques. At the end of this class, glove anesthesia is taught, which serves a dual purpose: It builds an incredible amount of confidence in the patient, and it gives her a method of pain control should an episiotomy be necessary at time of delivery.

The sixth and last class is a discussion session of possible complications that may occur and might necessitate changing the birthing plan. We discuss forceps and vacuum delivery, use of Pitocin, abnormalities of labor, and even cesarean section. Couples are taught that even though complications may occur along the way, it will be easy for them to make the necessary adjustments and remain in control.

Changing the patient's expectations about labor and delivery is vital to the success of this technique. Patients are encouraged through suggestion to look forward to their delivery as a joyous occasion. It is suggested that they plan this delivery as a celebration, bringing whatever they need to make it a happy birthday party. Changing expectations also reduces fear, tension, and pain.

Control is the most important aspect of the entire training process. The patient is taught to do whatever she feels necessary (within reason) to stay in control. At times this may mean taking an analgesic. Retaining control once the patient is admitted to the hospital requires a great deal of preparation on the patient's part and agreement of the staff to cooperate with the patient's requests. The staff must be trained to respond to hypnosis patients in a way that does not unintentionally sabotage all the work the patient and physician have invested. I require all nurses caring for my hypnosis-prepared obstetric patients to view a 45-minute tape about hypnosis and delivery. Preventing staff from giving the patient negative suggestions is a difficult problem that must be solved if hypnosis is to work well. In an effort to protect the moms from interference from well-meaning friends, family, and staff, I give patients the suggestion, "You can ignore negative comments from family, friends, and even staff that might interfere with your ability to have your baby your way."

Hypnosis provides many benefits to both the patient and physician. It converts a potentially stressful experience into an enjoyable shared endeavor for both parents and the physician; it can also greatly reduce the chances of cesarean section. The average rate of cesarean section in the United States is 20% to 30%. The rate for hypnosis patients is less than 5%. Needless to say, this reduction makes the hospitals and managed care groups very happy. A benefit to the baby is a significant reduction in exposure to medications during labor.

It is quite rare to see postpartum depression in a hypnosis mom, as a result of several factors. First,

---

Case study 7–4

At 4:00 PM, R.G., a 28-year-old gravida 2 para 1, arrived at the office having contractions 5 minutes apart. She had been having less regular contractions since approximately 9:00 AM but had spent most of the day attending to her routine chores, including the care of her young daughter. Upon presenting at the office, she was quite calm, comfortable, and completely in control. On occasion, she would close her eyes and drift into a relaxed state with a contraction. Pelvic exam revealed that her cervix was 4 to 5 cm dilated. Given the choice of hospitalization or observation, she opted for a trip to get a snack. When she returned an hour later, her cervix was 7 to 8 cm dilated, and she said she could feel the baby "moving down." She was sent to the hospital at this time, a 5-minute drive. Approximately 5 minutes after arriving on the labor floor, she delivered a 7 pound, 5 ounce baby girl over a midline episiotomy. The episiotomy was repaired under hypnoanalgesia. A retained placenta required manual removal and uterine curettage after delivery of the baby, which was also accomplished under hypnoanalgesia. R.G. then got off the delivery bed and walked out to recovery while her husband carried the baby.

Self-hypnotic techniques learned during class were used to contract the uterus in the postpartum period. Twenty-four hours after delivery, she went home. She received no medications during her hospital stay.

Case study 7–5

After every class, I.G. came over to me and said, "It's going to work for everyone else, but not for me." Now on her second baby, this Hispanic, Jewish mother-to-be was having great difficulty changing her expectations. She was an excellent hypnotic subject, having used hypnosis earlier in this pregnancy to control the nausea and vomiting that had plagued her entire first pregnancy. Her first delivery using Lamaze had not been a pleasant experience, to say the least. Her ethnic and cultural background made comfortable childbirth an unacceptable option. After each class I encouraged her to continue to practice and not worry whether or not she would be successful. Shortly after completing our classes, she called me at approximately 9 PM on a Saturday night and informed me that she was in labor; I told her that I would meet her at the hospital. I arrived at 9:30 PM; she arrived at 11:15 PM. When I asked I.G. what took so long to get to the hospital, she responded in a very calm, controlled manner that she needed to fix her husband meals for the next few nights since she was going to be in the hospital. Then, she needed to shower, shave her legs, and drop her daughter off at Grandma's before coming to the hospital. I suggested that we needed to check her progress. A pelvic exam revealed her cervix to be 9 cm dilated. We rapidly prepared her for delivery. Within a few minutes of admission, I.G. was in position ready to deliver. She began to push, and at this point looked between her legs and said, "Larry, I've got to scream." I said fine. I.G. let out a blood curdling scream and delivered the baby. After I placed the baby on her abdomen, she looked up at me again, and with a very straight face said, "See, I told you it wouldn't work for me." To this day, she still tells her family how she suffered during childbirth!

---

the delivery is an extremely rewarding experience for both parents. Second, relaxation techniques learned during classes can be effective in alleviating postpartum stress and allowing the mother to obtain much needed rest. Third, having been in control throughout the labor and delivery process gives the new mom much needed confidence during the postpartum period.

It is extremely important for physicians working with hypnosis-trained expectant mothers to realize that each patient will respond in her own way at time of delivery. The physician must not impose expectations for delivery upon the patient. Ethnic and cultural forces will mold patients' responses. Control, not painless childbirth, is the goal. If you attempt to make patients have their babies your way, you will be quite disappointed with the result.

Hypnotic Suggestions for Labor

Labor is a normal, physiologic process. The contractions of the uterus are no different than the contractions of any other muscle of the body.

Surely you will feel the power of your contractions, but they are nothing more than muscular contractions.

Remember that each contraction carries you closer and closer to the delivery of your baby through a normal vaginal delivery.

Each contraction will be perceived as you desire, not as others would have you perceive them.

Your unconscious mind will cause you to become relaxed with each contraction—the stronger your contractions become, the more deep your relaxation will be.

Your husband's voice will be as relaxing to you as mine. Your confidence in yourself and your partner will grow with each contraction.

You will look forward to each contraction, realizing that each one carries you closer and closer to the delivery of your baby.

Labor and delivery are exciting, enjoyable experiences that you can share with your partner in a relaxed, comfortable setting.

Remember that while you are in labor you are always in control.

You will find your husband's touch and voice to be relaxing and reassuring to you.

You will find that when your husband places his right hand on your left shoulder, you will become very deeply relaxed, when appropriate, without any effort on your part.

Just as you experience no discomfort when the muscles of your heart, intestine, or bladder contract, you will experience no discomfort when the muscles of your uterus contract because these are all normal physiological functions.

Breech Presentation

Breech presentations occur in approximately 3% of all term deliveries. Because of the present malpractice situation, the vast majority of these births are delivered via cesarean section. Several techniques have been suggested to convert the breech presentation to a vertex (cephalic—head down) position prior to the onset of labor. Among these are positioning the patient in knee-chest position, playing music between the patient's legs, external podalic version, and hypnosis. Of these, the most widely accepted method is external version, which entails manually manipulating the position of the baby through pressure placed on the baby through the abdominal wall. The success rate is approximately 50%.

Hypnosis has been suggested by one author and, although his results are impressive, his methods and statis-tical analysis are somewhat suspect (Dreher 1996). He proposes stress as a cause of breech presentation. (I am unaware of any scientific evidence to support this theory.) His treatment method is based on this proposal. Reducing stress, and positive suggestions for changing position of the baby, result in increased rates of spontaneous conversion, according to the author. Although I have had no experience with his method, I have found that the relaxation created with hypnosis significantly reduces the discomforts usually associated with external version attempts. This makes manipulation of the baby easier and most likely improves the success rate.

Whether hypnosis alone will prove to be a successful technique for conversion of breech presentations will require further study and replication of the aforementioned author's results.

Hypnosis has many uses throughout pregnancy. Both patient and physician can benefit from them. By making pregnancy safer and more rewarding for mom and her partner, the stress of pregnancy for patient and physician can be greatly reduced. An added benefit of the birth experience is the improved breastfeeding abilities of the relaxed, confident mother.

HYPNOSIS IN GYNECOLOGY

Female genital tract health and illness are tightly linked to women's psychological well being. The relationship is bidirectional: Emotional stress and trauma can cause or exacerbate gynecological disorders and gynecological disorders can cause emotional stress. Gynecological disorders can adversely effect psychic well being. Because of this tight relationship, hypnosis is an effective tool in a multitude of gynecological situations. Hypnotherapy can be used as a therapeutic and diagnostic modality, allowing the gynecologist to treat both the physiological and psychophysiological aspects of the patient's malady. Without this holistic approach, successful treatment of gynecological problems is difficult, if not impossible.

Menstrual Disorders

Menstrual disorders are most frequently caused by disturbances in the hypothalamic-pituitary-ovarian axis. Whether it is menstrual excess or inadequate menses, disturbance of the delicate balance of female hormones is usually the culprit. This hormonal milieu is incredibly sensitive to the woman's emotional state. Anovulation caused by any stressor (emotional or physiological) results in the absence of progesterone production, which leads to the ill effects of unopposed estrogen. This circumstance may result in menorrhagia, irregular menstrual bleeding, amenorrhea, and even endometrial hyperplasia and cancer.

Fear of pregnancy is one of the most common causes of amenorrhea, especially in teens. On the other hand, pseudocyesis (false pregnancy) is caused by an excess psychological need for pregnancy (Rakoff 1961). It is imperative that a gynecologist do a thorough physical and psychological examination when treating menstrual disorders.

Ideomotor questioning can be a very effective method of uncovering emotional stress that the patient may not be aware of on a conscious level. During treatment of amenorrhea, I ask the patient if she would like to have her period again soon. If the answer is no, further questioning may be necessary before a therapeutic plan can be devised. If the answer is yes, suggestions can be given to resume menstruation at a reasonable date in the near future. The suggestions may not be effective until the stress that precipitated the amenorrhea is adequately resolved. The source of the stress may be recent, since the last menses, or distant, from childhood.

Specific techniques and suggestions for resumption of menses have been described by several authors (e.g., Kroger 1977). In most of the techniques, suggestions incorporate specific sensory images from previous menses. These images are created by repeating information gleaned from questions answered by the patient describing previous periods. This information can be obtained with or without the use of hypnosis. A regression can be done to her last period. The patient is then asked to describe the physical and emotional experiences of that period. The suggestions are usually phrased in an indirect, though confident manner. "As you remember and feel these sensations, you may begin to wonder whether your period will begin in a few days or a week. You may wish to begin carrying a tampon with you so that you are prepared for its resumption." Using such suggestions can create a positive expectancy. Do not give the patient a specific date because this may create performance anxiety and failure.

Dysfunctional uterine bleeding, including menorrhagia (excessive flow), and intermenstrual bleeding may also have a psychogenic origin. It is not uncommon to see a woman begin a heavy flow immediately following a traumatic event. Death of a loved one, serious accident, or even an upcoming wedding may induce menstrual flow at an unexpected time. Just as anovulation can cause amenorrhea, prolonged anovulation can cause menorrhagia or metrorrhagia because of the unopposed estrogen effect. Cheek and LeCron have done a considerable amount of work in this area (Cheek 1968). Refer to their text for specific suggestions and effective techniques. Hypnosis is only an adjunct to the treatment plan; physical pathology must be adequately identified and treated using conventional therapeutic techniques to assure comprehensive treatment of the bleeding disorder. Resolution of the problem becomes a joint venture between the patient and physician. Hypnosis allows the patient to share in the responsibility and success of the treatment.

Premenstrual Syndrome (PMS)

Premenstrual syndrome (PMS) is a condition experienced by women sometime during the 10 to 14 days prior to their period. By definition, the symptom complex resolves with or shortly after the onset of menses. Symptoms of PMS are both physical and emotional. An estimated 40% to 90% of women suffer from one or more symptoms each month. Between 2% and 9% experience symptoms so severe that they are impacted either psychologially or physically. Psychological symptoms include irritability, depression, anxiety, emotional lability, anger, impaired concentration, suicidal ideation, and sleep and appetite disturbances (especially binge eating.) Physical symptoms may include abdominal bloating, breast tenderness, fluid retention, dysmenorrhea, fatigue, headaches, nausea, vomiting, diarrhea, impaired coordination, acne, constipation, backache, and pelvic pain. The mean age of onset is 33.8 years but may range from puberty through menopause. The cause is unknown, but most researchers believe the cause is a combination of changes in hormonal levels and disturbances in the neurotransmitters of the brain. Disturbances in serotonin, norepinephrine, and dopamine levels are believed to be a major factor causing the psychological components of the syndrome. Treatment regimens are as varied as the symptoms. Effectiveness of these regimens is also quite varied. Strategies have included nutrition and exercise changes, educational programs, stress reduction techniques, counseling, "relaxation training," hormonal manipulation (using oral contraceptives, progesterone, and estrogen), analgesics, tranquilizers, mood elevators, diuretics, and even total abdominal hysterectomy and bilateral salpingoophorectomy. Recently selective serotonin reuptake inhibitors (SSRIs) have been shown to be quite effective for controlling many of the psychological symptoms.

The most common complaint from women with PMS is "I feel as though I have lost control." The greatest gift that hypnosis bestows upon these women is the ability to regain control. When used in conjunction with the aforementioned multifaceted approach, hypnosis can potentiate all of their effects and give the woman a renewed sense of control. She can become an active participant in her own treatment. Self-hypnotic techniques can directly reduce anxiety, emotional lability, and anger while improving self-esteem and reducing depression. Control of dietary cravings for sweets may reduce symptoms brought on by their intake. These symptoms include irritability, fatigue, and headaches, all of which may be exacerbated by the reactive hypoglycemia following sugar ingestion.

Hypnotic techniques that have been shown to be effective in PMS treatment include ego-strengthening exercises, rapid induction of self relaxation, anger control through self-guided imagery, and direct symptom relief through pain control techniques. Biofeedback can be used to increase the patient's confidence concerning her control of body functions. Specific suggestions and techniques can be obtained from Dr. Cory Hammond's chapter in W. Keye's book, *The Premenstrual Syndrome* (Hammond 1988).

In a typical clinical example, a mother of three presents at the office with the chief complaint of "losing it" 1 week prior to each period. She complains of inability to control emotions and anger. Routine family stress leads to uncontrollable outbursts directed at children and husband.

The patient is given a PMS calendar to chart her symptoms and their exact timing and severity in relation to her period. She is also given an instruction sheet explaining PMS and describing changes in nutrition, exercise, and work schedules. At her return visit in 1 month, her calendar is reviewed and the effects of lifestyle changes are discussed. If the calendar confirms the PMS diagnosis, she is offered hypnosis as another adjunct to treatment. If she accepts, she is taught self-hypnotic techniques for rapid induction of relaxation. Usually a physical cue, such as pressing the thumb against the index finger, is used to induce light trance. She is instructed to use the cue any time she feels stress building. She is also taught to retreat to a private, safe place, and do imagery for stress reduction. The imagery, such as breaking large rocks into small ones with a hammer, allows her to release her anger without attacking family members. All of this can be taught in one or two sessions.

Dysmenorrhea

Dysmenorrhea (painful periods) can be quite disabling to women and can interfere with home, school, and business life. There are many ways to manage this problem, most of which entail taking oral medication. These medications may be analgesics (NSAIDs), muscle relaxants, or oral contraceptives. Occasionally, the problem may be so severe as to necessitate surgery. The extent of surgery may range from simple laparoscopic procedures to total abdominal hysterectomy.

It is important to ascertain the cause of dysmenorrhea, if possible. Physical or emotional problems, or a combination of both, may be the cause of the pain. History, physical exam, laboratory studies, ultrasound, and sometimes surgical procedures are necessary to elucidate the source of the pain. Hypnosis can be used as a diagnostic and therapeutic tool for dysmenorrhea.

Frequently, dysmenorrhea is a physical symptom of emotional stress. Traumatic events in a woman's early years may cause emotional scars resulting in physical pain. These traumas may have resulted from rape, incest, other forms of sexual abuse, or they may be the result of embarrassment occurring during adolescent years. In other cases, women have been conditioned to expect pain with periods through negative comments made by relatives or friends long before menarche. Whatever the source, treatment cannot be completely effective without eliciting the cause and dealing with it.

Hypnosis is an excellent tool for uncovering many of these causes. Through age regression techniques, anchoring, and ideomotor questioning, information that is not accessible to the conscious mind can be obtained. Once this information is obtained, treatment plans can be devised to resolve the unconscious source of pain. In some abuse situations referral for intensive psychiatric therapy may be required, whereas in other situations re-education and changing perceptions and expectations may be all that is necessary (this can be accomplished in both the waking and hypnotic state). Many times hypnosis can be used to reframe past traumas, remove self-guilt, and alleviate the need for self-punishment. The gynecologist's training and level of comfort will determine how much of this work is done in the gynecologist's office and how much is referred to a hypnotherapist.

Self-hypnosis can also be used for relaxation that raises the pain threshold. Patients can also learn hypnotic techniques for direct pain control if necessary. Hypnosis can significantly reduce the need for analgesic medications and the gastric irritation that frequently accompanies their use.

Sexual Dysfunction

Sexual dysfunction is quite similar to dysmenorrhea both in its cause and treatment. The source of either problem may be an early childhood trauma involving sexual abuse. Religious indoctrination may create guilt and negative expectations in a child, resulting in an unrewarding sexual life or quite painful periods. Once again, finding the cause is a very important part of resolving the problem. There are, however, several brief techniques for treatment of sexual dysfunction that ignore the cause and go directly to behavior modification techniques (Aroaz 1980). Hypnosis is again a very valuable tool in the treatment of this problem and can significantly shorten the course of therapy. Refer to the works of Dr. Corey Hammond for specifics of diagnosis and treatment of these problems, including effective hypnotic strategies and therapeutic suggestions (Hammond 1990).

Gynecologic Surgery

Hypnosis is an invaluable tool during major and minor gynecologic surgical procedures because it not only improves the outcome and reduces the need for many sedatives and analgesics but also has a much greater benefit to the patient. Hypnosis returns control of the situation to the patient and allows her to share in the responsibility and credit for her recovery. Hypnosis turns the surgical procedure into a team effort, improving the chances for success.

We use hypnosis preoperatively, intraoperatively, and postoperatively. Hypnosis is used as an educational tool preoperatively to reduce stress and increase positive expectations. Intraoperative suggestions while under anesthesia are used to reassure the patient that everything is going well and to create a positive attitude about recovery. Postoperatively, waking positive affirmations are given encouraging and complimenting the patient's ability to control and hasten her recovery. In the minor surgery setting, hypnosis removes the need for conscious sedation with medications, which significantly reduces postoperative recovery room time; therefore, the patient is allowed to return to normal activity soon after the procedure without a sedative "hangover."

Sexually Transmitted Diseases

Venereal warts, herpes, and HIV are all viral sexually transmitted diseases (STDs) with strong emotional interactions. Each of these infections causes considerable emotional stress in the victims, and that stress significantly increases the virulence and frequency of viral attacks. High stress levels tend to reduce the effectiveness of the immune system, which allows the human papilloma virus (HPV) (wart virus), herpes simplex virus (HSV), and HIV virus to escape the body's defense system. As a result, warts flourish, herpetic ulcers develop and spread, and T-cell counts drop precipitously.

Hypnosis can improve the immune response and can direct the system's attack on areas of viral activity. Herpes and condyloma sufferers can be taught self-hypnotic techniques for relaxation and stress reduction to decrease the number of outbreaks. Patients also learn visu-

---

Preparation of the Surgical Patient

Following is an outline of how I use hypnosis in gynecologic surgery:
Principles:

1. Keep all statements phrased in optimistic terms.
2. Avoid words like "if," "maybe," and "try."
3. Describe all planned surgery and mention possibilities of change of plan during procedure.
4. Remove fear.

Procedure
A. Introduction to hypnosis at preoperative office visit:

1. Relate how hypnosis improves recovery.
2. Dispel misconceptions.
3. Remove fear of hypnosis.
4. Discuss postoperative expectations.
B. Preparation in hospital the night before surgery:
1. Elicit and discuss fears and misconceptions about surgery.
2. Tour the expected path to operating room, including preoperative and postoperative areas and operating room.
3. Induction (usually Chiasson).
4. Rehearsal under hypnosis.
   a. Preoperative preparation, including IVs, enemas, medicine, catheter placement, and surgical preparation
   b. Stretcher ride; be as descriptive as possible
   c. Preoperative area
   d. Entrance into operating room
   e. Chemo-induction; taste of Pentathol or feel of epidural catheter placement or intubation
   f. Intraoperative sounds; discuss ability to retain hearing
   g. Awakening
   h. Transfer to recovery room
   i. Recovery room routine; deep breathing and no nausea
   j. Rapid recovery of bowel and bladder function after return to room
   k. Positive feeling to be experienced in postoperative period
   l. Control of postoperative discomfort
   m. Increased speed of wound healing

5. Intraoperatively, discuss surgery in positive terms and expectations, especially during induction and awakening from general anesthesia (a highly suggestible state).
6. In recovery room discuss case with patient whether awake or asleep; be very upbeat.
7. Reinforce suggestions for rapid recovery.
8. In patient's room, discuss case positively and reinforce suggestions for rapid recovery.
   Finally, your nursing staff will make it or break it for you. Train them well.

alization techniques for mobilizing the immune system to eliminate the warts and heal the ulcers. Hypnosis also can be valuable in controlling the pain of herpes and the itch of warts.

Difficult Patient

For many patients, a visit to the gynecologist is an intimidating, often traumatic experience. Negative expectations are learned at an early age and reinforced over many years. The gynecologist is rivaled only by the dentist when it comes to striking fear in the hearts of patients. Examining a patient who is embarrassed, scared, and possibly in pain can be a difficult and frustrating experience for both the doctor and patient. A technique that reduces the tension and discomfort during an examination can significantly improve the effectiveness of that examination and helps the patient have a positive experience.

Hypnosis can reduce patient anxiety and create a greater level of rapport between the patient and her gynecologist. Children and adolescents, usually the most difficult patients to examine, are excellent subjects for hypnotic techniques.

Music is a wonderful hypnotic technique that can be very effective in relaxing the patient long before you see her. Waiting room and exam room music can be quite soothing. When coupled with pleasant pictures and a room at a comfortable temperature, patient stress levels can be significantly lowered. Avoiding physical cues such as white lab coats, which heighten tension, also reduces the patient stress level. A soft voice and relaxed speech pace are indirect waking hypnotic suggestions to the patient that she can relax.

During the examination more formal hypnotic techniques, such as guided or unguided imagery, can be employed. Allowing the patient's conscious mind to leave the room during the exam can make the experience quite atraumatic for both patient and physician. Warming the speculum and using plenty of lubricant also helps. Having the patient focus on her breathing relaxes the mind and the abdominal muscles, a big advantage when doing a bimanual examination. Reducing the patient's anxieties and the discomforts usually associated with pelvic exams improves rapport between the physician and patient, which significantly improves the chance for successful treatment.

Infertility

Approximately 10% to 15% of couples attempting pregnancy experience infertility problems (Speroff 1994). In 80% of these cases a physiological cause for this problem can be found (Speroff 1994). The remaining 20% of infertile couples are left with no specific course of treat-

ment for their failure to conceive. Psychological factors have been long proposed as one of the causes of infertility in apparently physically normal couples. Anecdotal reports abound citing couples who escaped the performance anxiety and became pregnant while under no therapeutic regimen. One of the most frequent stories is about couples who give up trying to conceive, adopt a child, and within 1 year are pregnant. Another scenario is the vacation escape to the mountains with pregnancy ensuing from the mountain encounters. Stress certainly plays an important role in couples' ability to conceive.

The actual mechanism through which the psyche affects fertility is still controversial. Some believe stress adversely affects tubal motility (Kroger 1977). Others believe that ovulation is impaired, and cervical mucus becomes hostile to sperm because of hormonal imbalances.

Hypnosis, a proven stress-reduction technique, is an ideal therapeutic modality for helping the 20% of infertile couples in whom no physical defects could be detected. There have been several articles written on this subject. Gravitz recently reviewed the literature and described two cases in which hypnosis was successfully used to resolve infertility problems. In both cases the women became pregnant within 3 months (Gravitz 1995).

Hypnosis may be used to reduce performance anxiety. Visualization techniques may directly affect physiological functions. Direct suggestions describing the normal process of ovulation, ovum transport through the fallopian tubes, and implantation and nourishment of the fertilized egg have been shown to be quite effective (Gravitz 1995). Some feel that the reduction of stress provided by hypnosis reduces tubal spasm, allowing normal passage of the ovum through the fallopian tube (Leckie 1965). Reducing stress through hypnosis also allows the normal production of cyclic hormones (estrogen and progesterone), which are necessary to prepare the endometrium for implantation and create a "friendly" cervical mucus that will improve sperm migration into the uterus.

After years of failure, many infertile couples develop a negative mind-set about their ability to conceive. Hypnotic techniques can be used to create positive expectations. A more confident, optimistic couple will usually find sex more rewarding and less of a chore. This optimism may lead to more frequent intercourse, resulting in an increased chance of pregnancy.

Whatever its mechanism of action, hypnosis appears to be an effective therapeutic option for infertile couples, including the 80% with physiological problems.

Cancer

Endometrial, breast, cervical, and ovarian cancers account for a large number of female deaths each year.

Treatments for these malignancies include surgery, radiation, chemotherapy, and combinations of these regimens. Hypnosis can be used as an adjunct to each of these modalities (Levitan 1987) and can improve the body's immune response to the invading cancer (Olness 1981). Other therapeutic regimens become more effective when the patient's immune system is mobilized. Hypnosis can be used to improve patient expectation and increase the will to survive. Side effects of chemotherapy and radiation can be significantly reduced by using hypnosis.

HYPNOSIS AND THE OBSTETRIC–GYNECOLOGY PRACTICE

Malpractice Suit Prevention

Several years ago, I had a difficult delivery involving identical twins with twin/twin transfusion syndrome (shared circulation resulting in discordance in size and blood count). It was a complicated vaginal birth requiring a breech extraction of the second twin. Both babies eventually did quite well, but the second twin did require a blood transfusion. The patient was a hypnosis class graduate and did extremely well during the entire delivery. At her six-week checkup, the patient informed me that she had been contacted by a lawyer who informed her that there was money to be made from her complicated delivery. Not only did she refuse the offer, she reported the experience to me so that the lawyer's spy could be removed from the hospital staff.

Malpractice suits, and the fear of them, contribute greatly to reduced job enjoyment experienced by many physicians, especially obstetricians. We all realize that we are not judged on our techniques as much as on our results. No matter the cause, if the result is not perfect, it's our fault! Lawsuits have become an expected side effect of medical practice, adding stress to a profession that already has stress built into everyday practice.

One of the most common reasons given by plaintiffs for suing the doctor is lack of communication and rapport. When you use hypnosis in your practice, you are forced to communicate with your patients. Because of the increased interaction between physician and patient necessary to successfully incorporate hypnotic techniques into the treatment regimen, more time must be taken for communication. Without good rapport, hypnosis will not work.

Another important malpractice safeguard is the shared responsibility for treatment. Because hypnosis empowers the patient to become an active participant in the treatment of her problem or birth of her baby, she also shares in the responsibility for the success or failure of treatment. *Rehearsal of the surgical procedure or delivery under hypnosis is the ultimate informed consent.* In childbirth classes, rapport is also developed with the fathers, again reducing risks of misunderstandings. Patients trained in hypnosis are also more likely to comply with instructions, again improving the likelihood of a positive outcome. The improved rapport, the reduced risk of complication, and the happy, satisfied couple all reduce the risk of malpractice litigation.

Why did my patient turn down the lawyer's offer? I think that can be answered by quoting her statement after successfully delivering the second twin. As both babies lie in their warmers, she looked up at me and said, "See, I told you *we* could deliver these kids vaginally!"

Survival for the Obstetric–Gynecology Physician

Stress and the practice of obstetrics and gynecology are inseparable. Managed care, lawyers, life threatening illnesses, sleep deprivation, and financial pressures combine to make this specialty one of the most stressful in medicine. In Florida, the average age at which physicians drop obstetrics from their practices continues to decrease. Disability claims for OB–GYN physicians are at record levels. Physicians are retiring from medicine at earlier and earlier ages. Unless physicians find a way to reduce the stress, "burn out" is inevitable.

Hypnosis is not a panacea for doctor burn out, but it does offer an ounce of prevention when the pound of cure requires desertion from practice. Self-hypnotic techniques can rapidly reduce the stress of critical situations, allowing decision making to be more rational and effective. Removing the emotions of the moment may clarify the situation, enabling the physician to rapidly assess the problem and choose the proper course of therapy. The induction cue may be as simple as placing a stick of gum in the mouth or pressing the thumb against the index finger. An always available tranquilizer with no side effects. no clouding of intellect, and no possibility of addiction, hypnosis can be a life saver for the physician as well as the patient.

During those incredibly long, laborious days in the office when frustration with managed care intrusions, insurance company restrictions, and noncompliant patient encounters reach unbearable levels, self-hypnosis offers a quick relaxing escape to the beach or mountains. This hypnosis can be done between patients in the privacy of one's office. In a few minutes, the physician can re-energize and rejuvenate, making the rest of the day more pleasant and satisfying. Dissipating frustrations is more beneficial than unloading them on patients, staff, and family. Some physicians have found that scheduling specific times in the day for self-hypnosis is extremely effective. The time expended for hypnosis is more than made up for by the time saved working more efficiently in the revitalized posthypnotic state.

The effects of sleep deprivation can be obviated for short periods of time through short, self-hypnotic rest and relaxation periods. Rapid relaxation techniques also allow the OB-GYN physician to make the most of those periods when sleep is possible. It is a great advantage to be capable of rapidly reaching restful levels of sleep.

Being able to return to restful sleep following interruptive phone calls is a necessity.

The uses for hypnosis in obstetrics and gynecology are limited only by the physician's imagination. Hypnosis contributes immensely to patient care and satisfaction, and at the same time can lengthen the physician's career. OB-GYN physicians can benefit greatly by learning and using hypnotic techniques in their practices and personal lives.

REFERENCES

Aroaz DC: Clinical hypnosis in treating sexual abulia. American Journal of Family Therapy 8(1):48–57, 1980

Cheek DB, LeCron LM: Hypnosis in gynecology. *In* Cheek DB, LeCron LM: Clinical Hypnotherapy. New York, Grune & Stratton, 1968, pp 112–113

Chiasson SW: Hypnosis in other related medical conditions. *In* Wester W (ed): Clinical Hypnosis: A Multidisciplinary Approach. Cincinnati, Behavioral Science Center, 1984, pp 303–304

Crasilneck H, Hall J: Clinical Hypnosis: Principles and Applications, 2nd ed. Orlando, Grune & Stratton, 1985, pp 213–214, 352–353

Dreher H: Can hypnosis rotate a breech baby before birth? The Journal of Mind-Body Health 12(3):46–50, 1996

Fuchs K, Brandes J, Peretz BA: Treatment of hyperemesis gravidarum by hypnosis. Hanfauh 72:375–378, 1967

Fuchs K, Paldi E, Abramovich H, et al: Treatment of hyperemesis gravidarum. Int J Clin Exp Hypn 28:313–323, 1980

Garver RB: Self-hypnosis training. *In* Hammond C (ed): Handbook of Hypnotic Suggestions and Metaphors. New York, Norton, 1990, p 418

Goldman L: Control of hyperemesis. *In* Hammond C (ed): Handbook of Hypnotic Suggestions and Metaphors. New York, Norton, 1990, pp 303–304

Gravitz MA: Hypnosis in the treatment of functional infertility. Am J Clin Hypn 38:22–26, 1995

Hammond DC: A clinical approach of a psychologist to PMS. *In* Keyes WR (ed): The Premenstrual Syndrome. New York, W.B. Saunders, 1988, pp 189–198

Hammond DC: Hypnosis with sexual dysfunction and relationship problems. *In* Hammond DC (ed): Hypnotic Suggestions and Metaphors, lst ed. New York, Norton, 1990, pp 349–353

Kroger WS: Clinical and Experimental Hypnosis, 2nd ed. Philadelphia, Lippincott, 1977, p 232

Leckie FH: Further gynecologic conditions treated by hypnotherapy. Int J Clin Exp Hypn 13:11–25, 1965

Levitan AA: Hypnosis and oncology. *In* Wester W (ed): Clinical Hypnosis: A Case Management Approach. Cincinnati, Behavioral Science Center, 1987, pp 332–354

Little BC, Benson P, Bear RW, et al: Treatment of hypertension in pregnancy by relaxation and biofeedback. Lancet 1:865–867, 1984

Newton RW, Webster P, Binu PS, et al: Psychosocial stress in pregnancy and its relation to onset of premature labour. BMJ 2:411–413, 1979

Olness K: Imagery (self-hypnosis) as adjunct therapy in childhood cancer. American Journal of Pediatric Hematology and Oncology 1(3):313–321, 1981

Omer H: A hypnotic relaxation technique for the treatment of premature labor. Am J Clin Hypn 29(3):206–213, 1987

Rakoff AE, Fried P: Pseudocyesis: A psychosomatic study in gynecology. JAMA 145:1329–1342, 1961

Reed G: Childbirth Without Fear, 2nd ed. New York, Harper & Row Publishers, 1953

Roig-Garcia S: The hypnoreflexogenous method: A new procedure in obstetrical psychoanalgesia. Am J Clin Hypn 6:1–13, 1961

Speroff L, Kase NG, Glass RH: Clinical Gynecologic Endocrinology and Infertility, 5th ed. Baltimore, Williams & Wilkins, 1994, pp 809–816

Werner WE: The use of the hypnoreflexogenous technique in obstetric delivery. Am J Clin Hypn 6:15–21, 1963

8

Hypnosis and Pediatrics
Howard Hall

INTRODUCTION

Complementary and alternative medical practices are growing in popularity in not only the United States but also Europe, Australia, and New Zealand (Micozzi 1996). Relaxation techniques were among the most frequently reported unconventional therapies used by adult respondents in a recent survey (Eisenberg 1993). Relaxation plays an important role in many forms of hypnosis. For example, subjects given hypnotic inductions produce similar responses as do nonhypnotized subjects who follow relaxation practices (Edmonston 1981). The benefit and the effectiveness of relaxation-based therapies for the treatment of chronic pain and insomnia (NIH Technology Assessment Panel 1996) have been clearly documented. A physiological "relaxation response" as described by Herbert Benson (1975) may be evoked by a variety of techniques including hypnosis, progressive relaxation, transcendental meditation, autogenic training, Zen, and yoga. In pediatrics, hypnosis is now being employed in primary care settings to address the new morbidities (versus old morbidities, like infections) that include anxiety, invasive procedures, pelvic examinations, pain and headache management, habit disorders, emergency medical treatments, and chronic and terminal conditions (Sugarman 1996).

The use of hypnosis for medical conditions is not new. Historically, hypnosis was an early, psychologically based, alternative medical approach to healing, like early medical practices such as bloodletting and the pharmacological remedies of Materia Medica (Hall 1986). Contemporary views of hypnosis have moved away from metaphysical energy notions and have focused on psychological and cognitive factors (Orne 1971).

Research was supported in part by an NIDA Grant #DA07957. The assistance of Anne Brennan in preparing this manuscript is gratefully acknowledged.

Hypnosis techniques have been employed with children since ancient times. *Hypnosis and Hypnotherapy with Children* by Gardner and Olness brought attention to the unique aspects of doing hypnosis with children (Gardner 1981). The growing body of literature on hypnosis with children necessitated a third edition of that text, with coauthor Daniel Kohen (Olness 1996). In recognition of the diverse ways to use hypnosis with children, Wester and O'Grady made an added contribution to the field with an edited multi-authored book, *Clinical Hypnosis with Children* (Wester 1991). Prior to these more recent works, Milton Erickson, whom some consider the father of modern clinical hypnosis, wrote a chapter on pediatric hypnotherapy, reprinted from his collected papers (Erickson 1980), in which he reminds us that "Pediatric hypnotherapy is no more than hypnotherapy directed to the child with full cognizance of the fact that children are small, young people. As such, they view the world and its events in a different way than do adults, and their experiential understandings are limited and quite different from those of the adult. Therefore, not the therapy but only the manner of administering it differs" (Erickson 1980).

The term *hypnosis* in this chapter will describe a relaxation-based practice that might also include the use of imagery, suggestions, and some type of induction. *Hypnosis* may be a loaded term for some parents because of misconceptions and distortions that are perpetuated by the media. For some religious families the use of hypnosis might be unacceptable; some fundamentalists even go as far as to equate it with Satanic practices.

In adult hypnosis literature Martin Orne has offered the following definition: "Hypnosis is said to exist when suggestions from one individual seemingly alter the perceptions and memories of another" (Orne 1971). In its extreme form hypnosis is easily identified: "Appropriate suggestions will cause a subject to perceive an individual who is not actually there and behave as if he were, or if the subject is told to forget certain events that have transpired, he will suddenly seem unable to recall them" (Orne 1971). In the pediatric hypnotherapy field hypnosis has also been defined as an "altered state of consciousness that may have certain temporary beneficial effects, such as tension reduction, but is not itself designed for that purpose" (Olness 1996). The term *altered states of consciousness,* however, suffers from much ambiguity. The role and importance of such altered states in healing phenomena have recently been questioned (Hussein 1996). Also, it is well recognized that adults vary in their responses to hypnosis and their abilities to enter altered states as measured by standardized susceptibility scales (Bates 1993; Bowers 1976). The scales that measure hypnotic susceptibility have test–retest reliability ranges up to .90+. About 90% of individuals pass the motor dimensions of tests (e.g., suggestions that an extended arm is getting heavier), whereas only a small minority of individuals (about 20%) pass more difficult test items, such as the inability to smell ammonia when held under the nose (Bowers 1976). In this chapter, hypnosis is described as an alternative or complementary practice, particularly for the management of a variety of pediatric complaints and anxiety-based symptoms. This approach is consistent with the relaxation component of hypnosis that is used as an induction. Please note that this use of hypnosis is contrasted with a prescriptive approach when the practitioner attempts to determine which pediatric conditions would be appropriate for hypnosis. For example, from a prescriptive perspective, one might ask, "Could hypnosis treat an adolescent with chronic fatigue syndrome?" The viewpoint in this chapter rephrases the question to "Which symptoms of the chronic fatigue syndrome might respond to a relaxation-based hypnotherapy intervention: the headaches, the somatic symptoms, or the insomnia?" Hypnosis is considered to be a safe procedure, with negative aftereffects limited to headaches or drowsiness (Coe 1979; Coe 1995).

HYPNOSIS AND CHILD OR ADOLESCENT DEVELOPMENTAL CONSIDERATIONS

Hypnotherapy must always be used within a context of good clinical practice. A thorough assessment, with careful history taking, is mandatory before any treatment plan is developed. In a retrospective chart review of 200 pediatric patients seen at a behavioral pediatric clinic, 80 children were referred specifically for hypnosis (Olness 1987a). Of this subset of 80 children, 20 (25%) had an unrecognized organic condition such as diabetes, carbon monoxide poisoning, or hyperthyroidism. Hypnotizability is complex in children but assumed to vary across the age span, peaking around middle childhood years and then decreasing in late adolescence (Olness 1996). The decreased ability of adolescents to enter trance states is consistent with Piaget's stage theory of cognitive development in which the child moves from preoperational thought and the concrete operational period to Piaget's fourth stage of formal operations. At this later stage, thinking becomes more abstract and the child is able to reason deductively. Wall outlined developmental considerations when using a hypnotic intervention with children (Wall 1991). Sensorimotor approaches can be employed for the young infant, whereas story telling may be utilized for the young child. For the adolescent, more adult-like induction methods may be employed, but in a naturalistic or permissive manner that allows the individual to maintain control while setting boundaries (Wall 1991).

Adolescence is a period of tremendous change for the developing child, both physically as well as emotionally. There is a growing appreciation for the need to treat adolescents as a unique population within pediatrics, with specialties in Adolescent Medicine and even a Center for Adolescent Health at our university. Although the field of child hypnotherapy is growing, less attention has been given to the special needs of the adolescent (see case study of an adolescent psychiatric inpatient in Aronson 1986).

Most children enter into trance state following a hypnotic induction; however, this outcome with an adolescent is far less predictable (Olness 1996). Nonetheless, the ability or inability to enter into a trance state should not limit the use of hypnotherapy with adolescents. The adolescent should not have a lowered expectation about accomplishing a therapeutic goal with hypnosis in a timely manner, based upon the inability to enter a trance. This is particularly true if the goal is a relaxation-based treatment outcome. For the adolescent, the relaxation aspects of hypnosis are emphasized when offering it as a treatment option because it is the most reliable and predictable outcome, and it also provides a context for why hypnosis is being offered. Hypnosis is introduced to the adolescent patient as a means of self-regulating the body and emotions using relaxation. Children and their parents are told that hypnosis is a "skill and not a pill." Self-practice is introduced and, requested from the first session, reinforces the skill aspect of the intervention. The term *hypnotherapy* is widely used in the field and is also used in this chapter to indicate a therapy that might include other modalities to facilitate therapeutic goals (Kirsch 1994; Olness 1996).

Case study 8–1

Dysphagia or swallowing disorders are often seen in school-age children. Hypnotherapy approaches have been helpful in treating children with dysphagia and with food aversion (Culbert 1996). Hypnotherapy has also been helpful in reducing a gag and emesis response to pill swallowing (LaGrone 1993). A 13-year-old boy with sickle cell disease and chronic renal failure came to our practice. His medical condition worsened after he developed anxiety and a conditioned dysphagia to oral medication. The child had an extensive history of monthly hospitalizations for his renal condition, and he was required to take daily oral medications. He recently stopped taking his medication after once gagging while attempting to swallow a pill. This response resulted in a deterioration of his medical condition and necessitated an inpatient hospital admission.

My services were requested to help him start swallowing pills again. After developing a rapport, I informed him that he would be offered a way to learn to swallow pills again by controlling his body through self-hypnosis. The patient knew that he needed to take his medication in order to stay healthy. Next, an explanation was given for why swallowing pills was difficult now (i.e. his throat tenses up). His problem was also normalized by informing him of how people sometimes gag and then develop a phobic response. I also disclosed that I found it difficult to swallow pills as a young child. Next, a relaxation-based induction was done. He chose to imagine that he was one of the superheroes flying through the air and then controlling his body and swallowing pills. Suggestions were also given that he would be able to experience these positive feelings from self-hypnosis practice. He responded well to the induction and reported feeling relaxed afterward. Next, the patient was asked to do self-hypnosis while I was present (normally, if he were an outpatient, I would have asked him to go home and practice this on his own, pointing out that he might find particular ways of doing self-hypnosis that I would wish to incorporate). I next modeled for him by swallowing a small, coated breath mint. After this, he engaged in self-hypnosis and with some coaching he successfully swallowed a mint. Before he attempted to take his rather large tablets, he did another brief self-hypnotic induction with superhero imagery of swallowing pills. After this induction and again with some coaching, he successfully swallowed his medication. This event was witnessed by his pediatric nurses, who responded with genuine pandemonium. He had three more pills to swallow and he did a brief induction prior to each pill. Each success was reinforced by praises from his nurses and me. He successfully took all four of his required medications and was discharged at the end of the day with a follow-up appointment in a week.

The variety of behavioral change strategies that were employed illustrate the broad use for the term "hypnotherapy." Such approaches included social modeling, reinforcement, successive approximation, along with a hypnotic relaxation induction with imagery. He had no subsequent problems swallowing pills after that brief intervention.

Given marked individual variation in responses to hypnotic suggestions and ability to enter trance, the use of a broad range and blend of therapeutic modalities is good clinical practice. Incorporating hypnotherapy in a pediatric practice may facilitate needed behavioral modifications. We employed a broad spectrum behavioral-change approach to a conditioned pill-swallowing phobia.

PROCEDURE–PAIN MANAGEMENT

Hypnosis for Infants and Babies

At Rainbow Babies and Children's Hospital of University Hospitals of Cleveland, a clinical nurse specialist, Barbara Stephens, RN, MAN, and a child life clinical specialist, Mary Barkey, MA, CCLS, developed a program to help infants and young children get through painful medical procedures. Pain management for preverbal and very young children requires a completely different approach than working with a child who understands language. Some of the early approaches at our hospital forced a child to lie flat during a procedure. Barkey and Stephens developed what they term *positioning for comfort*. The infant or baby sits up with the parent or caregiver in close physical contact hugging the child in a secure, comforting manner. This physical contact promotes a sense of control for the baby and enables a health care worker to immobilize the extremities. Adapting the same low voice tone as used in formal hypnotherapy, this intervention (Stephens 1994) for an infant or young child promotes comfort and relaxation.

Hypnosis for Young Children

For children, there are a variety of distraction techniques that do not require a formal hypnotic induction. For example, blowing away the pain has been an effective distraction and pain reduction technique for children 4 to 7 years of age (French 1994). For children 3 to 6 years of age, reading favorite stories is another method (Kuttner 1988a). Distraction techniques that require the child to take an active role, such as looking at pop-up books or blowing bubbles, are effective for children between 7 and 10 years of age who undergo painful bone marrow aspirations (Kuttner 1988b). A colleague in general academic pediatrics who completed one of our hypnosis training courses (A. Richardson, personal communications, 1996) provides two examples

for the use of distraction in a general pediatric practice. The first is a 5-year-old child who required a PPD (purified protein derivative) Tine test. No mention of hypnosis was made, but the child was questioned about bunny rabbits. The pediatrician told the child she was going to lightly draw a bunny rabbit face on her arm with an ink pen. The child had an opportunity to choose on which arm she wanted the bunny. Next, a bunny was drawn with two ears, two eyes, and a mouth. The child was asked, "Wait a minute, something is missing. What is missing?" The child pointed out that the nose was missing. The pediatrician next said, "The bunny needs a nose. I am going to put a nose on the bunny." At this time the PPD test was done with the child very excited about completing the bunny face. The child was also asked to watch the bunny's nose over the next few days to see if it would get big or red. Please contrast this naturalistic distraction approach to the language of "This is going to sting."

The second example uses a blowing distraction technique for a 7-year-old girl who needed a genital exam because of itching. The patient was very anxious and her abdominal area was quite tense. The pediatrician asked the child to visualize a large birthday cake on her abdomen with 100 candles. The child was next asked to place her hand on her abdomen and blow out the candles. At first she did not blow very hard and was reminded that there were 100 candles and she needed to blow all of them out. After about 3 to 5 minutes, her abdomen softened and the exam was completed without difficulty. Such distraction techniques can be employed by the professionals working with children with a minimal amount of formal training but a great deal of imagination.

When my youngest daughter was 9 years old, she developed nausea and pain over her right lower quadrant of the abdomen. This pain occurred when we were out of town for a Thanksgiving dinner. Placing dinner on hold, we took her to the local emergency room to rule out appendicitis. Requiring both blood drawing and an intravenous drip for fluids, distractions were employed in a playful manner with the assistance of her favorite stuffed animal. First, she was told that the bunny needed to show us his arm so we could wipe it with some cool, clean alcohol. The bunny was swabbed and then my daughter's arm was wiped with alcohol. Next, a writing pen was used to model a blood draw, explaining that the bunny needed to give us a blood sample. Our daughter next had a needle placed in her vein; she had little anxiety. In a playful manner, it was joked that we wanted to see how well the bunny did with these tests. Next, the bunny's arm was taped to represent an intravenous catheter, and then an intraveneous catheter was placed in my daughter's arm. She rested comfortably for the time it took her to become hydrated. She was later discharged so that we could salvage the rest of the Thanksgiving day. It is interesting to note that she never developed any stress around needles or emergency rooms but did have some concerns the following year about becoming nauseated before Thanksgiving.

Sometimes, for the younger child, hypnosis may be introduced without a formal induction, explanation, or the child even being aware that hypnosis is utilized. For example, Milton Erickson describes an incident in which his 3-year-old son fell down a flight of stairs and split his lip. The child screamed and his lip bled profusely. Erickson responded emphatically and sympathetically, "That hurts awful, Robert. That hurts terrible. . . . And it will keep right on hurting. . . . And you really wish it would stop hurting. . . . Maybe it will stop hurting in a little while, in just a minute or two." Erickson developed rapport and embedded suggestions within a naturalist manner. He explains, "In pediatric hypnotherapy, there is no more important problem than so speaking to the patient that he can agree with you and respect your intelligent grasp of the situation as judged by him in terms of his own understanding." Next, Erickson focused on the bleeding. He stated to his son, "That's an awful lot of blood on the pavement. Is it good, red, strong blood? Look carefully, Mother, and see. I think it is, but I want you to be sure."

Next, "His mother picked him up and carried him to the bathroom, poured water over his face to see if the blood 'mixed properly with water' and gave it a 'proper pink color.' Then the redness was carefully checked and reconfirmed, following which the 'pinkness' was reconfirmed by washing him adequately, to Robert's intense satisfaction, because his blood was good, red, and strong and made water rightly pink.

"Then came the question of whether or not his mouth was 'bleeding right' and 'swelling right.' Close inspection, to Robert's complete satisfaction and relief, again disclosed that all developments were good and right and indicative of his essential and pleasing soundness in every way." This example by Erickson nicely illustrates how hypnotic suggestions can be used with a young child, without a formal induction and without an announcement that hypnosis is taking place (Erickson 1980).

Selecting Words

The use of language is very important and requires a delicate balance. You never lie to children about pain

by telling them it is not going to hurt, nor do you insist, in the name of honesty, that there will be pain. Most clinicians leave the range of possibilities open because every child is different.

Word selection is important when using hypnosis with adolescents and adults too. When I was a psychology intern at a teaching hospital in New Jersey, there was a request to see a young adolescent with leukemia who was terminal and in a great deal of pain. I offered to teach him relaxation and hypnosis to help manage some of his discomfort. To my surprise, he informed me that he was not interested. Someone else had attempted hypnosis with him, and it did not work. Apparently, someone had just learned hypnosis and wanted to use it clinically so he gave an induction and told the patient that the pain would go away. It did not go away and the patient was turned off to hypnosis.

An example of the importance of language was illustrated during an experience my oldest daughter had when she was 8 years old. She was starting to wake up from light intravenous anesthesia after oral surgery. I entered the room and gave the following suggestions, "You might be surprised how comfortable you feel, how well you will rest tonight. Tomorrow, you will continue to feel better and better." Please note no formal induction was done because she was already in a chemically altered state.

In the middle of these suggestions, the oral surgeon walked into the recovery room with a puzzled look on his face, shook his head, interrupted me, and said, "Oh no, she is really going to be in pain tonight. She is really going to hurt. . . ." At this point I held up my hands to stop him before he said anything more. I continued with my suggestions about how comfortable she would feel. Please note that I did not say she would feel no pain. My daughter would have accepted the surgeon's suggestions that she would be in a "great deal of pain tonight" had I not have intervened. She had a speedy, uncomplicated recovery with no major pain complaints.

MANAGEMENT OF ACUTE PAIN

Relaxation and hypnosis-based approaches are becoming more widely used to help children cope with medical procedures related to cancer treatments (Kuttner 1988b; Olness 1996). Sometimes the medical procedures are of greater concern to children than the disease itself. Initially, at our hospital, our oncology staff made frequent requests for hypnotherapy interventions to help children cope with painful procedures. Over time, oncologists requested that we provide inservice training to teach the oncology nursing staff how to incorporate these procedures into their practice. Four relaxation/imagery training sessions were conducted for the nurses at the cancer center with didactic instructions and lots of group practice by the participants with each other. The referrals for our service dropped dramatically following such training; the nurses now do the hypnosis themselves.

Burn patients are in acute pain. Burns represent a major cause of mortality (10%) and morbidity for children, with about 60,000 children hospitalized each year for burn treatment (Hrabovsky 1992). Dabney Ewin, a general surgeon and hypnotherapy practitioner, has done pioneering work in the use of hypnosis for the emergency room treatment of burn patients (Ewin 1986). (See Chapter 6.) Ewin points out that the acutely burned patient will be in a hypnoidal state from the trauma, and thus will be extremely suggestible because of the trauma-induced, dissociative state. Hypnosis has

been observed to have profound effects on decreasing the inflammatory reaction and pain sensation around the burn area. In their presumably dissociative trance, they are asked to notice how "cool and comfortable" the injured areas are. Such a simple intervention can be done while the medical management of the burn is being completed. Hypnotherapy may turn out to be one of the most promising areas for interventions with burn patients (Patterson 1996).

Acute Pain and Anxiety

A pediatrician consulted me because of a 10-year-old girl who was seen in the outpatient clinic. A cockroach had crawled into the child's ear while she was sleeping. The doctors could not retrieve it out of the ear. The child was in distress and they were interpreting the distress as nociceptive pain. Thus they were planning to contact the ENT specialist, otorhinologist, to numb the ear in order to remove the insect. When I met the child she

---

Case study 8–2

A 13-year-old girl with a 3-year history of chronic headaches was referred. She carried a diagnosis of mixed headache syndrome and suffered from both occasional migraine and more chronic tension headaches. She was referred for hypnotherapy by our pediatric neurologist after a thorough work-up. Each outpatient session began with an assessment where she provided a history of the frequency and intensity of her headache complaints. She presented with a current headache complaint of 5 on a 10-point scale. She was able to distinguish between the two types of headaches. Her tension headaches were described as being in the back of her head, her migraines were described as more intense, and sick headaches were accompanied by nausea and vomiting. She did acknowledge that stress resulted in headaches. She denied current symptoms of depression during the psychological part of the assessment. She also denied symptoms consistent with obstructive sleep apnea, although she did report occasional insomnia, which responded well to hypnotherapy relaxation.

A basic hypnotic relaxation induction was done with calm scene imagery with a count-down for deepening suggestions. Suggestions were given for increased comfort and relaxation. No suggestions were offered for altered pain sensations, although given her association of stress with headaches, the implications were clear that decreased stress should be associated with decreased headaches. She responded well to the induction with acknowledgment of increased relaxation and decreased pain intensity with a postinduction rating of 2 to 3 on the 10-point scale.

Because she reported tension in the back of her head, instructions were given to incorporate the "awareness through movement" practices of the Feldenkrais method and the conscious use of self approaches of the Alexander technique (Alexander 1955). It has been my impression that employing only passive relaxation approaches, including hypnotherapy, is not as effective for neck-related muscle tension as is the addition of body education/awareness methods. Instructions were also given for this headache patient to do home practice for self-hypnosis and for her to become more aware of her head and neck positions while sitting and standing. With the assessment, history taking, and interventions, a first session can take up to 1 hour, with all subsequent sessions scheduled for 30 minutes.

At her second appointment, a couple of weeks later, she reported decreased frequency and lower intensity of headaches. She presented with a current headache complaint rated 4 out of 10. Despite my recommendations, she had only practiced a couple of times and that was when she already had a headache. Her sleeping had improved; she could now fall asleep in under 30 minutes. Follow-up work was done with the Feldenkrais/Alexander methods while sitting and standing with a chair. Also, a booster hypnotic induction was conducted. By the fifth session, she no longer had headache complaints. She reported practicing the self-hypnosis on a regular basis and was becoming more aware of sitting and standing and she could comfortably manage any occasional headaches without needing further hypnotherapy sessions.

would not let anyone near her ear. Clearly, a cockroach in one's ear is not pleasant or desirable, but her anxiety level appeared to be the major factor in this case. Hypnotherapy would have been difficult to conduct with such a panicking child. The intervention involved having a child life worker spend about an hour with the child until she calmed down. The insect was easily removed. From a nociceptive viewpoint, numbing the ear would be the intervention, but it is doubtful that it would have facilitated removing the insect. At the behavioral level, pain and anxiety would present quite similarly. From the emotional dimension, anxiety was the issue that needed addressing before the child could be approached with a successful intervention.

Case study 8–3

A 17-year-old boy had a history of one-to-two headaches every couple of weeks. These headaches were sometimes accompanied by nausea and vomiting. He also reported photophobia and phonophobia. The headaches lasted from 4 to 5 hours. He denied problems with sleeping or depression. The patient was treated with five outpatient sessions of hypnotherapy with suggestions for relaxation. He was also given meditation instructions using the word "calmer." He reported practicing the self-hypnosis twice a day, every day. (This method is recommended to everyone but only occasionally does someone comply.) Each week, he reported decreasing frequency and intensity of headaches. By the fifth session, he was discharged, headache-free.

MANAGEMENT OF CHRONIC PAIN

Headaches

Hypnosis and other relaxation based therapies (Labbe 1995; Spinhoven 1988) have been effective primary treatments for migraine and tension headaches (Culbert 1994; Olness 1987b). In the pediatric population, the role of high hypnotic ability is not as clearly predictive of successful outcomes as with adults (Smith 1989). Recent thinking about hypnosis and pain management goes beyond altered states of consciousness and trance states to more cognitive–behavioral perspectives, such as appraisal processes with a focus on pain-coping strategies (Chaves 1994).

Neurologists and pediatricians frequently request hypnotherapy for children with headaches. A review of the last 50 patients referred for treatment of headache pain noted that the patients ranged in age from 8 to 17 years of age; approximately 60% were females and 40% males. The duration of headache complaints ranged from 2 to 108 months with a mean of 25 months. The four major categories of headaches were migraines (36%), tension (21%), mixed headaches (19%), and nonspecific headache diagnosis (24%). Patients were using a variety of medications ranging from Advil, Tylenol, Excedrin, Panadol, and Motrin IB to amitriptyline and Elavil. Following treatment with hypnotherapy, patients were rated in terms of decreases in the frequency and intensity of headache complaints. Over 80% reported major improvement. They had decreased frequency or intensity of pain complaints and some were headache free. Less than 20% reported no improvement. All of the migraine and mixed headache categories improved. Only one tension headache patient did not improve. All of the patients who did not improve had either one or

two hypnotherapy sessions. The other patients were seen up to five times.

Hypnotherapy as an Assessment Tool for Headaches

Similar to the studies of Olness and Libbey, who found unrecognized organic conditions for patients referred for hypnotherapy, a number of medical and psychosocial conditions have been identified within my headache population (Olness 1987a). When a patient's headaches do not respond to hypnosis intervention, it may be an indication that more diagnostic exploration is necessary. Obstructive sleep apnea must be ruled out for patients who wake up from headaches, for patients who stop breathing while sleeping, and for patients who snore. In some cases, referral for overnight cardiorespiratory polygraphic monitoring might be made. Neurally mediated syncope was identified for a couple of females with headaches and fainting, and confirmed with tilt testing. In such cases, management shifted away from hypnotherapy to conservative measures, including fluid loading and supplemental salt. Also, sexual abuse was identified in a couple of adolescent females with headaches as well as depression. Referrals to appropriate county agencies were done in those cases.

HYPNOTHERAPY FOR SYMPTOM CONTROL

Irritable Bowel Syndrome

Irritable bowel syndrome with abdominal pain, cramping, and a sense of urgency of stooling is a frequent gastrointestinal condition seen by pediatricians. A colleague who is a clinical psychologist and who completed one of our hypnotherapy workshops (C. Cunningham, personal communication, 1996) treated a 16-year-old adolescent with irritable bowel syndrome and a history of school avoidance since the first grade. The patient's family history was positive for gastrointestinal problems and for anxiety. She was initially seen in psychotherapy. When psychotherapy did not result in any gastrointestinal symptom improvement, relaxation-based hypnotherapy was added as an adjunct. The patient responded well to hypnotherapy; she reported decreased anxieties, decreased gastrointestinal symptoms, and increased school attendance. The useful suggestions offered during hypnosis were "Allow your body to become relaxed . . . organs relaxed, cells in organs relaxed . . . remember, you're in control."

Eosinophilic Granulomatosis Lung Disease

Hypnotherapy was requested for pain management for an 18-year-old man with a medical history of eosinophilic granulomatosis lung disease that was end-stage but diagnosed only three months before. This patient also had a history of reactive airway disease and had six spontaneous pneumothoraces that all required treatment with chest tubes. He was placed on numerous medications, including drugs for pain and anxiety. His frequent readmissions and increasing requests for pain medications precipitated a referral for hypnotherapy. It was clear that the patient had objective reasons for chest pain: nociceptive disease and procedure-based pain. However, it was also clear that he was very anxious, and his anxiety could lower his threshold for pain.

I introduced myself and explained that I could offer him a way to help manage his discomfort. (It is helpful to avoid the use of the word "pain.") A pain rating was requested by asking him to rate his discomfort from 0, no pain, to a 10, the worst pain he could imagine. He rated his chest pain as moderately severe, around a 6 out of 10. Next, he was asked to imagine a calm scene of his choice for the relaxation induction (e.g., beach or the woods). Then, a relaxation induction was conducted in which he was asked to allow his muscles to relax from feet to head. (My students have often asked me why I move from feet to head versus head to feet. My answer is not based upon any theory of relaxation but is simply the way I was taught.) The relaxation induction used permissive language such as "Allow your muscles to relax . . . loosen . . . let go tension . . .

gently." Then he was asked to imagine being in his comfortable place. (Please note that some individuals are not very visual so I do not request them to "see" but just imagine in any way that is meaningful to them.) Next, a count-down procedure, a deepening method, took place. I counted from 1 to 20 and he was asked to allow himself to become more relaxed and comfortable. No direct suggestions were given to eliminate pain. I assumed that if he could become more comfortable he would probably be in less pain. He was given the posthypnotic suggestions to practice this relaxation and to notice that he will find it easier and easier to become more and more comfortable. After the induction, he reported, much to his surprise, "That really worked." His postinduction pain rating had dropped to a 2. That night his requirement for pain medications significantly decreased. The entire induction took about 20 minutes.

Sickle Cell Anemia

One of the most characteristic clinical manifestations of sickle cell anemia is recurrent vaso-occlusive (V-O) pain (Platt 1991). Biofeedback and relaxation-based therapies have been employed to help manage sickle cell pain complaints (Cozzi 1987; Hall 1992c; Thomas 1984; Zeltzer 1979).

At the Rainbow Sickle Cell Anemia Center about 15% of the 250 patients (ages 0 to 35 years) suffer from recurrent V-O pain sufficient to warrant hospitalization more than two times a year (Hall 1992c). The goal of treatment is to avoid excessive narcotic use and to offer nonpharmacological hypnotherapy. Standardized pain assessments and nonpharmacological hypnotherapy pain management strategies are incorporated into the Rainbow Hospital's clinical paths for sickle cell V-O pain in children. The length of stay for sickle cell patients has been decreased for those on this care path.

A 9-year-old girl with sickle cell disease, and a history of missing more than 50 days of school within the past year because of pain-related complaints, was referred for hypnotherapy. She had extensive hospitalizations, necessitated when outpatient treatments failed to manage her pain with acetaminophen with codeine, naproxen, and hydromorphone. This patient was seen for monthly hypnosis and biofeedback sessions monitoring peripheral finger temperature. She was seen for a total of nine sessions. These sessions involved hypnotherapy with suggestions of increased relaxation and comfort, along with recommendations for home self-hypnosis practice. She started attending school regularly and even made the honor roll. She also required less pain medication. For her first year of therapy, she only had one major pain crisis and reported that she had one of her best winters in several years. She reported being able to manage mild skeletal complaints with acetaminophen with codeine and self-hypnosis.

There was a relapse 1 year later with 6 weeks of persistent pain, school absences, and daily Tylenol and codeine use. Two follow-up booster hypnosis sessions were given with suggestions of increased comfort and relaxation. Following this intervention, she returned to school and during her last physician visit she reported that she had not needed any analgesics (Hall 1992c).

Hemophilia

Hypnotic relaxation and imagery have been utilized in the management of pain and bleeding in hemophilia (Lebaron 1984; Olness 1996). The mechanism by which hypnotherapy might impact on this disease is unclear, but hypnotic susceptibility does not appear to be a factor (Lebaron 1984).

Gunshot Wound

The patient was a 17-year-old who was quadriplegic from a traumatic gun shot wound 1 year ago. He was a resident in an inpatient rehabilitation facility and was referred for hypnotherapy because of his poor adjustment at the treatment facility. With the aid of his nurses, he completed a symptom checklist (SCL-90R) (Derogatis 1994). The results of this assessment revealed extremely high levels of depression, greater than the 90th percentile. Phobias and anxiety were quite high, over the 80th percentile.

The patient could only communicate by nods, facial expressions, and vocal grunts. Although severely limited physically, he was able to acknowledge feelings of depression with suicidal ideations. My first intervention was not to conduct hypnosis, but to address the depression. He was placed on Prozac after this initial interview. Next, he was given an introductory hypnosis induction with suggestions of relaxation and calm scene imagery of being in a safe, pleasant place. It should be noted that because of the level of violence in the lives of some inner-city adolescents, finding a safe, comfortable place is often a challenge.

On his second visit, 1 week later, he presented with bright affect and reported practicing the relaxation on a daily basis. He had only been on the Prozac for 2 days by the time of this visit. He denied suicidal ideations at that time and was excited to do more hypnosis. A follow-up booster session was done with suggestions of sending his body signals from his brain, signals to move his muscles. He was informed that the experience of relaxation might be even greater than the first time he worked with me. This prediction is a high probability one because the second hypnosis session is almost universally better than the first.

For the third session, 2 weeks later, he started the session by saying, in an audible tone, "Hello." He was proud that he started to use his voice again. He also had gained 5 lbs and was progressing well. He now went quickly into a hypnotic state via relaxation. For anger management, he was instructed to imagine feeling angry and being assertive but not hurting anyone in his imagination.

Had his depression not been addressed through a careful history, it is doubtful that the hypnosis would have had such a positive impact. His response to therapy while on the antidepressant was very rapid, demonstrating the adjunctive usefulness of hypnosis in a very difficult case. Although pain was not a major problem in this case, hypnosis gave this person with limited physical movement the opportunity to encounter a broader range of experiences in his imagination. As he progressed and became more assertive and angry, hypnosis focused on allowing him to experience his anger in a less destructive manner. At the facility where he now stays he helps to look out for the younger patients and will use his call button if a younger patient needs help. Even with his physical limitations he is one of the most cognitively intact and helpful individuals at the facility.

Chronic Cough

Chronic coughing has been reported in the pediatric literature and has gone by a variety of names, including "psychogenic coughing," "habit cough," "psychogenic cough tic," "operant cough," and "nervous cough." It has also been known as the "barking cough of puberty" because it sounds similar to the "honking" of a wild Canadian goose (Grumet 1987). Sometimes the development of a cough habit follows a respiratory illness such as bronchitis; however, these patients demonstrate no bronchial constrictions nor do they have any objective laboratory evidence of disease. Typically, all pediatric patients with cough habits stop coughing during sleep (Gay 1987). Hypnosis and suggestion therapy have been successful in treating tic disorders (Kohen 1987; Olness 1996; Young 1991). Hypnosis has also been employed to treat habit coughs (Elkins 1986; Lokshin 1991; Olness 1996).

A 12-year-old girl was referred from our pulmonary clinic because of a 6-week history of chronic coughing. Her coughing was not associated with any wheezing or other breathing difficulties. The coughing bout was apparently preceded by mycoplasmal pneumonia with significant coughing episodes. She was initially placed on erythromycin but could not tolerate it, so it was later changed to Bactrim; this was given for 2 weeks. Monospot done after that was negative. Cold agglutinins were positive at 1:64. She was placed on 250 mg of tetracycline four times a day for 2 weeks. She continued to cough with increasing frequency at night. There was no family history of asthma or of any other allergies and she did not smoke. Her pulmonologist placed her on several cough suppressants that did not help. By the time she saw me she was on Hycodan cough syrup. This patient was referred for hypnotherapy to reduce her chronic cough habit.

During the initial assessment, she coughed throughout the session. Her psychophysiological profile revealed a great deal of sympathetic distress with galvanic skin recordings at the ceiling level of the recording range. Her heart rate was also quite high and variable.

The patient was given an introductory self-hypnosis induction with suggestions of increased relaxation. She did not cough while under hypnosis and instructions for self-hypnosis home practice were given and follow-up requested in one week. At the second session, she reported coughing less during the past week, but I did hear coughing in the waiting room and she did cough during the session. The patient reported having symptoms of panic that were not associated with any particular event. She revealed some stressful home situations, as well. She acknowledged feeling very sad about her family life and admitted that coughing sometimes distracted or interrupted some family arguments. The sessions were then structured so that the first half-hour involved individual psychotherapy and the latter half-hour hypnotherapy. A follow-up hypnosis induction was done with suggestions of increased relaxation and greater control over her coughing. Self-hypnosis home practice was encouraged.

For her third session 1 week later I observed no coughing from the waiting room, and she did not cough once during the session. She reported one panic attack that disappeared with self-hypnosis. The patient reported using hypnosis to reduce her feelings of stress and was able to identify a relationship between her coughing and stress at home. By the fourth session she was no longer chronically coughing. Although she did have a relapse with increasing school pressures, she used self-hypnosis to bring the coughing under control once

again. By the ninth session, about 7 months after she began hypnosis and psychotherapy, she no longer was coughing.

It should be noted that when I request home practice, I ask the child if his or her parent has chores for them to do. They generally indicate that they do. Then I ask the child if his or her parent "makes" them engage in one of their favorite activities such as playing a computer game. The child always says "no." "Good" is my response. "That is the way self-hypnosis practice should be. This is something you are doing for yourself and should not be viewed as a chore."

Sleep Disorders

Because sleep problems are very common complaints for children (Adners 1997), I always assess for any sleep-related difficulties, regardless of the presenting problems. Acute and chronic insomnia often respond to relaxation and hypnotherapy approaches, along with sleep hygiene instructions, in just a couple of sessions (Bechker 1993; Borkovec 1973; Elkins 1986).

First, a careful history is taken to rule out psychological factors such as depression, substance use or abuse, or any symptoms consistent with a breathing-related sleep problem such as obstructive sleep apnea. Then, sleep hygiene instructions are provided, and the child is requested to use the bed only for sleeping and only when tired. They are requested not to read, watch television, or eat in bed. A sleep diary is also given out with instructions to record the time they went to bed, approximately how long it took them to fall asleep, and when they woke up. They are also requested not to take naps, to discontinue caffeine, and to avoid vigorous exercise right before retiring.

A 12-year-old boy was referred with a 1-year history of anxiety-related stomach pain and diarrhea. He acknowledged feelings of depression but denied suicidal ideation. Recently, he developed symptoms of insomnia, and it took him longer than 1½ hours to fall asleep at night. Instructions for sleep hygiene were given along with a hypnotherapy relaxation induction with calm scene imagery of ice skating and suggestions of increased relaxation and sleepiness at night. Meditation instructions were also given, employing the word "calmer" to help diminish distracting thoughts at night. He was instructed to get out of bed and watch television or read something that would make him sleepy if he was not asleep in 30 minutes. When he became sleepy, he could get back in bed and again do the hypnosis relaxation. The wake-up time is very important, and he was told that getting up is one thing he could control, even if falling asleep was not yet under his influence. He was given a sleep diary. The following week, he reported falling asleep in 5 to 10 minutes with no further symptoms of insomnia. From my experience, it is rare for this treatment to take more than two to three hypnotherapy sessions. The patient's insomnia complaints responded very quickly to hypnotherapy (within one session), whereas it took about five sessions before he reported decreased gastrointestinal pain and diarrhea. On follow-up appointments he had no further problems with insomnia.

Hypnotherapy has been successfully employed with other sleep disorders such as nightmares or anxiety associated with falling asleep. The relaxation and self-control aspects of self-hypnosis are helpful in allowing children to become more comfortable going to bed. I have also had children construct a "dream catcher" above their bed. According to tradition, it captures the bad dreams in the net and allows the good dreams to get through. Hypnotherapy has also helped with night or sleep terrors, although the mechanism by which it impacts is unclear (Olness 1996). Koe successfully employed hypnotherapy with suggestions of decreased nocturnal sensory stimulation to eliminate night terrors in a 16-year-old boy with a history of this disorder since age 7 (Koe 1989).

I have treated a 15-year-old boy with a 1-year history of severe hypersomnolence and night terrors. Because of the intractable nature of this young man's complaints and the disruption to his family because of his symptoms, he had been seen by multiple specialists prior to being referred to me. They included a psychiatrist who prescribed antidepressants and a sleep specialist who conducted overnight polysomnograms and multiple sleep latency tests. None of the tests or specialists' evaluations demonstrated any abnormalities. Hypnotherapy was employed with suggestions that a part of his brain would help him to stay awake longer and help him with fewer night terrors. Also, suggestions were given that he would find it easier and easier to awaken after being asleep. He was instructed to practice self-hypnosis every night. He turned out to be a good hypnotic subject who was capable of arm levitation and deep subjective experiences. Therapy lasted with him for about a year, starting with weekly hypnotherapy sessions and, later, more psychotherapy sessions with hypnosis to explore emotional issues. His night terrors decreased during the first 6 months of the therapy followed by a decrease in his hypersomnolence. The mechanisms by which he improved were unclear, but he was very happy to have self-hypnosis skills during this difficult period. There is general agreement that relaxation-based approaches are effective treatments of insomnia (NIH Technology Assessment Panel 1996).

Enuresis

Nocturnal enuresis is a common pediatric concern. In our culture about 90% of children between 3 and 6 years of age learn not to urinate while sleeping (Schmitt 1990). Occasionally, children reach adolescence and still have problems with nocturnal enuresis. Before hypnosis treatment, patients have a physical by their physician to rule out any possible organic factors. Hypnotherapy has been successfully employed to treat children and adolescents with primary nocturnal enuresis (Olness 1996; Baumann 1991). There is also some suggestion that hypnotic strategies for enuresis are more effective for children older than 5 to 7 years of age than imipramine (Banerjee 1993).

In a typical session the patient is given a drawing and explanation of how the bladder works, followed by an introductory hypnotic induction with suggestions that a section of his brain will wake him when he has a full bladder (Olness 1996). Results are usually evident after just a few sessions.

Encopresis

There is consensus that given the physiological aspects of encopresis, hypnotherapy alone is not the primary treatment of choice for a child with fecal soiling (Baumann 1991; Olness 1996). As with every condition, a careful assessment of the patient is needed, with a thorough medical examination. When a child is referred to me for hypnotherapy because of soiling problems, the parents are often angry at the child for what they see as intentional behavior. Consequently, the first step of treatment is to educate the parents and obtain a medical evaluation for constipation problems. Hypnosis is not discussed at this point. After confirming the constipation diagnosis, the child's pediatrician makes diet recommendations and advises how to clean out the stool. Given its mechanical nature, encopresis responds well to this type of physical intervention alone. Occasionally, hypnotherapy and anorectal biofeedback may be needed to strengthen the muscles in the lower part of the rectum (Owens-Stively 1986).

Test Anxiety

Many children and adolescents have extreme reactions to test situations. I recently treated a 16-year-old sophomore in a private high school, referred by a neuropsychologist. She was a typical student needing help to manage anxiety in test situations. This patient's academic stress dated back 5 to 6 years. Her grade point average had recently dropped. Cognitive testing had ruled out any possible attention deficits or learning disabilities. A psychophysiological assessment of her baseline anxiety was conducted. Her heart rate levels were quite labile, ranging up to around 140 beats per minute while she rested in a recliner chair.

An introductory hypnotherapy induction was conducted with calm scene imagery of her being on the beach and suggestion of increased relaxation. She reported feeling somewhat relaxed following this introductory session. Instructions for home practice were given and follow-up requested for a series of 4 to 6 visits. During later sessions, while under hypnosis, she was asked to imagine herself taking a test and remaining calm. Also, I asked her to recall a successful experience in her life and associate that with taking tests. By the sixth session, 2 months after treatment began, she reported major improvements in multiple areas: Her test grades went up, her anxiety was decreased, and she had better recall of information.

Neurally Mediated Syncope

A cardiologist referred a 9-year-old girl with a positive tilt test for neurally mediated syncope. This patient had no history of headache complaints, but psychosocial stressors were remarkable for the parents being separated. Three hypnotherapy sessions were conducted with suggestions for increased relaxation and control over fainting. She reported practicing about four times a week. She had an excellent response to this brief intervention with no further symptoms of fainting.

Attention Deficit/Hyperactivity Disorder

Hypnotherapy has relaxation-enhancing properties and thus can help manage anxiety symptoms experienced by children with Attention Deficit/Hyperactivity Disorder (ADHD) (Olness 1996). It should be noted that hypnosis does not in any way preclude the use of psychotropic medications and may be employed productively with Ritalin therapy. Hypnotherapy may also be used to help manage anger symptoms for a child with ADHD, as shown in the following example of an 8-year-old boy. He was a second grader in a class for severely behaviorally handicapped children. He was on 15 mg of Ritalin twice

a day. Psychosocial stressors were remarkable for his parents being divorced for 3 years.

During his first session, the patient was somewhat shy but later warmed up during the interview. He acknowledged problems with anger management and told of an incident that occurred when his teacher corrected him for making a spelling error. He became very angry, started to cry, and then began knocking over books in the classroom. His actions escalated until he was sent to the principal's office and sent home. A Conners' rating scale, completed by his teacher, revealed conduct problems at the 98th percentile.

In his therapy, the patient was invited to learn a way to be the "boss of his anger." He mentioned that he enjoyed playing Nintendo games so the theme of a "control panel" was employed in hypnotherapy. A relaxation induction was conducted in which he was requested to relax from feet to head. Next, imagery was employed in which he was asked to imagine being at a Nintendo control panel that was connected to his brain and could help control his anger and behavior. He was also asked to squeeze his right thumb against the pointer finger and imagine a red stoplight and say to himself, "Stop!" Multiple sensory stimuli were used to help him manage his behavior. He was told that the more he practiced, the easier it would be to "stop" his behavior. Then he was instructed to relax and think of alternative behaviors he could engage in other than acting out. Instructions were also given to practice twice a day, after school and at bedtime.

He was seen in follow-up 1 week later with glowing reports from his parents and teachers regarding major improvements in his behavior. He reported, however, that he only practiced once at home. Consequently, a follow-up hypnotherapy induction was done reinforcing the red light/stop technique. Meditation instructions were also added in which he was asked to repeat the word "calmer" to help him become even more relaxed. At his third follow-up, a couple of weeks later, his behavior continued to be outstanding. Follow-up 1 year later indicated that school had gone very well; he had had only one incident in which he became angry. Two hypnotherapy booster sessions were conducted to reinforce the red light control technique, and he continued to report that he rarely practices the technique at home.

Substance Abuse

There is growing concern regarding both high and increasing use of cigarettes, alcohol, and illicit drugs by children and adolescents. A 1995 *Monitoring the*

Future Survey of various drug use by eighth graders, tenth graders, and high school seniors revealed a disturbing pattern. Since 1991, an increasing number of adolescents use illicit drugs at an earlier age. More than 48% of high school seniors reported using illicit drugs, 41% used marijuana/hashish, 64% reported using cigarettes, and over 80% reported using alcohol (NIDA 1995). Many people drink alcohol as a method of managing stress and anxiety. (Hester 1995). Also, elevated levels of anxiety have been observed among substance-abusing individuals (Cox 1990; Singer 1995; Walfish 1990). In addition, both chronic and acute use of stimulants, such as cocaine, have been linked to the onset of panic disorder (Geracioti 1991). Speedball users (those who co-inject cocaine and opioid) have been found to have elevated anxiety and depressive mood scores (Malow 1992). To the extent that anxiety plays a role in drug use, anxiety reduction interventions may reduce substance abuse. Relaxation training may be a useful part of a multimodal intervention program for cocaine dependence. Learning to manage negative emotional states has also been identified as an important issue by patients in relapse prevention treatment programs for cocaine dependence (Lovejoy 1995).

Baumann employed hypnotherapy with adolescents who used marijuana, LSD, methedrine, barbiturate, and heroin (Baumann 1970). His approach to hypnotherapy for this patient population was to use hypnosis to self-induce and "revivify" a "good trip" or to hallucinate a more intense "good" drug experience. Although Baumann found that this approach did not cure the addictions, his patients were able to experience the self-induced hypnotic drug experience. Case reports have been published where hypnotherapy was helpful in successfully recovering from cocaine (Page 1993) and other chemical dependency (Orman 1991).

HYPNOTHERAPY AND CULTURAL SENSITIVITY

The hypnotherapist and the patient may be from different cultures, but it is important to use culturally sensitive treatment approaches with children and adolescents (Canio and Spurlock 1994). Before the induction, the therapist and patient should agree upon language that communicates the appropriate meanings to the patient.

I routinely ask a child to imagine a calm place or a safe place, but it is often difficult for children from violent settings to find such a place in their minds. Homicide is the leading cause of death for African-American males ages 15 to 44 (U.S. Department of Health and Human Services 1986). When I work with inner city children who have witnessed violence, there are times when I avoid the "safe place" or "calm scene" imagery and just give relaxation instructions.

SUMMARY

The effectiveness of mind/body hypnotic and relaxation-based interventions needs to be researched and investigated in controlled clinical trials. It would also be helpful for the field to have more reports of side effects from hypnotherapy interventions and more information about why some conditions are resistant to hypnotherapy, such as somatic complaints of adolescents with chronic fatigue syndrome.

AIDS is pushing the field beyond the mind/body framework. Research into the potential of healing energy phenomena may open up a new arena for alternative/complementary healing approaches, bringing the field back to a place that Mesmer might have originally envisioned.

REFERENCES

Adners TF, Elben LA: Pediatric sleep disorders: A review of the past 10 years. J Am Acad Child Adolesc Psychiatry 36(1):9–20, 1997

Alexander FM: Constructive conscious control of the individual. Bexley, Kent, Integral Press, 1955

Aronson DM: The adolescent as hypnotist: Hypnosis and self-hypnosis with adolescent psychiatric inpatients. Am J Clin Hypn 28(3):163–169, 1986

Banerjee S, Srivastav A, Palan BM: Hypnosis and self-hypnosis in the management of nocturnal enuresis: A comparative study with imipramine therapy. Am J Clin Hypn 36(2):113–119, 1993

Bates LB: Individual differences in response to hypnosis. In Rhue JW, Lynn SJ, Kirsch I (eds): Handbook of Clinical Hypnosis. Washington, DC, American Psychological Association, 1993, pp 23–54

Baumann F: Enuresis and encopresis in a pediatric practice. In Wester, WC, O'Grady DJ: Clinical Hypnosis With Children. New York, Brunner/Mazel Publishers, 1991, pp 258–263

Baumann F: Hypnosis and the adolescent drug abuser. Am J Clin Hypn 13(1):17–21, 1970

Bechker PM: Chronic insomnia: Outcome of hypnothereapeutic intervention in six cases. Am J Clin Hypn 36(2):98–105, 1993

Benson H: The Relaxation Response. New York, Avon, 1975

Borkovec TD, Fowles DC: Controlled investigation of the effects of progressive and hypnotic relaxation on insomnia. J Abnorm Psych 82:153–158, 1973

Bowers K: Hypnosis for the Seriously Curious. New York, W.W. Norton & Company, 1976

Canino IA, Spurlock J: Culturally Diverse Children and Adolescents. New York, The Guilford Press, 1994

Chaves JF: Recent advances in the application of hypnosis to pain management. Am J Clin Hypn 37(2):117–129, 1994

Coe WC, Peterson P, Gwynn M: Expectations and sequelae to hypnosis: Initial findings. Am J Clin Hypn 38(1):3–12, 1995

Coe WC, Ryken K: Hypnosis and risks to human subjects. Am Psychol 34(8):673–681, 1979

Cox B, Norton G, Swinson R, et al: Substance abuse and panic-related anxiety: A critical review. Behav Res Ther 28(5):385–393, 1990

Cozzi L, Tryon WW, Sedlacek K: The effectiveness of biofeedback-assisted relaxation in modifying sickle cell crisis. Biofeedback and Self-Regulation 12:51–61, 1987

Culbert TP, Kajander RL, Kohen DP, et al: Hypnobehavioral approaches for school-age children with dysphagia and food aversion: A case series. J Dev Behav Pediatr 17(5):335–340, 1996

Culbert TP, Reaney JB, Kohen DP: Cyberphysiologic strategies for children: The clinical hypnosis/biofeedback interface. Int J Clin Exp Hypn XLII (2):97–117, 1994

Derogatis LR: SCLs-90-r: Symptom checklist-90-r. Minneapolis, National Computer Systems, Inc., 1994

Edmonston WE: Hypnosis and relaxation: Modern verification of an old equation. New York, John Wiley & Sons, 1981

Eisenberg DM, Kessler RC, Foster C, et al: Unconventional medicine in the United States: Prevalence, costs, and patterns of use. New Engl J Med 328(4):246–252, 1993

Elkins GR, Carter DB: Hypnotherapy in the treatment of childhood psychogenic coughing: A case report. Am J Clin Hypn 29(1):59–63, 1986

Erickson MH: Pediatric hypnotherapy. In Rossi EL (ed): Innovative Hypnotherapy by Milton H. Erickson. New York, Irvington Publishers, Inc., 1980

Ewin DM: Emergency room hypnosis for the burned patient. Am J Clin Hypn 29(1):7–12, 1986

French GM, Painter EC, Coury DL: Blowing away shot pain: A technique for pain management during immunization. Pediatrics 93(3):384–388, 1994

Gardner G, Olness K: Hypnosis and Hypnotherapy With Children. New York, Norton, 1981

Gay M, Blager F, Bartsch K, et al: Psychogenic habit cough: Review and case reports. J Clin Psychiatry 48(12):483–486, 1987

Geracioti TD, Post RM: Onset of panic disorder associated with rare use of cocaine. Biol Psychiatry 29:403–406, 1991

Grumet GW: Psychogenic coughing: A review and case report. Compr Psychiatry 27(1):28–34, 1987

Hall H: Hypnosis, suggestion and the psychology of healing. Advances 3(3):29–37, 1986

Hall H, Mumma G, Longo S, et al: Voluntary immunomodulation: A preliminary study. Int J Neurosci 63:275–285, 1992c

Hester RK, Miller WR: Handbook of Alcoholism Treatment Approaches: Effective Alternatives, 2nd ed. Massachusetts, Allyn & Bacon, 1995

Hrabovsky EE: Cutaneous emergencies: Burns. In Reece RM (ed): Manual of Emergency Pediatrics, 4th ed. Philadelphia, W. B. Saunders Company, 1992, pp 30–32

Hussein JN, Fatoohi LJ: The role of ambiguous terminology of consciousness in misunderstanding healing phenomena. Frontier Perspectives, 6(1):27–32, 1996

Kirsch I, Lynn SJ, Rhue J: Introduction to clinical hypnosis. In Rhue JW, Lynn SJ, Kirsch I (eds): Handbook of Clinical Hypnosis. Washington, D.C. American Psychological Association, 1994

Koe GG: Hypnotic treatment of sleep terror disorder. Am J Clin Hypn 32(1):36–40, 1989

Kohen DP, Botts P: Relaxation-imagery (self-hypnosis) I Tourette syndrome: Experience with four children. Am J Clin Hypn 29(4):227–237, 1987

Kuttner L: Favorite stories: A hypnotic pain-reduction technique for children in acute pain. Am J Clin Hypn 30(4):289–295, 1988a

Kuttner L, Bowman M, Teasdale M: Psychological treatment of distress, pain, and anxiety for young children with cancer. J Dev Behav Pediatr 9(6):374–381, 1988b

Labbe EE: Treatment of childhood migraine with autogenic training and skin temperature biofeedback: A component analysis. Headache 35:10–13, 1995

LaGrone RG: Hypnobehavioral therapy to reduce gag and emeseis with a 10-year-old pill swallower. Am J Clin Hypn 36(2):132–136, 1993

Lebaron S, Zeltzer L: Research on hypnosis in hemophilia: Preliminary success and problems: A brief communication. Int J Clin Exp Hypn 23(3):290–295, 1984

Lokshin B, Lindgren S, Weinberger M, et al: Outcome of habit cough in children treated with a brief session of suggestion therapy. Annals of Allergy 67(6):579–582, 1991

Lovejoy M, Rosenblum A, Magura, et al: Patients' perspective on the process of change in substance abuse treatment. J Subst Abuse 12(4):269–282, 1995

Malow R, West J, Corrigan S, et al: Cocaine and speedball users: Differences in psychopathology. J Subst Abuse 9:287–291, 1992

Micozzi MS: Fundamentals of complementary and alternative medicine. New York, Churchill Livingstone, 1996

NIDA: Monitoring the Future Survey on Drug Abuse. Rockville, Office of the National Institute on Drug Abuse, 1995

NIH Technology Assessment Panel on Integration of Behavioral and Relaxation Approaches into the Treatment of Chronic Pain and Insomnia: Integration of behavioral and relaxation approaches into the treatment of chronic pain and insomnia. JAMA 276(4):313–318, 1996

Olness K, Kohen DP: Hypnosis and hypnotherapy with children, 3rd ed. New York, The Guilford Press, 1996

Olness K, Libbey P: Unrecognized biologic bases of behavioral symptoms in patients referred for hypnotherapy. Am J Clin Hypn 30(1):1–8, 1987a

Olness K, MacDonald JT, Uden DL: Comparison of self-hypnosis and propranolol in the treatment of juvenile classic migraine. Pediatrics 79(4):593–597, 1987b

Orman DJ: Reframing of an addiction via hypnotherapy: A case presentation. Am J Clin Hypn 33(4):263–271, 1991

Orne MT: The simulation of hypnosis: Why, how, and what it means. Int J Clin Exp Hypn 19(4):183–210, 1971

Owens-Stively J: Childhood constipation and soiling: A practical guide for parents and children. Minneapolis, Minneapolis Children's Medical Center Behavioral Pediatrics Program, 1986

Page RA, Handley GW: The use of hypnosis in cocaine addiction. Am J Clin Hypn 36(2):120–123, 1993

Patterson DR, Goldberg ML, Ehde DM: Hypnosis in the treatment of patients with severe burns. Am J Clin Hypn 38(3):200–212, 1996

Platt OS, Thorington BD, Brambilla DJ, et al: Pain in sickle cell disease. New Engl J Med 325(1):11–16, 1991

Schmitt BD: Nocturnal enuresis: Finding the treatment that fits the child. Contemporary Pediatrics September:70–97, 1990

Singer L, Arendt R, Minnes S, Farkas K, et al: Increased psychological distress in postpartum, cocaine-using mothers. J Subst Abuse 7(2):165–174, 1995

Smith MS, Womack WM, Chen ACN: Hypnotizability does not predict outcome of behavioral treatment in pediatric headache. Am J Clin Hypn 31(4):237–241, 1989

Spinhoven P: Similarities and dissimilarities in hypnotic and nonhypnotic procedures for headache control: A review. Am J Clin Hypn 30(3):183–194, 1988

Stephens B, Barkey M: Positioning for comfort. Paper presented for ACCH Children and Hospitals Weeks, Hurt Alert Day, March 22, 1994

Sugarman LI: Hypnosis in primary care practice: Developing skills for the "new morbidities." J Dev Behav Ped 17(5):300–305, 1996

Thomas JE, Koshy M, Patterson L, et al: Management of pain in sickle cell disease using biofeedback therapy: A preliminary study. Biofeedback and Self-Regulation 9:413–420, 1984

U.S. Department of Health and Human Services: Report of the secretary's task force on black and minority health, vol 5. Homicide, suicide, and unintentional injuries. Washington, D.C., U.S. Government Printing Office, 1986

Walfish S, Massey R, Krone A: Anxiety and anger among abusers of different substances. Drug and Alcohol Dependence 25:253–256, 1990

Wall V: Developmental considerations in the use of hypnosis with children. *In* Wester WC, O'Grady DJ (eds): Clinical Hypnosis With Children. New York, Brunner/Mazel Publishers, 1991, pp 3–18

Wester WC, O'Grady DJ: Clinical Hypnosis With Children. New York, Brunner/Mazel Publishers, 1991

Young MH: Ties. *In* Wester WC, O'Grady DJ (eds): Clinical Hypnosis With Children. New York, Brunner/Mazel Publishers, 1991, pp 97–112

Zeltzer L, Dash J, Holland JP: Hypnotically induced pain control in sickle cell anemia. Pediatrics 64:533–536, 1979

9

Hypnosis in Radiology

Elvira V. Lang
Eleanor Laser

INTRODUCTION

Pharmacological management of pain and anxiety in the radiology department has limited effectiveness, serious side effects, and high cost. Hypnotic methods have the potential to be a more reliable, safer, and less costly adjunct or alternative. Hypnotic methods suitable for use in radiology are not fundamentally different from applications in other areas. Successful implementation, however, requires a thorough understanding of the setting, the conventional approaches to management of pain and anxiety, the implications of a change in practice, and the potential barriers to be anticipated. Familiarity with these issues is needed for designing a custom-tailored approach that is time-efficient and acceptable to patients and staff. We will lay the foundation of this knowledge, then follow with specific methodology.

THE SETTING

Radiologists are specialists of diagnostic imaging (diagnostic radiologists) and image-guided therapy (interventional radiologists). Although the designation "radiologist" originally entailed the use of x-rays, some modern techniques are free of radiation. Great strides have been made in developing new modalities such as computerized tomography (CT), ultrasound, power duplex, magnetic resonance imaging (MRI), nuclear scintigraphy, positron emission tomography (PET), endoscopy, and virtual representations. Interventional radiologists perform minimally invasive procedures by advancing instruments and devices under image guidance through small incisions or natural body openings. Interventional radiologists treat diseases that traditionally required open surgery: They may open blocked arteries or bile ducts, treat tumors, remove kidney stones or gallstones through the skin, drain pus, or obtain tissue samples.

Interventional radiologists have to face patients' anxiety and address the effects of painful stimuli.

The most recent National Hospital Discharge Survey of the Centers for Disease Control in 1993 lists 5.6 million diagnostic radiological tests and 8.7 million minimally invasive procedures (Centers for Disease Control and Prevention/National Center for Health Statistics 1995). Because of the large number of examinations and the high cost of equipment, radiology departments are geared toward a fast examination time of patients. Patients are typically greeted by a receptionist, directed by another staff member to undress and put on a hospital gown, then are brought into an examination room. Some patients may not have been told by their referring physicians the need for, or nature of, the examination. Patients may or may not personally meet a radiologist. The diagnostic radiologist gains information about the patient's status from a requisition form that is often sparse. He or she then interprets the images, often without seeing the patient. Sometimes the diagnostic radiologist meets the patient first and only when obtaining consent (such as for a contrast medium injection) or when questions arise regarding the indication or interpretation of the examination. Interventional radiologists are more involved: They explain the upcoming procedure, evaluate the patient, and perform the procedure.

Imaging patients often have to wait (waiting room, dressing room, preparation room, examination room, "checking of the images," and production of a report). Stations are often staffed by different personnel. Imaging takes varying amounts of time: seconds for a chest radiograph, 10 to 20 minutes for a CT scan, and 15 to 90 minutes for an ultrasound, MRI, or PET examination. Interventional procedures can last from 15 minutes to 8 hours. Most diagnostic examinations and procedures are performed on awake patients because cooperation is important. Patients are required to refrain from moving and to hold their breath upon instruction because motion deteriorates image quality. Immobilization often takes place in a darkened room (to enhance visibility on TV screens), in a cooled room (to keep the imaging computers functioning), or in the tightly confined space of an MRI, CT, or PET scanner. The MRI examination additionally entails a loud hammering sound, contributing to the unfamiliarity of the experience. Because of exposure to radiation or magnetization, personnel may leave patients alone in the imaging equipment while moving to the adjacent control room. Communication with the patients takes place via a microphone speaker when the connecting door is closed or through loud voice interactions when the door remains ajar.

Patients' Perceptions

Although short, the visit in the radiology department often determines diagnosis or prognosis, and the neces-

sity and efficacy of treatment. Evaluation of symptoms, and even a "routine" preventive check-up, can directly challenge the notion of bodily integrity and immortality. It is not surprising that as many as 78% of patients in a radiology waiting room experience heightened anxiety and fears (Brennan 1988; Cragg 1991; Flaherty 1989; Morris 1987; Peteet 1992; Quirk 1989a; Smith 1990). As with patients awaiting surgery (Graham 1971), patients undergoing radiological procedures named fear of the unknown as the prevailing source of anxiety, followed by the fear of diagnosis (cancer in particular), fearful curiosity about technology, anticipation of discomfort, and limitation of motion during a lengthy examination (Brennan 1988; Morris 1987; Peteet 1992; Quirk 1989b). Concerns about the competency of staff, complications, and fear of death are less frequent (Graham 1971). The "high-tech" environment, although cherished, can be daunting (Campion 1993; Hartley 1988). Being immobilized or being left alone in a darkened room adds to the emotional charge. Preoccupation with disease is supplemented by fears of losing control to technology or personnel and by feelings of abandonment. Some distress may be compatible with imaging and treatment, but some patients frankly panic, making diagnosis or intervention impossible. An estimated 1.5% to 20% of patients scheduled for MRI examinations experience severe panic attacks that may or may not respond to medication (Avrahami 1990; Bydder 1983; Flaherty 1989; Hricak 1984; Kilborn 1990; Klonoff 1986; Nixon 1986; Sallevelt 1993). These examinations then have to be aborted. Unfortunately, the psychological distress created can persist and even trigger persistent claustrophobia (Fishbain 1989; Kilborn 1990). A patient with a distressing experience, who requires another examination, may develop cumulative fear, making adequate diagnosis impossible. Also, patients who had successful prior interventional procedures and return for equivalent interventions tend to require more medication than during prior visits (Lang 1994).

Patients may associate strikingly theatening images with the visit to the radiology department, such as being entombed, overpowered, or mutilated (Hartley 1988; Lang 1994; Lang 1996; Smith 1990). Whether or not these perceptions parallel reality is irrelevant to the experienced emotion. This frightening situation can elicit a dissociated, hypnosis-like state in which patients are highly susceptible to suggestions. Although ancient rituals and interactions with the healer, priest, or medicine man heavily relied on the power of words and images in the diagnostic and healing process (Sanders 1991), "modern" health care providers are little aware of mind/body interaction and the impact of their statements. What health care workers say to patients in this state of high suggestibility is critical. Every word is amplified. Seemingly harmless, well meant statements can assume paradoxical meanings. For example, "Soon, it's all over" may elicit allegorical notions of death. Thus health care workers unknowingly direct the patient's auto- or self-hypnotic experience.

NEED FOR ANALGESIA AND ANXIOLYSIS

Diagnostic tests and interventional procedures can include painful or uncomfortable stimuli such as injection of contrast media, rectal probing for an enema, dilatation of tissues, or pressure from extended immobilization on a firm table. Patients may suffer from pre-existing painful conditions. Pre-existing pain has been associated with increased levels of anxiety during MRI examination and a significantly higher incidence of panic attacks and interruptions of examinations (Kilborn 1990). Writhing, accelerated breathing, increased heart rate, and restlessness introduce blurring of images and may make accurate manipulation of instruments impossible (Friday 1990; Lang 1994; Neuhaus 1993). Pain and anxiety can elevate the blood pressure. Subsequently, the risk of stroke, cardiac strain, and bleeding from treatment sites also increases. Fear of pain and anxiety intensify pain perception and can initiate a self-reinforcing spiral of increasing pain and anxiety. Treating physicians may then become fearful themselves and give excessive amounts of sedatives and narcotics (Essinger 1993; Graham 1971). Anxiety that transmits from the patient to the operator can undermine dexterity, clear thinking, and the stamina required for lengthy interventions. Less experienced or less determined physicians may then unnecessarily abort a procedure or take unwise shortcuts to be relieved of the patient's distress.

Pharmacological Management of Pain and Anxiety

The customary approach for management of acute pain and anxiety in the radiology department is the use of intravenous sedatives and narcotics (intravenous conscious sedation) (Cragg 1991; Essinger 1993; Lang 1996). Narcotics decrease the perception of the intensity of pain (Gracely, McGrath, & Dubner, 1979). Sedatives decrease anxiety, reduce the level of "unpleasantness" of pain (Gracely 1978), and potentiate the action of narcotics. These drugs can have serious side effects, including respiratory and cardiovascular depression, bradycardia, chest wall rigidity, and contraction of the

sphincter muscles of the bladder and bile duct. By extrapolating data obtained by a study with more than 21,000 patients undergoing endoscopy with intravenous conscious sedation (Arrowsmith 1991) with the estimated 8.7 million invasive procedures performed annually in U.S. nonfederal hospitals (Centers for Disease Control and Prevention/National Center for Health Statistics 1995), one would expect at least 47,000 patients to suffer serious cardiorespiratory complications and 2600 patients to die each year from sequelae of intravenous conscious sedation.

Intravenous conscious sedation has limitations. Experienced personnel know that high anxiety levels can override even massive doses of medication. Highly anxious patients typically remain restless and experience disproportionate pain throughout a procedure. At the end of the examination or procedure and when the patient is removed from the imaging suite, adrenergic stimulation ceases, and the full drug effects break through. Patients can then slide into a coma-like state, causing significant concern for the recovery team.

Users of intravenous conscious sedation have to weigh the risks of oversedation against the risk of improperly treated pain. This dilemma partly may be the reason for the wide variety of medication schedules that are given in different hospitals for the same procedure (Fig. 1). Dosage schedules include various weighting of sedatives and narcotics; some use nonspecific criteria (Allan 1989; Miller 1987), and others use induction of drowsiness or slurred speech (Cragg 1991; Hendrix 1985; Roberts 1993). Even mean maximum recommended midazolam dosages for vascular interventions range from 2.5 to 10 mg (Conrad 1989; Hiew 1995; Miller 1987). *A study of 214 patients undergoing lower extremity arteriography at three different hospitals revealed that the particular institution was the most important determinant in the amount and type of drugs used, even when the same physicians were attending* (Chen 1996).

Because of the wide variation in customary drug use with no clean-cut criteria or rationale, we investigated the relation between drug use and patients' pain perception and anxiety levels in 34 consecutive patients undergoing invasive procedures at the University of Iowa Hospital and Clinics (UIHC). Patients indicated their pain and anxiety levels at the beginning and every 20 minutes during the procedures on 0 to 10 visual analog scales. Figure 2 shows that most drug deliveries occurred when patients indicated relatively low pain and anxiety. On the other hand, high pain or anxiety levels were not necessarily associated with drug deliveries.

Patients with little pain and anxiety at the onset who received intravenous medication tended to do well. When pain or anxiety levels were high, drugs often were either not given or had little effect. Withholding of drugs ensued in particular when blood oxygen saturation

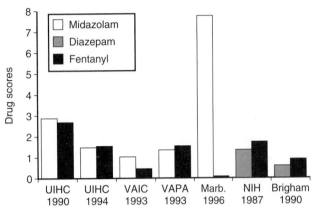

Figure 9–1. Effect of institution on drug use during IV conscious sedation. Average total drug use per peripheral lower extremity arteriogram. Drug scores are given in units: 1 mg of midazolam = 1 unit; 5 mg of diazepam = 1 unit; 50 μg of fentanyl = 1 unit. University of Iowa Hospital and Clinics (UIHC) 1990 data from Cragg et al (Cragg et al, 1991); Brigham and Women's Hospital data from Mandle et al, 1990; Veterans Affairs Medical Center, Palo Alto (VAPA) data from Lang & Hamilton, 1994; Veterans Affairs Medical Center, Iowa City (VAIC) and UIHC 1993 data from Chen et al, 1996; NIH data from Miller & Wall, 1987; and Marburg data from Wagner et al, 1996. VAPA 1993 and UIHC 1994 averaged approximately the same amount of drug whereas the VAIC averaged about half that amount. This difference is despite the fact that (1) patients' status of health and complexity of procedures were similar in the three institutions, (2) the procedures at UIHC averaged about half the time as the procedures at the two other hospitals, and (3) the same attending physicians performed many of the procedures. Drug use at UIHC was significantly higher in 1990 under the direction of a different section chief, although the procedure protocol, equipment, and patient demographics were the same.

(customarily measured during intravenous conscious sedation) was low because of earlier drug deliveries, or when pain was felt not to be procedure related. There was no correlation between total amounts of fentanyl or midazolam administered and the individual patient's pain and anxiety scores averaged over the course of the procedure. Reasons for medicating patients seemed to be in decreasing order of importance: (1) fear of anxiety, (2) fear of pain, (3) anxiety, and (4) pain.

Factors affecting delivery of intravenous conscious sedation are poorly understood and researched. Consequently, there are no standards or guidelines available to establish and improve practice. Medication is subjective and, as pointed out previously, tends to reflect institutional philosophy rather than patients' need (Chen 1996). Nevertheless, health care workers can be very passionate about what they feel is right in pain management even when confronted with data contradicting their beliefs. A first step toward patient-oriented pain management is willingness of health care workers to recognize their own bias. Efforts to change pain management have to take these barriers into account, which applies to changes in the practice of pharmacological analgesia and becomes paramount for nonpharmacological methods.

POTENTIAL OF HYPNOTIC TECHNIQUES

The perception of pain depends on many variables, including the situation, the meaning to the individual, expectations for relief, anxiety, and perception of control (Beecher 1956; Chapman 1986; McGrath 1983; Melzack 1970; Pennebaker 1977). Many of us happily accept bodily insults and temperature challenges during outdoor recreational activities that, if experienced in another context, would be unacceptable. People willingly go up on ski lifts in subzero temperature, but shiver when their bedroom thermostat goes below 70°F. Even if a painful or frightening stimulus cannot be removed, a change in perception can nevertheless take the "hurt" out of the experience. Some patients, confronted with pain and distress, resort to their own cognitive "nonpharmacological" means of coping, such as imagination of pleasant scenes, distraction, relaxation, self-hypnosis, or meditation (Anand 1961; Chaves 1974; Hilgard 1977; Quirk 1989a; Spanos 1981; Spanos 1984; Spanos 1979).

Reduction of anxiety decreases pain and symptoms (Barber 1959; Barber 1960; Hilgard 1969; Hill 1952a; Hill 1952b; Martin 1991; Shor 1962). Hypnosis as a means of anxiety reduction has proven highly beneficial for patients undergoing MRI examinations (Friday 1990) and was shown to reduce drug use during coronary angioplasty (Weinstein 1991). In these studies, however, *additional* physicians/psychologists were needed for about 30 minutes, and this is impractical in most settings. Tapes promoting relaxation have been used to reduce

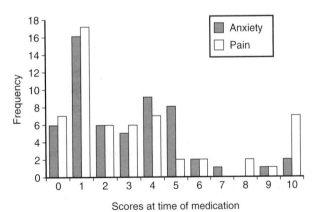

Figure 9–2. Pain and anxiety scores at time of medication. Pain and anxiety levels prior to delivery of IV conscious sedation were recorded. The frequency (number of observations) of individual pain and anxiety scores at the time of drug delivery was plotted. Pain scale: 0 = no pain at all; 10 = worst pain possible. Anxiety scale: 0 = most comfortable possible; 10 = terrified.

drug use during dental surgery (Corah 1979), gastrointestinal endoscopy (Wilson 1982), and femoral angiography (Mandle 1990). Tapes, however, have a 13% rejection rate (Feher 1989) and can result in the withholding of needed drugs in nonreceptive patients. Also, presence of a "live therapist," who is a member of the treating team, is believed to be superior (Blankfield 1991). Self-hypnotic techniques including relaxation training and imagery, applied by members of an interventional radiology team, were highly effective in reducing pain and drug use during invasive procedures (Lang 1994; Lang 1996). In a prospective randomized study with patients undergoing invasive procedures, hemodynamic instability and procedure interruptions were significantly less frequent when patients had self-hypnotic relaxation (Lang 1996). Overall, self-hypnotic relaxation greatly increased procedural safety by reducing the occurrence of drug-related complications.

The Concept of Nonpharmacological Analgesia

The Clinical Practice Guidelines for Acute Pain Management, published by the United States Department of Health and Human Services (Acute Pain Management Guideline Panel 1992), recognizes the limitations of intravenous conscious sedation and suggests that use of nonpharmacological analgesia methods be included in the repertoire of acute pain management. Because there are no guidelines for how these methods should be employed, we undertook to identify methods that regular staff members of a radiology department can apply in a safe fashion. These methods were elaborated during four training courses with different interventional radiology team members and encompass a spectrum of hypnotic techniques (Lang 1996b). We chose the designation *nonpharmacological analgesia* as a descriptive, generally acceptable term to allow for the individual adaptation of the techniques that are presented in the "Methodology" section of this chapter.

Economic Impact of Managing Pain and Anxiety

Managing patients' anxiety and pain materially affects the health care budget. If a patient receives any amount of intravenous conscious sedation, stringent monitoring requirements and a full set of conscious sedation policies in accordance with the standard of care must be followed (Association of Operating Room Nurses 1992; Lang 1996; Steinbrich 1993). The patient's history must be taken, an anesthesia plan must be developed, and a dedicated observer who is not allowed to engage in any other activities must remain with the patient for the duration of the examination and afterward for at least

30 minutes after the last drug dose. The patient requires a responsible adult to accompany him or her home and is not permitted to drive, operate machinery, or conduct important legal business for the next 24 hours. Avoiding these inconveniences and costs to patient and hospital by use of nonpharmacological means is a highly economical alternative.

Based on data obtained from 34 consecutive patients treated in the Interventional Radiology Suite at the University of Iowa Hospital and Clinics, materials and observation requirements for intravenous conscious sedation added an average of $140 to every interventional radiology procedure. If it were possible to reduce the need for intravenous conscious sedation to 25% of all procedures and to reduce the need for procedure interruptions from 35–50% to 14%, as was the case for a randomized trial (Lang 1996), the average cost for procedure analgesia and anxiolysis could be reduced from $140 to $39 per case, a very substantial saving. The economic impact becomes obvious when extrapolating this cost reduction to the millions of procedures performed annually.

The time slots on MRI, CT, or PET scanners are tightly booked and are expensive. When a patient panics, and the examination cannot be concluded, the department loses $400 to $3000 in charges. When intravenous conscious sedation is used to overcome the patient's panic, costs incur as pointed out previously.

Ethical considerations alone are a professional imperative for reducing patients' suffering. The recent emphasis on enhancing patients' comfort levels is additionally driven by the increasing economic importance of patients' satisfaction surveys. Such surveys are used by third party payers to determine choice and reimbursement of health care facilities. Therein lies a great incentive for introducing behavioral therapy in the radiology department.

METHODOLOGY

Overview

The goal of nonpharmacological analgesia in radiology is to induce a pleasant state of temporary dissociation in the time available. Patient contacts with individual personnel in the radiology department are relatively short. There is no time for lengthy intervention. Fortunately, a small investment of attention delivered up front can go far toward interrupting the spiral of distress. If, on the other hand, a patient's emotional needs are neglected, attention likely will be required later, often in the form of costly interruptions at inopportune moments. Nonpharmacological analgesia starts from the moment the patient is met. It is appropriate at every stage: while walking with the patient down the hallway, while inserting intravenous access or an enema tip, while positioning the patient on the procedure table, while applying antibiotic solution and draping the patient, and during the procedure. One staff member can take over for another without interruption of work flow.

Hypnotic methods span a continuum from correct use of suggestions at one end to deep hypnotic analgesia on the other. Time constraints, prevailing anxiety, and invasiveness of intervention have to be taken into account when applying nonpharmacological analgesia. Appropriate choice of words may be all that is needed to provide comfort for a noninvasive examination in a patient with low anxiety levels. Patients who panic at the sight of equipment, as well as those who undergo invasive procedures, require more treatment. Imagery is particularly useful in highly anxious patients (Lang 1994). As has been found in phobic patients (Frankel 1976), individuals with the most vivid fears are likely to be those with high levels of hypnotizability, high imagery potential, and, therefore, high susceptibility to suggestions. We speculate that persons capable of dissociating from reality by imagining a worst-case scenario also possess superior ability to dissociate and can imagine a pleasant scenario, if guided appropriately (Lang 1996a). On the other hand, a poorly hypnotizable patient may lack the ability to create vivid fears, may appear stoic, and may benefit from simple distraction.

The methods can easily be integrated in the work flow so that time is not wasted. Rapport is essential for all subsequent interventions. Therefore, we first address rapport skills and expression of empathic attention, then follow with imagery and self-hypnotic relaxation.

Rapport Skills

Personnel should be nonthreatening and should be able to adjust to the patients' preferred mode of verbal and nonverbal communication. Radiology personnel may meet a patient for the first time either in a clinic office, on the ward, in the reception area, the preparation room, in a hallway, or the procedure suite. Patients may be ambulatory, in a wheelchair, in a hospital bed, or on a gurney. The patient should be greeted while still in street clothes if at all possible or at least while covered by some clothing or drapes. It is advisable to find out how the patient wishes to be called: by first name, last name, or a nickname.

Assuming body positions at different heights or placing barriers between the patient and the health care provider (such as tables or desks) imposes a relationship of superiority/inferiority. Towering over a seated patient or over a patient on a gurney or examination table tends to portray the health care worker in a dominating, controlling fashion. Bending over or sitting down and adjusting to the patient's level makes a difference. Some patients may seek closeness and physically move toward the health care workers, others need space. It is important to respect and adjust to this preference and not to misinterpret it as "coming on" or "withdrawal." If a patient's demeanor is quiet, slow, or reflective, a busy, chipper attitude of the health care worker can raise an emotional barrier. If, on the other hand, the patient is excited and gesticulates wildly, a display of reserved calm is unwarranted and may annoy the patient. *Initial matching of the patient's body posture, demeanor, or level of activation by the health care worker establishes necessary rapport so that the next steps of the process can be successfully accomplished.* Subsequently, patients are guided to a more serene and relaxed demeanor by transition from the matched behavior toward the desired state.

Distressed patients may be breathing rapidly or in a shallow, constricted fashion. Following the patient's breathing pattern for a few breaths and then leading toward a relaxed deep inspiration and expiration can be very effective. This technique works well when verbal communication is not immediately possible, as with trauma patients, patients under oxygen masks, or intubated patients. A deep inspiration by the staff, followed by a gentle long expiration, indicates to the patient that the staff has time and is not hurried.

In addition to matching the body signals, it is desirable to match the patients' language. The health care worker can match volume, tone, and tempo, and then guide toward a relaxed level.

Correct Use of Suggestions

Anticipation of discomfort, abdication of control, or enhanced anxiety can alter awareness and greatly increase susceptibility to suggestions (Barber 1962; Blankfield 1991). Health care providers can purposefully build on this pre-existing suggestible state by using positive suggestions, evoking a desired ideation and experience, and thereby enhancing the patients' feeling of well-being (Erickson III 1994).

The heightened suggestibility of patients prior to and during procedures makes choice of words crucial. Phrases designed to reassure patients can produce the opposite effect. "We will put you out" may evoke allegorical notions of death rather than comfort. Words with negative emotional content, such as "pain" or "hurt," reinforce anxiety and fear and thereby worsen the experience of pain. Even disclaimers such as "you will feel no pain" tend to evoke seemingly paradoxical effects

(Barber 1962; Blankfield 1991). There is a misconception that catastrophizing an upcoming event will ease the experience. In procedure suites one may hear a variety of phrases: "Pain and pressure now"; "Bee sting now"; "You may throw up"; "The contrast dye will burn like hell"; "What shall I tell you, this really hurts"; or "Don't gag."

We use the following alternative phrases for negatively loaded suggestions: Prior to application of local anesthetic, we say, "Please concentrate on a feeling of numbness spreading through the tissues" or "I will be giving you the numbing medicine; you may feel coolness or some tingling." Prior to contrast medium injection, we say, "You will feel warmth spreading throughout your body" or "This may feel like the rising sun in your belly." Prior to an MRI scan (if you know that the patient likes music) we might say, "You will hear a rhythmic noise like a metronome. You can think of your favorite melody for accompaniment."

Provision of Perception of Control

Fear of loss of control to the disease, to personnel, or to technology can be daunting. Therefore, it is important to give patients at least some perception of control. This perception can be provided by swift response to requests and asking the patient what he or she wishes (e.g., "Please let us know at any time what we can do for you to make you more comfortable"). The patient needs to be anchored in a sense of security and should be reassured that his or her requests will be taken seriously and will be acted upon. Fulfilling of seemingly unimportant requests can mean very much for the patient, establish trust, and improve the entire interaction.

Self-Hypnotic Relaxation and Imagery

Hypnosis is defined as a state of focused concentration. Absorption in the self-hypnotic process permits dissociation from or reframing of a (painful) reality. It is, in fact, the purposeful utilization of a process that happens naturally. Examples of self-hypnosis in everyday life are absorption in a movie or daydreaming. Relaxation, imagery, and hypnosis are interrelated and are not separable in the nonpharmacological analgesia process. Imagery and self-hypnotic relaxation can be easily introduced even when time is limited. "Where would you rather be" or "Imagine a safe (pleasant, happy, comfortable) place" and instructions to focus on the sights, sounds, smells, feelings of this place may be all that is needed for induction. *Focusing the patient's attention by combining an imaginative experience with relaxation breathing constitutes the essence of medical hypnosis.*

The goal of hypnosis is to allow the patient's mind

Case study 9–1

A 73-year-old diabetic patient with peripheral vascular disease and threatening limb ischemia arrived on a gurney at the door of the procedure suite. He was angry, insulted the staff approaching him, and complained about not having had breakfast. One staff member stated that she didn't have breakfast either. The patient felt mocked, didn't believe the staff, and refused to go on with the procedure. The staff became increasingly distressed and the attending physician was called. The attending asked "What do you want?" The patient said: "I want food now." The attending produced a box of attractive candies received as a gift the day before. The patient chose a chocolate figure, then agreed to undergo the procedure. When asked if anything else could be done, he demanded "silence" which was granted. He did not eat the candy, but rubbed it on his chest throughout the 2-hour procedure, and remained stable without medication. In a way, the candy elicited effective self-hypnosis by assuming the significance of a transitional object (a symbol that reinforces a comfortable, safe self-experience) (Winnicott, 1953).

The patient was given some control. Since *he* could choose whether he eats, the act of eating suddenly was less important, and *he* could choose the safer alternative of fasting. Admittedly, eating the candy could have limited anesthesia options. The risk, however, seemed acceptable as compared to delaying the procedure and thereby decreasing the chances for a successful revascularization and increasing the odds for an amputation. It is important that such decisions are made with the attending physician and are included in the risk assessment.

---

to transport to a safe and happy place while the patient's body is cared for in the examination suite. The patient is assisted to become associated with his or her preferred setting. The process can be interactive (the patient participates verbally in communication), or staff reads a script guiding the patient's experience based on knowledge of the patient's preferences. To do the latter well, staff profits from having talked to the patient during procedure preparation and having learned about occupation, hobbies, or the like. If, with more expertise, or for particularly painful procedures (such as biliary drainages or transjugular portosystemic shunts) a deeper state of hypnosis is desired, cues such as ideomotor signals can provide valuable feedback.

Poor Example

The anesthesiologist who provided stand-by for an arteriogram in a patient with suspicion of pheochromocytoma (a condition in which contrast medium injection can elicit severe hypertension, hypotension, and possibly death) did not establish a sufficient relationship with the patient. Instead, he indulged in his own trip-to-the-Hawaii-beach-imagery in great detail with no regard for the patient's interests. The patient happened to be afraid of water but was never given a chance to say so.

Good Example

A 19-year-old patient with a liver transplant and stricture in the bile chooses to go to a park of her childhood and to take a friendly stroll. The staff instructs, "Imagine you are *here* now in the park, in your body, looking out through your eyes. What do you see? Are there any sounds? Can you feel the air on your skin? Is it warm or cold? Are there any smells? How does it feel to be here?" All sensory aspects are addressed in the process.

Once the patient is associated with the preferred place, a deep relaxed breath of the staff can help integrate relaxation breathing with the experience. The patient can be asked "Are you in your body or do you see yourself?" The goal is to give patients an immediate bodily experience of the safe and pleasant environment. When patients experience distressing imagery, it is important to have them see themselves from a distance (as on a screen) and to dissociate from their bodies. The patient is associated with the pleasant situation and dissociated from the unpleasant situation.

Guidance toward imagery that involves little or no movement is best suited for use in the radiology department. Physical action imagery such as skiing, swimming, or running can induce motion and interfere with a procedure or imaging. For example, a patient, whose preferred place was at home, started to rock as if on his favorite rocking chair, making accurate placement of an angioplasty balloon in his diseased legs difficult.

Deepening of the hypnotic state can be achieved by words, including the notion of drifting further "down": a *down* blanket, fish that are caught further *down and down* in the water, walking the path further *down* into the forest, and so on. Deepening can be sustained with a simple "good," or "hmmm" from time to time. Patients who are having their own hypnotic experience can be left without interference for 5 to 20 minutes if

---

Case study 9–2

A 50-year-old woman with a liver transplant needed drainage of her bile ducts (usually a very painful procedure). Her liver was very hard and required forceful advancement of needles and instruments. The patient had chosen a walk in the woods and was guided to become a tree (trees don't move). Potentially painful advancement of instruments was integrated as if the visit of a woodpecker and was well tolerated.

---

no significant changes in the procedure are anticipated. When potentially painful procedure stimuli arise, deepening and appropriate suggestions should be used.

About half of the patients we see present with vivid distressing imagery. The goal is to dissociate the person from the threatening experience. Some strategies include the following:

- Moving the distressing feeling out and away from the body.
- Viewing the threatening image from greater and greater distance.
- Making it less threatening or removing it altogether.
- Converting it into something manageable.

If, for example, the answer to the question "How do you feel" elicits "As if two vultures are coming down to get me," options include having the vultures fly into the sunset and disappear behind the horizon, having the patient grow into something bigger than the vultures and chase them away, having the vultures become smaller, transforming the vultures into a small photograph in the distance and giving the patient the power to turn the viewing light on and off, or transforming the threatening vultures into an ally by turning them into a cozy, warm down bed.

Use of ideomotor signals can be useful in the procedure room. Ideomotor responses are believed to tap a deeper level of consciousness than is possible with verbal communication (Hammond 1988). The staff teaches the patient to indicate "yes" or "no" by moving a particular finger. The motion of the finger can be very subtle, a minimal motion, or a little twitch. Determination of this mode of communication becomes valuable when talking could interrupt a deeper state of hypnosis or when a patient may not want to speak. Choice of a finger also is helpful when nodding of the head would disturb imaging, such as during MRI or PET scans.

SAMPLE SCRIPT

An example for progressive muscle relaxation, relaxation breathing, and self-hypnosis is given in the following script. The reading of the script can be started when the patient is placed on a gurney in the holding area or on the procedure table. One half to two thirds of the script can already be read while the patient is prepped, draped, and connected to the monitoring equipment.

I would like to invite you to begin, either with your eyes open or closed, by allowing your body to relax and rest comfortably against the table. Now slowly take a breath in through your nose . . . hold . . . then exhale out through your mouth. Once again, take a deep breath in through your nose . . . hold it . . . then exhale through your mouth.

Now, as you continue this deep, relaxing breathing, I would like you to notice how just the act of breathing alone can help your body to relax and feel more comfortable. I would like you to continue the breathing, slowly taking a deep breath through your nose, and out through your mouth, and continue focusing on the sound of my voice, and allow yourself to relax completely, feeling calm and comfortable and fully at ease.

As you focus on the sound of my voice, and on your breathing, I would like to do an exercise with you to show your body the difference between tension and relaxation. We can do this by focusing on some of the smallest muscles in your body: the muscles in your eyes. I would like you to continue focusing on your breathing, in through your nose, out through your mouth. And now I would like to invite you to focus on the muscles in your eyes. Tense those muscles as hard as you can. Really allow them to become tight and hard. That's right, really tense. Tighten your eye muscles.

In a moment I am going to count to three, and when I get to three, you will be able to release all the tension in your eyes, allowing them to become fully relaxed and at ease. One . . . really feel the tension . . . two . . . tight, tight, tight . . . three. Now, allow your eye muscles to become completely relaxed and limp. Good

Now, notice the sensation of this relaxing feeling. You might experience this as a feeling of warmth, or you might see a calming white light. Now allow this relaxing sensation to flow from your eyes, up into your eyebrows, and now up over the top of your head. Continue breathing deeply, and with each breath, allow the relaxation to spread . . . over the top of your head, now down the back of your head, over your ears, and down into your neck. Let this pleasant and soothing sensation now cause your whole head and neck to become completely relaxed and at ease.

With each breath you inhale, you inhale relaxation. And with each breath you exhale, you exhale any tension and let go whatever you want to let go of. Good.

Now, allow the sensation to spread down your shoulders . . . down your arms and your hands, and right down to the tips of your fingers. Let the relaxation spread across your back, and down through your abdomen . . . into your legs, and down through your calves, to the tips of your toes. Good.

And now, to show how successful you are at relaxing, I'd like to ask you if there's any place in your body that would like to feel even more relaxed than it already is (wait for response). So take a very deep breath . . . hold this breath . . . now exhale. This is called a signal breath. It is your way of signaling your body to allow yourself to become even more fully relaxed and comfortable. When you take your signal breath, imagine that you are inhaling relaxation and comfort, and allow that breath to focus on the very spot of your body that you would like to feel even more relaxed. Now inhale relaxation, and allow the exhaled breath to go right to that spot, and breathe any tension right out through the skin at that spot. Let the relaxation and calm replace any feeling of tightness, discomfort, or tension.

Now any time during the procedure that you would like to feel more relaxed and more comfortable, you will be able to remember to use your signal breath to breathe calming relaxation to that spot to help you feel completely at ease.

You will notice lots of noises around you during the procedure; people will be talking and moving, the equipment will make noises, and the lights will go on and off quite often. As you are aware of these things, you will be able to allow them to take you even deeper into a state of complete relaxation and comfort.

While the procedure is under way, you may have questions about what's going on around you. You know that you can remain in your fully relaxed state of calm, and still be able to ask whatever questions you would like. I will try to answer them for you, or I will find out the answers for you.

When the procedure is over, or whenever you decide, you can return to your regular alert state by simply counting from one to three, either in your head or out loud. When you do this, you will find that even in your alert and fully attentive state you will continue to benefit from the calming sense of relaxation you now feel. And you can return to this place of calm whenever you like, by simply closing your eyes for a moment, counting back from three to one, and taking your signal breath.

Case study 9–3

A 68-year-old patient who developed extensive scarring of her bile duct after gallbladder surgery is dependent on a percutaneous tube to drain bile into the intestines. She is well known to the service and usually comes with her family for her routine bimonthly tube change. Because she seemed anxious and was very concerned about hurting during the tube change, we tried self-hypnosis. She relaxed somewhat but something prevented her from deepening. Upon initial questioning she denied that something bothered her. Imagery was continued and she engaged in her favorite pastime, quilt-making. She had been a seamstress. Finally, she asked whether the "stitch" (the suture) that holds her tube in place could be tied on top, not on the bottom of the tube. The interventional radiologist assured her that the knot would be placed on top and that the threads would be shortened. She immediately relaxed. At the end of the procedure, the family was called in, and the new tube stitch was shown. Subsequent tube changes were remarkably pain-free in this patient.

This example highlights that seemly unimportant details can have significant meaning to the patient. Patients may be too shy to voice such concerns. (Incidentally, it seemed that the family members who usually do the dressing changes were unaware of the problem with the stitch.) For the meticulous seamstress who took great pride in her perfect stitches, a nonperfect stitch around her tube was bothersome. Asking the physician (and questioning the competence) seemed daunting but fortunately was overcome. She felt acknowledged and safe in letting go of conscious control because her concern had been attended to. This experience also highlights that a one-time investment of nonpharmacological analgesia can interrupt the spiral of distress and have positive effects on subsequent interventions.

TROUBLESHOOTING

Resistance to Imagery

Some patients may claim that they are incapable of imagery, which does not necessarily mean that they cannot be guided toward imagery-based mental activities. In these cases alternative words or inductions can be used. "Do you dream?"; "Would you like to have a nice dream during this procedure?"; "Where would you rather be?"; "Is there any place you always wanted to go?"; "What do you like to do?"; "Do you have fantasies?" In general, patients will follow with some type of description in which they can be directed to experience all sensory dimensions. Some patients may choose scenes that are action oriented. For example, they may choose to go fishing and take the entire operating team with them, or go gambling to Las Vegas, or visit with friends. Topics from small talk can be brought up and the patient can be instructed to elaborate on the event. One patient, for example, told the story of his honeymoon that occurred 50 years ago and described many details in an imagery-like process. It is worthwhile to search for a wording or a concept for imagery that is acceptable to the patient.

Another patient, a young male veteran who resisted all other approaches, was finally asked to describe his home. Arriving at the kitchen, he was instructed to list the contents of his refrigerator. He suddenly showed interest and described all the food there in great detail and all the dishes he could prepare, becoming fully absorbed in a self-hypnotic process.

Resistance to Self-Hypnosis

To let go into a state of relaxation and self-hypnosis requires trust. The process of relaxation or imagery may be under way when something prevents progress. In this situation it is best to ask, "What do you want?" or "What is stopping you?" Some patients reveal their concerns faster than others.

CONCLUSIONS

Nonpharmacological analgesia in the radiology department is a worthwhile endeavor that enhances the patient's experience and satisfaction with service provided. Increased procedure safety and improved resources utilization are additional potential benefits. Implementation of hypnotic techniques in medicine requires a paradigm shift. Radiologists have repeatedly pioneered new diagnostic and therapeutic modalities that subsequently have been adopted by other specialties. The radiology department is an ideal setting to introduce mind-body therapy into conventional "high-tech" medicine.

REFERENCES

Acute Pain Management Guideline Panel: Acute pain management: Operative or medical procedures and trauma. Clinical practice guideline. AHCPR Pub. No. 92-0032. Rockville, MD, Agency for Health Care Policy and Research, Public Health Service, U.S. Department of Health and Human Services, 1992

Allan MWB, Lawrence AS, Gundawardena WJ: A comparison of two sedation techniques for neuroradiology. Eur J Anaesthesiol 6:379–384, 1989

Anand BK, China GS, Singh B: Some aspects of electroencephalographic studies in yogis. Electroencephalogr Clin Neurophysiol 13:452, 1961

Arrowsmith JB, Gerstman BB, Fleischner DE, et al: Results from the American Society for Gastrointestinal Endoscopy/U.S. Food and Drug Administration collaborative study on complication rates and drug use during gastrointestinal endoscopy. Gastrointest Endosc 37:421–427, 1991

Association of Operating Room Nurses: Proposed recommended practice: Monitoring the patient receiving IV conscious sedation. AORN J 56:316–324, 1992

Avrahami E: Panic attacks during MR imaging: Treatment with IV diazepam. AJNR Am J Neuroradiol 11:833–835, 1990

Barber TX: "Hypnosis," analgesia, and the placebo effect. JAMA 172:680, 1960

Barber TX: Toward a theory of pain: Relief of chronic pain by prefrontal leucotomy, opiates, placebos, and hypnosis. Psychol Bull 56:430, 1959

Barber TX, Hahn KW Jr: Physiological and subjective responses to pain-producing stimulation under hypnotically suggested and waking-imagined "analgesia." J Abnormal Soc Psychol 65:411–418, 1960

Beecher HK: Relationship of significance of wound to pain experienced. JAMA 161:1609–1613, 1956

Blankfield RP: Suggestion, relaxation, and hypnosis as adjuncts in the care of surgery patients: A review of the literature. Am J Clin Hypn 33:172–186, 1991

Brennan SC, Redd WH, Jacobsen PB, et al: Anxiety and panic during magnetic resonance scans. Lancet 27:512, 1988

Bydder GM: Clinical nuclear magnetic resonance imaging. Br J Hosp Med 29:348–356, 1983

Campion EW: Why unconventional medicine? [editorial]. N Engl J Med 328:282–283, 1992

Centers for Disease Control and Prevention/National Center for Health Statistics: Vital and health statistics. Detailed diagnoses and procedures, National Hospital Discharge Survey, 1993. Series 13, No 118. Hyattsville, MD, Public Health Service, U.S. Department of Health and Human Services, 1995

Chapman CR, Turner JA: Psychological control of acute pain in medical settings. J Pain Symptom Manage 1:9–20, 1986

Chaves JF, Barber TX: Cognitive strategies, experimental modeling, and expectations in the attenuation of pain. J Abnorm Psychol 83:356–363, 1974

Chen F, Lang E, Berbaum K: Radiology 201:315, 1996

Conrad M: Excellent anxiolytic effect achieved with low doses of versed [Letter to the editor]. Radiology 170:579, 1989

Corah NL, Gale EN, Illig SJ: The use of relaxation and distraction during dental procedures. J Am Dent Assoc 98:390–394, 1979

Cragg AH, Smith TP, Berbaum KS, et al: Randomized double-blind trial of midazolam/placebo and midazolam/fentanyl for sedation and analgesia in lower extremity angiography. AJR Am J Roentgenol 157:173–176, 1991

Erickson III JC: The use of hypnosis in anesthesia: A master class commentary. Int J Clin Exp Hypn 42:8–12, 1994

Essinger A, Ravussin P: Analgesia and sedation in the hands of the interventional radiologist. In Steinbrich W, Gross-Fengels W (eds): Interventional Radiology: Adjunctive Medication and Monitoring. Berlin, Heidelberg, New York, Springer, 1993

Feher SDK, Berger LR, Johnson JD, et al: Increasing breast milk production for premature infants with relaxation/imagery audiotape. Pediatrics 83:57–60, 1989

Fishbain D, Goldberg M, Labbe ED, et al: Long-term claustrophobia following magnetic resonance imaging. Am J Psychiat 145:1038–1039, 1989

Flaherty JA, Hoskinson K: Emotional distress during magnetic resonance imaging. N Engl J Med 320:467–468, 1989

Frankel FH, Orne MT: Hypnotizability and phobic behavior. Arch Gen Psychiatry 33:1259–1261, 1976

Friday PJ, Kubal WS: Magnetic resonance imaging: Improved patient tolerance utilizing medical hypnosis. Am J Clin Hypn 33:80–84, 1990

Gracely RH, McGrath P, Dubner R: Nacrotic analgesia: Fentanyl reduces the intensity but not the unpleasantness of painful tooth pulp sensations. Science 203:1261–1263, 1979

Gracely RH, McGrath P, Dubner R: Validity and sensitivity of ratio scales of sensory and affective verbal pain descriptors: Manipulation of affect by diazepam. Pain 5:19–29, 1978

Graham L, Conley J: Evaluation of anxiety and fear in adult surgical patients. Nurse Res 20:113–122, 1971

Hammond DC, Cheek DB: Ideomotor signaling: A method for rapid unconscious exploration. In Hammond DC (ed): Hypnotic Induction and Suggestion: An Introductory Manual. Des Plaines, American Society of Clinical Hypnosis, 1988, pp 90–97

Hartley BS: Ode to an MR machine: To the patient beware! Radiology 168:582, 1988

Hendrix GH, Gensini GG, Ludbrook PA, et al: A comparison of diazepam and midazolam for conscious sedation in patients undergoing cardiac catheterization and angiography. Anesthesiol Review 12:70–73, 1985

Hiew CY, Hart GK, Thomson KR, et al: Analgesia and sedation in interventional radiological procedures. Australasian Radiology 39:128–134, 1995

Hilgard ER: Pain as a puzzle for psychology and physiology. Am Psychol 24:103, 1969

Hilgard ER: The problem of divided consciousness: A neodissociation interpretation. Ann New York Acad Sci 296:48–59, 1977

Hill HE, Kornetsky CH, Flanary HG, et al: Effects of anxiety and morphine on discrimination of intensities of painful stimuli. J Clin Invest 31:473, 1952a

Hill HE, Kornetsky CH, Flanary HG, et al: Effects of anxiety associated with anticipation of pain: Effects of morphine. Arch Neurol Psychiatry 67:612, 1952b

Hricak H, Amparo EG: Body MRI: Alleviation of claustrophobia by prone positioning. Radiology 152:819, 1984

Kilborn LC, Labbe EE: Magnetic resonance imaging scanning procedures: Development of phobic response during scan and at one-month follow-up. J Behav Med 13:391–401, 1990

Klonoff EA, Janata JW, Kaufman B: The use of systemic desensitization procedure to overcome resistance to magnetic resonance imaging (MRI) scanning. J Behav Ther Exp Psychiat 17:189–192, 1986

Lang EV: Intravenous conscious sedation. J Vasc Interv Radiol 9(3):407–412, 1996

Lang EV, Hamilton D: Anodyne imagery: An alternative to intravenous sedation in interventional radiology. AJR Am J Roentgenol 162:1221–1226, 1994

Lang EV, Joyce JS, Spiegel D, et al: Self-hypnotic relaxation during interventional radiological procedures. Effects on pain perception and intravenous drug use. Int J Clin Exp Hypn 44:106–119, 1996

Lang EV, Laser E: Communicating with the patient. Luxury or necessity? Academic Radiol 3(9):786–788, 1996

Lang EV, Laser E: Training interventional radiology personnel in nonpharmacologic analgesia. Radiology 201:214, 1996b

Mandle CL, Domar AD, Harrington DP, et al: Relaxation response in femoral angiography. Radiology 174:737–739, 1990

Martin JB, Ahles TA, Jeffert R: The role of private body consciousness and anxiety in the report of somatic symptoms during magnetic resonance imaging. J Behavior Ther Exp Psychiat 22:3–7, 1991

McGrath PA: The role of situational variables in pain control. Anesth Progr 30:137–146, 1983

Melzack R, Wall DD: Psychophysiology of pain. Int Anesthesiol Clin 8:3–34, 1970

Miller D: Letter to the editor. Radiology 164(1):284, 1987

Miller, DL, Wall R: Fentanyl and diazepam for analgesia and sedation during radiologic special procedures. Radiology 162:195–198, 1987

Morris KJ, Tarico VS, Smith WL, et al: Critical analysis of radiologist-patient interaction. Radiology 163:565–567, 1987

Neuhaus C, Leppek R, Christ G, et al: Monitoring of vital functions in the course of interventional radiology procedures. In Steinbrich W, Gross-Fengels W (eds): Interventional Radiology: Adjunctive Medication and Monitoring. Berlin, Heidelberg, New York, Springer, 1993, pp 79–96

Nixon C, Hirsch NP, Ormerod EC, et al: Nuclear magnetic resonance: Its implications for the anaesthetist. Anaesthesia 41:131–137, 1986

Pennebaker JW, Burnam MA, Schaeffer MA: Lack of control as determinant of perceived physical symptoms. J Pers Soc Psychol 35:167, 1977

Peteet JR, Stomper PC, Murray-Ross D, et al: Emotional support for patients with cancer who are undergoing CT: Semistructured interviews of patients at a cancer institute. Radiology 182:99–102, 1992

Quirk ME, Letendre AJ, Ciottone RA, et al: Anxiety of patients undergoing MR imaging. Radiology 170:463–466, 1989a

Quirk ME, Letenre AJ, Ciottone RA, et al: Evaluation of three psychologic intervention to reduce anxiety during MR imaging. Radiology 173:759–762, 1989b

Roberts SP, Hargreaves J, Pollard BJ: The use of midazolam and flumazenil for invasive radiographic procedures. Postgrad Med J 69:922–926, 1993

Sallevelt PEJM, Barentsz JO, Hekster YA: Magnetic resonance imaging in patients with claustrophobia: Results of treatment with intramuscular clorazepate. Eur Radiol 3:335–356, 1993

Sanders S: Clinical self-hypnosis. The power of words and images. New York, The Guilford Press, 1991

Shor RE: Physiological effects of painful stimulation during hypnotic analgesia under conditions designed to minimize anxiety. Int J Clin Exp Hypn 10:183, 1962

Smith A: MRI—a patient's perspective. N Engl J Med 322(12):856, 1990

Spanos NP, Brown JM, Jones B, et al: Cognitive activity and suggestions for analgesia in the reduction of reported pain. J Abnorm Psychol 90:554–561, 1981

Spanos NP, Hodgins DC, Stam HJ, et al: Suffering for science: The effects of implicit social demands on response to experimentally induced pain. J Pers Soc Psychol 46:1162–1172, 1984

Spanos NP, Radtke-Bodorik HL, Ferguson J, et al: The effects of hypnotic susceptibility suggestions for analgesia, and the utilization of cognitive strategies on the reduction of pain. J Abnorm Psychol 88:282–292, 1979

Steinbrich W, Gross-Fengels W: Interventional Radiology. Adjunctive Medications and Monitoring. Berlin, Heidelberg, New York, Springer, 1993

Wagner HJ, Nowacki J, Klose KJ: Propofol versus midazolam for sedation during PTA. JVIR 7:673–680, 1996

Weinstein EJ, Au PK: Use of hypnosis before and during angioplasty. Am J Clin Hypn 34:29–37, 1991

Wilson JF, Moore RW, Randolph S, et al: Behavioral preparation of patients for gastrointestinal endoscopy: Information, relaxation and coping style. J Hum Stress 8:13–23, 1982

Winnicott DW: Transitional objects and transitional phenomena. Int J Psychoanal 34:89–97, 1953

10

Oncology

Alexander A. Levitan

"The secret of the care of the patient is in caring for the patient."
Francis Weld Peabody (1927)

As technical advances in the field of oncology become increasingly dependent on complex scientific undertakings and equally sophisticated scientific equipment, it is imperative that the human element not be lost when caring for individuals facing a life-threatening illness. Hypnosis is uniquely positioned not only to establish a therapeutic relationship with cancer patients but also to make a significant and material impact on the eventual outcome of the disease. As defined earlier in this textbook, hypnosis is an altered state of consciousness that could begin at the instant a deviation from customary wellness occurs (Brown 1991). From the moment a woman discovers a questionable lump in her breast or a man discovers one in his scrotum, an altered state of consciousness ensues. At that moment, far too often, negative self-hypnosis results. By the time patients seek a consultation from their primary physician because they discovered one of cancer's warning signs, they may have already experienced a litany of negative suggestions both from within and without. Despite incredible progress in the field, the diagnosis of cancer is almost universally regarded as a sentence of death. How, then, can any individual react to this possible diagnosis without experiencing an alteration of the usual and customary state of mentation?

It is imperative that each health care provider initially making contact with the patient is trained in at least the rudiments of hypnosis and knows the extreme susceptibility of these patients to all suggestions enunciated by perceived authority figures. Far too often, individuals with little or no hypnotherapeutic training make negative statements at moments of patient vulnerability. Those statements can have a persistent negative effect. It must be remembered that under circumstances of stress or altered mental states, ambiguous statements have a greater propensity to be interpreted as predictive of a negative outcome. For example, a patient may hear the statement, "You'll have to live with it," and conclude that if the pain or symptom goes away, he or she will die. This situation can happen in the realm of chemotherapy when, inadvertently, the expectation of nausea can be communicated to the patient. The patient may believe that in order for the chemotherapy to be effective, emesis must occur because he or she has been told the well-meaning statement, "Don't worry if you vomit; it just means that the therapy is working."

NONVERBAL COMMUNICATION

Communication occurs in many forms, not the least of which is nonverbal. All of us have had the experience of observing a total stranger from a distance and knowing immediately whether we liked or disliked that individual and whether, if permitted the choice, we wished to have any other interaction with him or her.

How does this occur? From the moment a human infant can distinguish between self and nonself, nonverbal communication begins between the individual and caregivers. The infant quickly learns which facial expressions and body postures result in rewards and which have the opposite effect. It is extremely important for successful therapists to be attuned to the body language of their patients (clients) as well as to their own nonverbal communications (Gravitz 1981).

Those individuals who choose not to touch or even shake hands with a cancer patient are reinforcing the far too frequently held patient belief that they have become untouchable. It is much better to greet the patient with outstretched arms, palms up, and clasping both of their hands, welcoming the patient into an environment of care, concern, and protection. Numerous studies have documented the distinct therapeutic advantage of human touch as augmenting outcomes in undertakings as diverse as obstetrical pain, hemoglobin increase, and healing in general (Levitan 1986; Samarel 1992). It is beyond the realm of this chapter to discuss the role of Oriental healing practices, such as xi-gong and acupressure, both of which are dependent upon touch, but few would dispute the value and relevance of healing practices that have survived over 10,000 years of human experience. Only now are scientific studies documenting the sophisticated mechanisms by which these practices heal (Rossi 1994; Steggles 1997; Besedovsky 1996).

In addition to nonverbal communication, the circumstances under which a referral for hypnotherapy occurs have a significant effect on outcome. If hypnosis is advocated as a highly effective intervention specifically proven to have application to the clinical issue in question, it will be far more effective than if suggested as a last-ditch alternative that in all likelihood won't work anyway. For this reason, it is sometimes useful to instruct the personnel scheduling patients for hypnotherapy to be positive about the likelihood of benefit to the patient in question. Similarly, it can be very useful to bracket the patient presenting for therapy of a particular problem with two other patients, each of whom has attained success in dealing with the issue at hand. Patients have a way of talking with each other in the waiting room, and affirmations of success from patients scheduled to see the hypnotherapist both before and after the new patient could be very helpful in setting up a positive expectancy. Alternatively, new patients may request the telephone numbers of successfully treated patients, with the latter's permission, for individual inquiry.

BEGINNING THE THERAPEUTIC INTERVENTION

All patients present for hypnotherapy with a variety of presuppositions, both positive and negative (Torem 1992). On intake, it is useful to garner comprehensive understanding of the extent and nature of the disease in question, to know the reasons for the referral for hypnotherapy, and more importantly, to know the patient's understanding of what has occurred and will occur as therapy progresses. It is important that misconceptions are corrected as soon as possible, lest the patient assume that the therapist has corroborated them. Helpful questions can be as simple as, "What is your understanding of what is going on now and where we go from here?"

If for any reason the therapist's fund of information does not include a comprehensive understanding of the disease process in question or the anticipated therapeutic course, then it is incumbent on the therapist to contact the referring physician and, if necessary, use the resources of a research library. Uncertainty or overt ignorance about the disease in question on the part of any member of the therapeutic team can be devastating to the patient. All medical personnel dealing with the patient should be prepared to admit ignorance when necessary and have a willingness to search for the answer to any questions.

Having clarified the patient's fund of information and expectancies from hypnosis, it is then appropriate for the hypnotherapist to define a time line and an approach to dealing with the issues in question. The patient may have been referred for hypnosis because of a specific problem such as nausea or anticipatory emesis, or the patient may be well read in the field of alternative medicine and wish assistance in imagery and lifestyle modification in an attempt to shrink the tumor itself (Bovbjerg 1991; Bridge 1988; Cohen 1996; Ruzyla-Smith 1995).

It is important for the patient to appreciate that he or she may have already experienced negative hypnosis as a consequence of society's negative perception of cancer therapy and outcomes. Far too often patients equate the diagnosis of cancer with impending death, even though the vast number of malignancies can be very effectively treated and often cured. It is the constant influence of these negative suggestions, often enunciated by highly respected personal authority figures, which has such a pernicious effect on the patient's psyche.

To counteract the effect of these past repetitive negative suggestions, I make it a practice to suggest that the patient take a moment for self-hypnosis at least once an hour, if only for a few seconds each time. Often taking a moment to focus attention inwardly while taking a deep breath and allowing all unnecessary tension and stress to leave with exhalation is all that is required. A useful metaphor is that of a computer program, jointly written by the therapist and patient, which automatically runs each time the patient takes a moment to practice self-hypnosis if only for a few seconds—similar to the response of a running computer when the "Enter" key is pressed.

An alternative and equally effective strategy that I often employ in the first session is to block the effect of negative suggestions. Because most patients present to the therapist's office in an existing alternative state of consciousness, that state may be utilized to their advantage and obviate the need for a formal induction. Thus I can easily instruct the patient as follows: "Should anyone say anything to you that is negative or less than helpful, it will have no effect. It will be as if those comments, or even self-doubts, were expressed in a language that is foreign to you and that you do not understand. If anything, they will facilitate your success and make it easier for you to obtain your objectives." I call this "Reversing the Negatives."

I've found it a useful practice to request that patients bring a blank audiotape cassette to the first session so that it may be recorded for their subsequent use. Should the patient forget to do this, I usually have a supply of tapes containing drug company messages that are easily recorded over by applying a small piece of scotch tape to the apertures on the portion of the cassette making contact with the recording heads. By recording the initial session, Erickson's suggestion that "my voice will go with you" is made easily accessible for the patient. Patients periodically report that they have difficulty achieving the depth of trance during self-hypnosis practice that they were able to attain during the initial hetero-hypnosis. This problem is obviated when they use the tape recording made during the first session. Some patients have used the tape repetitively, even going so far as to listen to it each night while falling asleep;

others are comforted by merely having the tape in their possession.

It is prudent to point out that the best induction tape accessible to patients is the one they carry within themselves. It is indeed important for the therapist to remember that the patient is inducing the trance, because all hypnosis is self-hypnosis, and the therapist is merely facilitating a native ability present in almost every one of us (Brown 1991).

Indeed, it is useful for the therapist to appreciate that all forms of hypnotic induction are merely rituals employed to attain the degree of relaxation and receptivity to suggestions necessary for effective therapy. In truth, if we were really effective as therapists, we would be able to look the patient in the eyes and, with conviction, say the word "change," and the desired therapeutic outcome would be attained. Because this outcome usually cannot be accomplished without multiple therapeutic sessions and a variety of appropriate interventions directed at the desired therapeutic outcome, it merely speaks to the ineptitude of our current therapeutic abilities.

Practitioners should learn to *inquire about comfort rather than pain* and to be careful to suggest that a patient "achieve" an objective rather than "try to achieve" an objective, the latter having the implicit suggestion of potential failure. It is also useful for patients to interdict negative and counterproductive thoughts when these thoughts initially present themselves. It is not uncommon for a patient to have a problem of long duration resolved at a hypnotherapeutic session, much to the patient's amazement and delight, only to have the problem recur at a later time. It is impossible for a problem of many years' duration to be resolved by a single therapeutic session. Indeed, the negative self hypnotic suggestion is then acted upon and realized.

Before a long-standing problem is permanently resolved, often there is an exacerbation of the symptom and then it disappears. I have found it useful to anticipate this event and analogize it to the phenomenon of that of a candle that flares up before finally burning out consequent to the consumption of all available wax. "Anticipating a relapse" is a useful therapeutic ploy and should be explained to the patient as an indication that the therapeutic intervention is being directed at the appropriate area of psychological sensitivity and bodes a favorable therapeutic outcome. This anticipation of a flare in symptoms avoids the problem of the occasional patient who experiences an increase in symptoms and thus becomes discouraged with the therapeutic process and discontinues seeing the therapist.

An alternative and equally effective approach to long-standing problems is to encourage an exacerbation during the therapeutic session and to allow the patient to experience the effect of hypnotherapy in relieving the particular symptom in question. An example is the patient with anticipatory emesis who becomes increasingly nauseated as the day of the office or chemotherapy appointment approaches. A useful strategy is to ask the patient to gauge the severity of the problem on a numerical analog scale from 1 to 10 at the initial office presentation. Customarily, unless the patient is a hysteric, the numerical rating is in the range of 3 to 8. Hypnosis is then induced and the patient is asked to visualize the circumstance that augments the presenting symptom. The severity of the symptom increases with negative suggestion, and at a point when the patient is appreciably distressed by the symptom, he or she is given permission to use the newly learned hypnotherapeutic technique to allow the symptom to relent. In this manner, the patient appreciates that it is possible to have an impact on the symptom. If through adverse circumstance visualization of the patient's symptom goes from a rating of 4 to 8 and then back to 4 again, the patient has learned that it is possible to significantly impact the intensity of the symptom.

It is precisely by making the symptom worse that patients can be taught the benefit of self-hypnosis to allow the symptom at a minimum to return to its baseline level from its exacerbated state. More commonly, the symptom is significantly improved over the baseline state as reported by the patient during the initial inquiry.

SPECIFIC THERAPEUTIC INTERVENTIONS

Pain and Needle Phobia

All cancer patients should be taught the technique of glove anesthesia and regional anesthesia because they are frequently subjected to invasive procedures such as venapuncture, repetitive finger sticks, various biopsies, and endoscopies. All of us have at one time or another experienced our arm or leg "falling asleep" as a consequence of pressure on the nerve or vascular supply of the extremity for a protracted period of time. It is easy to suggest that this sensation may recur under hypnosis without the additional experience of any adverse associated sensations such as the "pins and needles" feeling often described in association with a "sleeping" extremity. I have found it useful to suggest that the patient visualize the extremity as transparent, and then subsequently to visualize colored nerves or wires beginning in the fingertips (or toes), joining other nerves further up the arm (or leg) to form a sturdier cable network, eventually leading to the brain, in which a series of switches controlling each and every part of the body

can be found. I suggest that the patient visualize a light of whatever color the patient prefers, indicating over each switch whether the switch is "on" or "off." I then suggest that the patient turn off the pain switch to the extremity or region in question, and then allow the light over the switch to extinguish along with pain perception in the specific area. It is not necessary to suggest that any other sensations be extinguished. Thus, patients can retain tactile, temperature, or other perceptions without experiencing any awareness of pain. The patients will not assume that because they are aware of the tactile sensation associated with the procedure that they have been unsuccessful in blocking pain awareness. A useful phrase is, "You will feel me touch you, but you need have no pain, no bleeding, no swelling; when the needle is withdrawn it will be as if no puncture had ever occurred."

Alternative and additional pain interdiction strategies include the circumferential or regional injection of a powerful imaginary anesthetic, or the drawing up over the extremity of a magic glove, stocking, or cloth containing the most powerful contact anesthetic. Other useful visualizations include soaking the hand in ice water or packing it in snow until awareness of pain ceases. Headache sufferers have found it useful to visualize standing under a cooling shower or waterfall that washes away all awareness of pain from without and within.

If a more extensive procedure requiring hypnoanesthesia or hypnoanalgesia is required, it is useful to visualize and rehearse the procedure once or twice utilizing the previous techniques before the procedure is actually performed. It is also useful to ratify the patient's success in controlling pain in the area by testing with a sharp object such as a sterile needle. The needle can be passed through a skin fold, ratifying both pain and bleeding control as well as the immediacy of healing.

As an interesting aside, hypnoanesthesia, when employed for medical or religious purposes, has almost never been associated with secondary infection regardless of the procedure involved.

Nausea Control

With the recent advent of more effective anti-nausea medications, chemotherapy- and radiation therapy–induced nausea has become much less of a problem. Nevertheless, many patients do experience some degree of nausea and possibly emesis in association with their therapy.

I may offer a variety of therapeutic suggestions to the patient after inducing a state of hypnosis.

(1) Visualize the body as a house with many rooms, each with individual light switches and controls (Levitan

1987). I suggest that the patient finds that room in the house controlling the sensation of nausea and turns off the light switch in that room. Then I suggest that the patient allows the sensation to be extinguished and then quietly closes the door, so that no other parts of the body are disturbed.

(2) A similar approach is to suggest that the nausea switch in the brain to that part of the body be turned off in a similar fashion to that employed for pain control.

(3) I also suggest visualization of a lake or body of water experiencing a turbulent storm with high waves and whitecaps. I then suggest that a gradual parting of the overlying storm clouds occurs. Then there is an initial perception of a few rays of bright sunlight, progressing to the gradual disappearance of all storm clouds and associated disappearance of all turbulence on the water's surface. Only a smooth, glass-like surface remains.

(4) A similar visualization, which is equally effective for pain control, is that of a bright red, flaming sun slowly sinking into a western horizon with its colors changing from red to pink to lavender, and to purple-blue, and eventually ending with the wonderful stillness and quiet associated with the period immediately after sunset.

(5) Another visualization that is applicable to a variety of symptom interventions is the concept of "an emotional snapshot." In the case of the symptom of nausea it is suggested that the patients visualize or recall a particular experience in which they were going out to a lovely restaurant for a dinner associated with a special occasion. The patients should visualize the anticipation of the experience, dressing specially to go the the restaurant, arriving at the restaurant and being delighted with the décor and the location of their particular table, as well as their dinner companions. They are then presented with the menu for selection of their choice of foods. As they read through the multiplicity of delicious choices, a delightful anticipatory hunger develops as the patient wonders how each dish will taste, predicated on its description in the menu. The patient is asked to take "an emotional snapshot," freezing in memory this feeling of anticipatory hunger that excludes any alternative negative gastrointestinal sensation. Whenever patients experience even a forewarning of the possibility of nausea occurring it is suggested that they reach for the emotional snapshot of the delightful anticipatory hunger, thereby replacing any pending alternative sensation. It is almost as if a slide projector is advanced to the next slide, replacing one scene on the screen with another. This technique can be used to replace sensations of anxiety with those of security, sensations of pain with those of comfort, sensations of loneliness with pleasant memories of the warm company of others on special occasions, and in general reverse any number of negatives associated with cancer or its therapy.

(6) Under some circumstances, this dissociative technique is useful. A magic mirror can be passed through the middle of the person's body allowing awareness and sensation to remain contentedly on one side of the mirror, while on the other side of the mirror all unpleasant sensations, such as nausea, anxiety, and fear, remain confined.

Anticipatory Emesis

Aversive conditioning occurs as a consequence of the Pavlovian conditioning and learning associated with a negative experience. If patients experience nausea and vomiting subsequent to each visit to the outpatient chemotherapy center, they will obviously not look forward to the next experience and will often experience increased nausea in the days prior to their chemotherapy appointment (Jacknow 1994). Also, if a patient associated a certain food with the chemotherapy-related nausea, he or she may be reminded of this nausea the next time the particular food is served, whether or not it is associated with concomitant chemotherapy (Redd 1982; Morrow 1982). Amnesia for any antecedent negative experience is a useful strategy to apply in association with the previously mentioned problems. Indeed, if one is psychologically experiencing chemotherapy for the first time, it is impossible to have nausea occur as a consequence of a prior experience. Useful verbalizations offered to the hypnotized patient include, "Feel free to remember to forget, or even to forget to remember, any previous chemotherapy sessions, so that each time you will comfortably experience the treatment for the very first time."

A useful visualization for the same situation would be to place a memory on the top shelf of a dusty cabinet in the back of an attic at the very top of a house and then lock the cabinet, tiptoe out of the attic, and shut off the light, closing the door and forgetting all about it along with all the other myriad things stored in the attic.

Anxiety and Claustrophobia

Just as amnesia can be of great assistance in eliminating anticipatory symptoms, *education and familiarity can reduce the anxiety often associated with unfamiliar interventions and experiences*. If a patient is familiarized in detail with what is likely to occur during a pending therapeutic or diagnostic intervention, that patient will often be much more comfortable during the actual procedure. Hypnotherapeutic future projection techniques accomplish this very effectively. After inducing hypnosis, the patient is advised that he or she can speak comfortably and naturally and that each word said will act to deepen the state of relaxation that he or she experiences. This suggestion is made to counter the normal trance lightening effect that verbalization has on the hypnotic experience.

The patient is then asked to visualize the procedure or circumstance involved, and inquiry is made as to how he or she feels. If a patient expresses specific concerns, attention is focused on giving suggestions to correct the problem. For example, in patients expressing claustrophobia in association with computed tomography (CT) or magnetic resonance imaging (MRI) studies (Lang 1996), it is desirable to first completely acquaint them with what is likely to occur so there is no anxiety relative to the unknown. Next, it may be necessary to psychologically uncover some elements of the cause of their anxiety about confined spaces and reframe or hypnotherapeutically modify their memories of such experiences so that those memories will not apply to the present circumstances (Genuis 1995).

Another suggested visualization technique is to recall a camping experience in which the patient first had the opportunity to delightedly use a sleeping bag. Memories of comfort, security, and warmth can be elicited along with the recollection that the air around the patient's nose and face was somewhat cool, as customarily is the case with ventilation provided in the CT or MRI enclosure.

Another technique is to have patients experience, while in hypnosis, sliding comfortably into a warm fragrant bubble bath. Then patients can visualize relaxing their necks on a specially provided pillow while delightedly soaking in the tub with eyes closed.

Time distortion can be accomplished under hypnosis, which can make the procedure seem to last only a few moments in time before it is over. Specific suggestions I've found useful include "Time will pass extremely quickly," and "The procedure will be completed even before you realize it has begun." Alternatively, for patients experiencing intermittent episodes of discomfort, I suggest that "The intervals between discomfort will be long and luxurious, and the duration of any discomfort will be so brief that it is barely noticeable."

It is also possible to provide a relaxation tape to be played for the patient during the course of the procedure. It is also useful to train CT and MRI technologists in the rudiments of hypnotherapeutic suggestions so that they can communicate more effectively with their patients.

THE USE OF IMAGERY TO PROMOTE HEALING

The new information developing in the burgeoning field of psychoneuroimmunology suggests that self-hypnosis and imagery can be used to benefit not only symptoms associated with cancer therapy but also the outcome as well. David Spiegel's study reported in 1989 in *Lancet* showed significant augmentation of survival in a control group of patients receiving psychological intervention. Multiple studies are currently underway to replicate this result. As a consequence of Spiegel's study, cancer patients frequently contact practicing hypnotherapists for assistance in the techniques directed at influencing regression of their malignancy and its response to therapy, hopefully resulting in cure.

Initial work in this field was done by Carl and Stephanie Simonton and was publicized in their popular book, *Getting Well Again* (Simonton 1978). Scientific validity was added to this approach by Robert Ader, based on his animal conditioning experiments (Cohen 1979; Bovbjerg 1982). *It is now almost universally accepted that the mind can have an effect on neuroendocrine function* (Anderson 1996; Fife 1996). See Chapter 4 on psychoneuroimmunology in this book.

The basic imagery approach currently utilized to mobilize intrinsic healing and immunologic stimulation directed against the malignancy is as follows: Hypnosis is induced and the patient is asked to visualize and describe the nature, extent, and location of the malignancy should he feel that any residual disease exists. This visualization is periodically reframed to portray any existent cancer cells as disorganized, nonpurposeful cells whose continued growth imperils their own existence as well as that of the host. The patient is then asked to visualize his or her own healing resources, which have been operating all their lives to heal injuries on the exterior as well as in the interior of their bodies. These resources, including particularly the immune system, are depicted as organized, vigilant, and resourceful. The immune cells are visualized as outnumbering the defenseless cancer cells. The immune cells can readily detect the cancer cells and surround them by virtue of their greatly superior numbers. The immune cells wall off all cancer cells and initiate their rapid and complete destruction. Once all the cancer cells are destroyed, the surveillance process continues and prevents the recurrence of any further malignant cells.

For those patients currently undergoing chemotherapy or radiation therapy, it is suggested that they visualize the drugs or radiation directly affecting the existing cancer cells, causing them to shrivel up and die, and their breakdown products eliminated from the body through the action of the normal macrophage cells (Levitan 1987; Levitan 1992). Thereafter, it is useful to see the normal surrounding tissues repairing themselves and filling in the void left by the dead cancer cells with totally normal tissue. As has been pointed out earlier, I believe it is more effective for the patient to practice self-hypnosis for a few seconds once an hour using the previous visualizations as opposed to devoting a lengthy period of time once a day in a "white knuckle" attempt to achieve maximal depth of trance for a more favorable outcome.

ANXIETY ABOUT DEATH AND THE DYING PROCESS

Because death is an experience that is unknown to all of us, it is understandable that its anticipation can be associated with anxiety. Merely discussing the topic when appropriate can defuse a considerable amount of the normally associated fear. Patients should be assured that current pain technology allows us to keep patients comfortable at all times, even if on occasion drowsiness occurs as a side effect. It is important to emphasize that although we cannot prevent death *we can always prevent suffering,* even if it means the use of continuous infusion pain medication that is unlimited for all cancer patients.

For patients in whom a more specific insight into the dying process is desirable, the technique of death rehearsal has proven to be highly effective (Levitan 1985; Levitan 1991). In this technique, patients are asked to future project to a time when their death is imminent and to describe in detail both their feelings and the circumstances in which they find themselves. Any negative feelings or descriptions are reframed to help patients understand that they will not be alone and that dying is as natural and simple a process as being born. If patients describe those around them as being sad, this description is reframed as an expression of love and concern over the physical loss of the patient with the

understanding that their love and legacy of shared memories remains immutable. If the patient expresses concern about unfinished business or unresolved conflicts, it is suggested that these be resolved, and specific methods for accomplishing this are suggested with the additional visualization of a successful outcome. If patients experience anxiety over the specifics of the dying process, they are asked to visualize moment by moment what occurs at the specific time of their death and, if needed, this is reframed into a soothing, welcoming, comforting process. Patients are also encouraged to visualize circumstances following their death in order to appreciate the impact their life has had on the lives of others. By hypnotically rehearsing the dying process, patients do not find it as foreign and anxiety provoking when it actually occurs because they have already gained a familiarity with the experience itself.

CONCLUSION

A knowledge of hypnotherapy and its utilization is extremely valuable in dealing with the oncology patient. It teaches the therapist how to positively communicate with the patient, while inadvertently avoiding any negative suggestions. *Because most hypnotherapists experience trance themselves while doing hypnotherapy,* a greater degree of comfort in the therapist makes communicating with seriously ill and dying patients less stressful. As with all positive therapeutic interventions, once one has been of assistance to one patient in a material way, the value of hypnotherapy is permanently established in the therapist's armamentarium. My personal belief is that the principles of hypnotherapy and its associated communication skills are the "art" of medicine.

REFERENCES

Anderson JA: The immune system and major depression. Adv Neuroimmunol 6:119–129, 1996

Besedovsky HO, Herberman RB, Temoshok LR, et al: Psychoneuroimmunology and cancer: Fifteenth Sapporo Cancer Seminar. Cancer Res 56(18):4278–4281, 1996

Bovbjerg DH: Psychoneuroimmunology: Implications for oncology? Cancer 67(3):828–832, 1991

Bovbjerg DH, Ader R, Cohen N: Behaviorally conditioned suppression of a graft-versus-host response. Proc Natl Acad Sci USA 79:583–585, 1982

Bridge LR, Benson P, Pietroni PC, et al: Relaxation and imagery in the treatment of breast cancer. BMJ 297(6657):1169–1172, 1988

Brown P: The Hypnotic Brain: Hypnotherapy and Social Communication. New Haven, Yale University Press, 1991, pp 85–122

Cohen N, Ader R, Green N, et al: Conditioned suppression of a thymus-independent antibody response. Psychosom Med 41:487–491, 1979

Cohen S, Herbert TB: Health psychology: Psychological factors and physical disease from the perspective of human psychoneuroimmunology. Annual Review of Psychology 47(1):113–142, 1996

Fife A, Beasley PJ, Fertig DL: Psychoneuroimmunology and cancer: Historical perspectives and current research. Adv Neuroimmunol 6:179–190, 1996

Genuis ML: The use of hypnosis in helping cancer patients control anxiety, pain, and emesis: A review of recent empirical studies. Am J Clin Hypn 37(4):316–325, 1995

Gravitz M: Non-verbal hypnotic techniques in a centrally deaf brain-damaged patient. Int J Clin Exp Hypn 29(2):110–116, 1981

Jacknow DS, Tschann JM, Link MP, et al: Hypnosis in the prevention of chemotherapy-related nausea and vomiting in children: A prospective study. J Dev Behav Pediat 15(4):258–264, 1994

Lang EV, Joyce JS, Spiegel D, et al: Self-hypnotic relaxation during interventional radiological procedures: Effects on pain perception and intravenous drug use. Int J Clin Exp Hypn 44(2):106–119, 1996

Levitan AA: Hypnosis and oncology. *In* Wester II WC (ed): Clinical Hypnosis: A Case Management Approach. Cincinnati, Behavioral Science Center, Inc. Publications, 1987, pp 332–356

Levitan AA: Hypnotic death rehearsal. Am J Clin Hypn 27(4):211–215, 1985

Levitan AA: Hypnotic death rehearsal. *In* Sheikh AA, Sheikh KS (eds): Death Imagery: Confronting Death Brings Us to the Threshold of Life. Milwaukee, American Imagery Institute, 1991, pp 95–108

Levitan AA: The use of hypnosis with cancer patients. Psychiatric Medicine 10(1):119–131, 1992

Levitan AA, Johnson J: The role of touch in healing and hypnotherapy. Am J Clin Hypn 28(4):218–223, 1986

Morrow GR, Morrell C: Behavioral treatment for the anticipatory nausea and vomiting induced by cancer chemotherapy. New Engl J Med 307(24):1476–1480, 1982

Peabody FW: The care of the patient. JAMA 88:877–882, 1927

Redd WH, Andersen GV, Minagawa RY: Hypnotic control of antici-
patory emesis in patients receiving cancer chemotherapy. J Consult Clin Psychol 50(1):14–19, 1982

Rossi EL: New theories of healing and hypnosis: The emergence of mind-gene communication. European Journal of Clinical Hypnosis 3:1–14, 1994

Ruzyla-Smith P, Barabasz A, Barabasz, et al: Effects of hypnosis on the immune response: B-cell, T-cells, helper and suppressor cells. Am J Clin Hypn 38(2):71–79, 1995

Samarel N: The experience of receiving therapeutic touch. J Adv Nurs 17:651–657, 1992

Simonton OC, Matthews-Simonton S, Creighton J: Getting Well Again. Los Angeles, JP Tarcher, 1978

Spiegel D, Bloom JR, Kraemer HC, et al: Effect of psychosocial treatment on survival of patients with metastatic breast cancer. Lancet 2(8668):888–891, 1989

Steggles S, Maxwell J, Lightfoot NE, et al: Hypnosis and cancer: An annotated bibliography 1985–1995. Am J Clin Hypn 39(3):187–200, 1997

Torem MS: Hypnosis: Lingering myths and established facts. Psychiatric Medicine 10(1):1–11, 1992

11

Hypnosis and Its Usefulness in Managing Patients with Respiratory Problems

Marcia J. Wagaman

THE PATIENT WITH ASTHMA

"You cured me! I don't even know I have asthma anymore."

"I use much less medication."

"I have more freedom."

"I control my asthma now instead of it controlling me."

"I'm more aware of my body and take care of my asthma sooner instead of waiting until it gets real bad."

"This is the first time in years that I've had a cold and not had to take antibiotics."

These are some of the comments I have heard from patients after adding hypnosis to their therapeutic regimen. Hypnosis can decrease anxiety, increase comfort, reduce symptoms, and decrease the need for medication.

SOCIOECONOMIC ASPECTS

Hypnosis with asthma patients is given the most attention in this chapter because it is the respiratory problem for which hypnosis has been and is used the most frequently. Asthma has affected approximately 7% of Americans at some point in their lives (Davis 1972, cited in King 1980). In 1979, a report from a National Institutes of Health (NIH) Task Force indicated that 8.9 million Americans had asthma (NIAID Task Force 1979, cited in Cluss 1985). During 1980 to 1987, the

Portions of this chapter are based on work done as part of the author's doctoral program at Union Institute.

prevalence rate of asthma in the United States increased 29% to an estimated 10 million. In 1987, asthma was listed as the primary diagnosis for 6.5 million out-patient visits, for more than 450,000 hospitalizations, and the cause of death for 4580 people in the United States.

In addition to, and probably resulting from, the physical suffering and the threat of death, the asthma patient is frequently forced to contend with a variety of psychological, psychosocial, and economic problems. Among these are increased absenteeism from school or work, loss of income, unemployment, alcohol abuse, depression, anxiety, denial, significant medical expenses, and family or social loss and disruption. In 1988, asthma-related health care costs were greater than 4 billion dollars in the United States (NIH 1991). Families have spent 2% to 30% of their total income in efforts to control the disease (Vance and Taylor 1971, cited in Cluss 1985). Additionally, chronic intractable asthma in a family member may result in family disruption or divorce (NIAID Task Force 1979, cited in Cluss 1985).

PSYCHOBIOLOGY OF ASTHMA

Our understanding of asthma has evolved from considering it to be a disorder of nervous or psychological origin (Alexander 1987), to an allergic-induced physiologic response resulting in bronchoconstriction, to a chronic persistent inflammatory disease involving many interacting cells and mediators (Barnes 1989a; Barnes 1989b). The precise immunologic mechanism of this inflammatory process has not yet been elucidated; it is most likely multifactorial, and it is unlikely that a single cell or mediator will be identified as the sole culprit (Ackerman 1989; McFadden Jr 1992).

Asthma was once thought to be primarily a nervous disorder and was referred to as "asthma nervosa." This viewpoint became obsolete, however, following recognition of the allergic phenomenon (Alexander 1987). Although some still clung to the idea of a primary emotional cause by differentiating between "allergic asthma" and "emotional asthma," Wistuba found no significant difference between allergic and nonallergic asthmatics in personality, psychosocial, or behavioral analysis (Wistuba 1986). Parker and Lipscombe (cited in Cluss 1985) evaluated parental overprotectiveness of asthmatics and found it to be a consequence of the illness rather than an antecedent. Matus and Bush evaluated the contribution of psychological adjustment to the prediction of asthma symptoms and found that, although predictability significantly increased when family and child adjustment ratings were considered along with the pulmonary function factor forced expiratory volume in 1 second (FEV_1), the single best predictor of attack frequency was the pulmonary function factor maximum midexpiratory flow (Matus 1979).

Even in allergic patients, some studies have shown both that the amount of allergen required to produce an effect is less under conditions of increased stress, and that the degree of pulmonary compromise to a given stimulus can vary with the emotional state of the subject. These results suggest a multifactorial and probably an interactive relationship involving the degree of airway inflammation at the time, the effect of the state on the autonomic nervous system, or the effect on the immune system (Clarke 1983).

As early as 1970, Purnell and Weiss (cited in Brown and Fromm 1987) stated that most often anxiety, depression, frustration, and anger were results of an asthma attack rather than the cause. In 1984, Spittle and Sears, after failing to find a substantial relationship between illness severity, serum IgE, and various psychological and social factors, concluded that there is insufficient support for asthma as a psychosomatic disorder, an opinion also shared by Creer and Steptoe (both cited in Maes 1988).

The National Asthma Education Program of the NIH (1991) has defined asthma as a lung disease with the following characteristics: (1) airway obstruction that is reversible (but not completely so in some patients) either spontaneously or with treatment; (2) airway inflammation; and (3) increased airway responsiveness to a variety of stimuli.

Clinical manifestations include increased use of accessory muscles of respiration, shortness of breath, chest tightness, wheezing, and coughing. Precipitating factors include both allergens (extrinsic asthma) and nonallergenic stimuli (intrinsic asthma). The latter includes viral infection, exercise, environmental irritants, physical irritants (such as cold air, changes in air flow as can occur from laughter and emotion), a heavy meal, idiosyncratic reactions to drugs and chemicals (such as aspirin, sulfites, and MSG), and stress (NIH 1991; Weiner 1987). Activation of the vagus nerve or autonomic imbalance manifesting in an increased parasympathetic reflex may contribute to the paradoxical response in stress-sensitive asthmatics (Ader 1991).

WHY HYPNOSIS?

Medical noncompliance with treatment is estimated to be greater than 50% in patients with asthma. Reasons for noncompliance can be drug related such as awkward regimens, real or imagined side effects, or fear of side effects. Reasons may also be nondrug related such as underestimation of severity of the disease, rebellion or anger, attitudes toward ill health, cultural factors, stigmatization, miscommunication, misinterpretation, or a poor doctor–patient relationship (NIH 1991; Randall 1992). Conversely, exceptionally high anxiety about breathing difficulties can result in excessive use of medication, even when no bronchoconstriction is present (Kinsman 1980).

Although expectations of controlling asthma with nonpharmacological means alone are probably unrealistic, the addition of nonpharmacological techniques to traditional therapy may enable some patients to be managed on lower doses of steroids or less frequent use of bronchodilators. Results of various trials of self-regulating techniques in the control of asthma have been inconsistent and equivocal. One explanation may be that most of these methods use *deep relaxation, which may be counterproductive for asthma relief by decreasing sympathetic activity too much and promoting parasympathetic dominance.* Hypnosis does not have to incorporate deep relaxation, yet it does produce heightened suggestibility, and it can utilize the phenomenon of posthypnotic suggestion. Thus hypnosis may be more valuable than relaxation techniques in the control of asthma (Mather 1975).

HYPNOSIS AND ASTHMA

Review of Literature

Numerous investigators have reported successfully inducing both bronchoconstriction and bronchodilation in asthmatics by means of suggestion, without utilizing hypnosis. Some have administered aerosolized solutions by inhalation, both with and without added pharmacological agents, accompanied by suggestion related to the desired experimental effect of the solution (Butler 1986; Horton 1978; Luparello 1968; McFadden 1969; Neild 1985; Philip 1972; Spector 1976; Strupp 1974). In 1970, Weiss et al (cited in Strupp 1974), however, did not confirm those results in more severely ill patients using peak expiratory flow rate as assessment, nor did Isenberg et al (Isenberg 1992b). Placebo effects have also been reported in two studies. Godfrey and Silverman (cited in Butler 1986) found that bronchoconstriction induced by treadmill exercise could be partially reversed by placebo. In accordance, Butler and Steptoe report that a suggested bronchoconstrictive response to the inhalation of distilled water could be abolished by pretreatment with placebo (Butler 1986).

Some authors report having induced bronchoconstriction by hypnotic suggestion without inhalation. Thorne and Fisher showed that response to a hypnotically suggested asthma experience was associated with hypnotic susceptibility and not with a history of previous asthma. Subjects who responded appeared to be suffering an asthma attack and reported the experience as seeming "real" to them, but measurements of FEV_1 and FEV_3, although different from presuggestion values, were not similar in slope to those seen in true asthmatics (Thorne 1978).

These findings would be consistent with the observations of Neal Miller during the beginning of his work with biofeedback. Three subjects of high hypnotizability were given the suggestion, under hypnosis, of increasing temperature in one hand while simultaneously decreasing temperature in the other hand. No actual temperature change occurred; however the subjects were convinced that one hand was hot and the other was cold. In other words they had hallucinated temperature change in the absence of objective change (Hall 1989). This phenomenon was also observed by Locke et al (cited in Hall 1989), who studied the ability of untrained subjects with high hypnotizability scores to alter their immune response to delayed-type hypersensitivity antigens. Although no objective change was demonstrated, subjects reported that they felt they had produced the changes. The possible contribution of several factors needs to be considered when reviewing the studies of suggestion alone.

Waking Suggestion and Hypnotic Ability

A review regarding the effects of suggestion and emotional arousal on pulmonary function in asthmatics (Isenberg 1992a) estimated that across the studies of asthmatics, only 35% to 40% showed bronchoconstriction to both suggestion and stress; because of methodological considerations the estimations might be more conservatively, and accurately, estimated as closer to 20%. Because this response does not appear to be consistent in the majority of asthmatics, one wonders if this could be attributed to the phenomenon of waking suggestion in subjects with moderate to high hypnotic ability, as described by Bowers (1976). Some people do not need the benefit of a formal induction in order to respond to suggestions. In a study using both asthmatic and nonasthmatic subjects, Thorne and Fisher found that physical response to a tape recorded hypnotically suggested that experience of asthma was predicted by hypnotic susceptibility assessed by the Harvard Scale and not by a history of previous asthma. Hypnotic susceptibility has also been hypothesized to predict response to placebo, particularly when suggestion is given regarding expected effects (Wickramasekera 1980).

Temperature of Inhaled Solution

The inhalation of cold air serves as a stimulus for bronchoconstriction in the asthmatic airway (Simonsson 1967). Lewis et al found that 9 out of 30 asthmatics, but no normal subjects, bronchoconstricted in response to normal saline inhalation accompanied by suggestion. This response was abolished, however, when the solution was warmed to 37°C (body temperature) (Lewis 1984).

Tonicity of the Solution

Some of the investigators used distilled water instead of normal saline solution, and some added pharmacologic agents to the solution. Hypertonic or hypotonic solutions can induce bronchospasm in asthmatics. This reaction is exemplified in the study by Chin and Nussbaum in which bronchoconstriction after the inhalation of a hypotonic solution composed of distilled water and sodium cromolyn (a drug used in the treatment of asthma) was corrected by the addition of normal saline (Chin 1992).

Hyperventilation

In 1968, Sterling demonstrated bronchoconstriction resulting from hypocapnia secondary to hyperventilation. The procedure of aerosol inhalation involves taking a prolonged series of deep breaths, thereby involving some degree of hyperventilation in the process itself. The degree of hyperventilation varies with the technique of the individual. Additionally, there is some evidence that stretch receptor activity in airways, as may occur as a result of deep breathing during the aerosol inhalation, may trigger bronchoconstriction (Garfinkle et al 1979 and Orelick et al 1975, both cited in Isenberg 1992a). Hyperventilation can also occur in association with emotion, which may provide an explanation for emotion precipitating bronchoconstriction. In accordance, hyperventilation could result from anticipatory anxiety and fear in response to the suggestion, and the consequent expectancy of precipitating an asthma attack.

Mechanical Irritation of the Airways

Rapid respiratory maneuvers or changes in airflow have been shown to cause increased airway resistance in asthmatics. In turn, stimulation of cough receptors by any means, including mechanical irritation, produces reflex bronchoconstriction (Simonsson 1967).

Bronchial Hyper-reactivity

Although it does not happen consistently, it is not unusual for an asthmatic to develop some reflex broncho-

spasm in response to aerosol administration. In addition to the previously mentioned contributing factors, the response at any point in time, with or without suggestion, is most likely influenced a great deal by the degree of bronchial hyper-reactivity present. In fact, Horton et al (cited in Janson-Bjerklie 1986) found significant correlation between the degree of bronchial hyper-reactivity and airway response to suggestion. The lack of bronchial hyper-reactivity may also account for the lack of response of nonasthmatics.

Neural and Psychological Factors

The possible association between emotion, changes in the air flow, hyperventilation, and bronchospasm has already been discussed. Horton et al (cited in Janson-Bjerklie 1986) observed that bronchoconstrictive response to suggestion was not only significantly related to the degree of bronchial hyper-reactivity but also to physiologic measures (blood pressure and pulse) of emotional reactions to bronchoconstrictive suggestions; it was unclear, however, whether emotional response was the cause or effect of the bronchospasm. Janson-Bjerklie et al found the response to suggestion of bronchoconstriction when inhaling normal saline could not be predicted by report of perceived response to emotional triggers of asthma; therefore, she questions whether the use of suggestion is valid in studying the roles of psychological factors and emotional arousal in the provocation of asthma, in that emotional arousal and suggestion may not be comparable stimuli or may operate via different mechanisms (Janson-Bjerklie 1986). It has been postulated that emotions may activate the autonomic nervous system or the vagal nerve, triggering bronchospasm (Clarke 1983). It has also been proposed that suggestion triggers neural activity in the central nervous system, resulting in emotional arousal secondary to expectation and consequent bronchoconstriction via the autonomic nervous system (Janson-Bjerklie 1986). This proposal would be consistent with the concept of bronchoconstriction in response to suggestion or certain stimuli as being a conditioned response. An example of this was provided by MacKenzie in 1885 when he described production of both symptoms and physical findings of "rose cold" in response to an artificial rose. The placebo response is considered to be a classic conditioned response by some (Lang and Rand 1969, cited in Butler 1986; Wickramasekera 1980). This finding would be in agreement with Goldstein (1960) and Morris and O'Neal (1975) who argued that expectations predict the response to treatment (both cited in Butler 1986).

Maher-Loughnan et al have reported three studies, two of which were controlled. The first, published in

1962, used hypnotic suggestions for symptom removal and ego strengthening in nine sessions distributed over a period of 6 months, in 27 asthmatic subjects who were assessed for both ease and depth of trance. Patients were also instructed in the use of self-hypnosis. The control group of 28 subjects received a new bronchodilator drug; no assessment of hypnotizability was performed on this group. Assessment was primarily subjective in that patients kept daily recordings of degree of wheezing and of frequency of bronchodilator use. Frequency of bronchodilator use was greatly reduced in the hypnosis group by the sixth month, versus only slight changes in the control group. Wheezing decreased by 50% within 3 months in the hypnosis group. In a few patients, vital capacity, peak flow, and FEV_1 were assessed at each visit also. No significant changes in pulmonary function were observed in either group. All degrees of asthma fared well, but those with mild disease showed much greater improvement than those with medium or severe disease. Patients who were easily hypnotized and achieved medium or deep trance made the most progress. Blood and sputum were examined for eosinophilia also. No change was demonstrated, but the number of patients with high counts was too small to be considered an adequate sample. The second study, published in 1968, used hypnotic suggestions for easing tension and free breathing during monthly sessions, along with daily self-hypnosis for 1 year in 91 patients who were assessed for "depth" of hypnosis. Eighty-five control subjects utilized breathing exercises aimed at progressive relaxation, again with no hypnotizability assessment. Although downward trends in subjective assessments of wheezing and bronchodilator use and upward trends in FEV_1 were all greater in the hypnosis group, only reduction of wheezing attained significance. Clinical assessment by independent physicians at the end of the year was also significant; asthma was considered to be "much better" in 59% of the hypnosis group versus 43% of the control group. In 1970, subjective improvement was reported in 82% of 173 preselected patients in response to similar hypnotic suggestions in the third report, which was not controlled.

Two more controlled studies emerged in the 1980s. Ben-Zvi et al assessed the efficacy of hypnosis in attenuating exercise-induced asthma in 10 stable asthmatics who served as their own controls. Hypnotizability was assessed using the Hypnotic Induction Profile of Spiegel; all subjects fell in the mid range (2 to 3 out of a 0 to 5 scale). Seven out of ten patients responded to hypnosis; of these, four failed to respond to placebo (saline with non-hypnotic suggestion). The three patients responding to placebo had a similar or greater attenuation with hypnosis. Hypnosis resulted in a 15.9% decrease in FEV_1 compared with a 31.8% decrease on control days (Ben-Zvi 1982).

In 1986, Ewer and Stewart assessed responses to six weekly sessions of hypnotherapy in 39 patients, using daily patient diaries and both pulmonary mechanics and methacholine challenge tests before and after the treatment. Hypnotic ability was assessed by the Stanford Hypnotic Clinical Scale. Hypnotherapy consisted of suggestions for progressive relaxation, ego enhancement, a method for self hypnosis, guided imageries, and symptom induction and resolution. The control group met weekly with a nurse who reviewed their daily recordings. The treatment group showed significant improvement in both peak expiratory flow rate and maximum expiratory flow rate at 50% vital capacity following the course of treatment. The highly hypnotizable subjects in the treatment group also showed significant improvement in daily symptoms, activity limitations, frequency of bronchodilator use, and response to methacholine challenge. Treatment group subjects with low hypnotizability and control subjects failed to demonstrate significant change in any of these parameters.

Wagaman et al (conference abstract, 1997b) has reported significant decreases in medication requirements in 14 patients with moderate to moderately severe asthma treated with hypnosis, compared with the control group of seven patients who required medication increases.

Edwards reported using short-term hypnotherapy daily over several days with six patients hospitalized for severe asthma but who were not in any apparent danger of dying. Suggestion was for gradual remission of the asthma and free breathing. One failed to respond and one responded poorly. Two experienced complete remission subjectively but not objectively, and two had complete remission both subjectively and objectively (as measured by vital capacity and FEV_1). Edwards emphasized that hypnosis may result in patient improvement physiologically (decreased airway resistance) or psychologically (decreased *awareness* of airway resistance) (Edwards 1960).

Morrison reported a series of 33 patients followed for 18 months who were not relieved by conventional therapy but showed a decrease in both hospital admissions and medication requirements after hypnosis. Steroid therapy was able to be discontinued in 27%, and all drugs were discontinued in three patients. Twenty-two patients demonstrated improved pulmonary function tests over the long term. Once again, subjective improvement without objective improvement was noticed in some participants. Hypnotic ability was not evaluated, and type of suggestion was not specified (Morrison 1976).

Several authors have used hypnotherapy with asthmatic patients who were unresponsive to conventional treatment and who had coexisting psychological issues. White treated 10 patients with hypnotic suggestions for easier breathing, decreased tension, decreased bronchospasm, and increased compliance using 7 to 10 sessions over 4 to 6 months. Six patients suffered from various degrees of anticipatory anxiety directly related to the asthma attacks ranging from marked anxiety to agoraphobia, three were depressed, and one was psychopathic. All were followed from 12 to 17 months. Six demonstrated improvement in both psychological symptoms and life activities, along with fewer attacks. Total hospital admissions for the group fell from 14 for the previous year to a low of four during the follow-up period. Three of the six showing improvement also used bronchodilators less frequently; no patient had an increase in usage. No patient was totally free from bronchospasm, and there was no significant change in long-term respiratory functions. Overestimation of subjective improvement correlated with depth of hypnosis (White 1961). Hanley (1974) and Brown (1965) have published information concerning the use of hypnotic symptom rehearsal and hypnotic exploratory techniques, such as regression with reframing and hypnoanalysis, to modify and treat the psychological components that complicate, maintain, and exacerbate asthma and other chronic illnesses.

Future Research

Various unresolved issues deserve further consideration and investigation when reviewing the studies of suggestions via hypnosis.

Timing of Pulmonary Function Tests Relative to the Type of Suggestions Given

Most suggestions were for relaxation, ego strengthening, and symptom removal; many studies did not assess objective measures, and of those that did, most pulmonary functions were performed at a time when patients were not experiencing an acute attack. Because suggestions were directed at symptom removal (bronchospasm) and not at the basic underlying pathology, one would not expect baseline values to be affected. It is possible that pulmonary function testing performed before and after hypnosis at the time of an acute attack might have reflected a change. This possibility also raises the question as to whether suggestions directed at resolving the underlying pathology (inflammation) would be more efficient at improving long-term baseline values. Although Morrison had speculated about the role of a possible neurochemical mechanism in the hypnotic treatment of asthma as early as 1976, only two case reports have utilized any type of suggestion relating to biochemical alteration. Both reported clinical and subjective improvement, but only one measured pulmonary function. Although monthly assessment of pulmonary function

was unchanged, daily peak flow did increase. Again, even the biochemical suggestions in this case were directed at acute symptom removal and not at underlying pathology (Madrid 1991; Neinstein 1992).

Although I have administered suggestions for resolution of inflammation and appropriate immune function without demonstrating a significant difference compared to suggestions for symptom reduction alone, the number of subjects and the duration of the study may have been too small for detection (Wagaman 1997b).

Hallucination of Change in the Absence of Objective Change

As cited earlier in this chapter, highly hypnotizable individuals may experience this phenomenon. I have also seen this occur in both a low and a moderately hypnotizable patient, although it is difficult to distinguish how much was attributable to hypnosis and how much to denial because both patients were symptomatic at the time. Numerous authors have expressed concern that this disparity between subjective improvement and objective improvement might be dangerous. If the patient's awareness of the actual severity of airway compromise is diminished, the patient may delay seeking appropriate help (Ben-Zvi 1982; Edwards 1960; Ewer 1986; Morrison 1976; White 1961). Also, it may give the patient an exaggerated (false) sense of coping ability. Morrison recounted the tale of a patient who had been hypnotized and apparently felt well enough to go out shopping but collapsed walking to her car and died in status asthmaticus. Cause and effect cannot be assumed of course because sudden death in severe asthmatics does occur (Morrison 1976).

Deep Relaxation May Not Be a Good Choice for Asthma Relief

If the patient experiences symptoms at the time of the hypnotic intervention, suggestions for deep relaxation may not offer relief of asthma.

When patients relax under hypnosis, there may be a relative decrease in tidal volume because of slower, more shallow breathing. Morrison noted that those patients in whom pulmonary function parameters worsened immediately following hypnosis appeared to be in a rather relaxed state, and he speculated a residual effect on the respiratory muscles (Morrison 1976).

During an acute exacerbation, functional residual capacity rises due to air trapping, and the patient breathes close to his or her total lung capacity. This hyperinflation enables patients to keep their airways open, permitting gas exchange to occur. Patients use accessory muscles to maintain hyperinflation (National Institutes of Health 1991). Asthma is paradoxical in that bronchodilation is enhanced by the stress-related hormones (adrenaline and cortisone) and possibly opposed by acetylcholine. Although results were inconsistent not only in different subjects but also in multiple trials with the same subjects, Sachar et al demonstrated decreases in plasma 17-hydroxy corticosteroid concentration to unusually low levels in 6 out of 24 experiments following a deep hypnotic trance. The trance lasted for 90 minutes, the subjects were reclining, and the suggestions they received emphasized relaxation, peace, tranquillity, and so forth. The values occurred only at the end of trance and tended to rebound to normal levels 90 minutes later (Sachar 1965). The fact that the decreases were inconsistent and unpredictable may also suggest some sort of artifact unrelated to the actual hypnotic trance. During a pilot study, however, hypnotic trance relaxation was followed by a 1-hour period of hypnotically suggested anxiety during which levels increased in three out of four subjects. This result would appear to indicate that the levels were associated with the type of suggestion and not with the trance state. Given the possibility that suggestion for relaxation could have this effect on some individuals, such suggestions may not be desirable for asthmatics, particularly during an exacerbation. These observations also may lend support to the influence of the central nervous system on the body's biochemistry. Deep relaxation, which decreases sympathetic activity and promotes parasympathetic dominance, may be counterproductive in asthma (Weiner 1987). This reaction may explain the equivocal results of attempts to use other methods of deep relaxation in the treatment of asthma (Cluss 1985; Erskine-Milliss 1979; Erskine-Milliss 1981; Richter 1982).

Sinclair-Gieben has reported a case that illustrates this point. Hypnosis was used as a last resort with a 60-year-old hospitalized man who appeared to be dying of status asthmaticus, unresponsive to treatment. The patient was unable to respond to suggestions for relaxation, as he required all his accessory muscles for breathing and was in a severe panic state. He responded immediately, however, to direct suggestion of cessation of wheezing and free and easy breathing. Audible wheezing stopped and almost no bronchospasm could be detected on auscultation. The patient's color also began to improve after a few minutes. Hypnosis was reinforced on alternate days for 10 days with continued improvement (Sinclair-Gieben 1960).

The Effect of Hypnosis on Patient Psychology and Personal Style

Although several publications have described the influence of both personal style and secondary psychological effects on asthma and other chronic illnesses (Dirks et al 1977, Dirks 1980, and Kinsman et al 1982, all cited in Brown 1984; Brown 1965; Hanley 1974), few of the aforementioned studies assess the effect of hypnosis

on these dimensions. As suggested by LeBaron and Zeltzer, hypnosis and other behavioral techniques may prove to be most useful to asthmatics by reducing anxiety and increasing coping and compliance (LeBaron 1983).

Hypnotizability

Hypnotic susceptibility is considered by some to be a good predictor of response to various psychological and behavioral interventions, even when the treatment is not (overtly) hypnotic, particularly for patients with immune system or other psychophysiological disorders (Bower and Kelly 1979, cited in Murphy 1989; Hall 1983; Wickramasekera 1988). Some investigators have suggested that response to relaxation therapy specifically may be linked to hypnotizability (Benson 1981; Kornfield 1985; and Miller and Cross 1985, cited in Murphy 1989). In an experiment in relaxation therapy for asthma, however, Murphy et al found only borderline significant correlation of hypnotic susceptibility scores with improvement in methacholine challenge testing (Murphy 1989). This finding was similar in both the relaxation and control groups. The amnesia item of the Harvard Group Scale of Hypnotic Susceptibility, however, was a strong predictor of improvement of self-reported asthmatic symptoms. This result suggests, once again, that the relationship between hypnotizability and physiological change may be lower than that between hypnotizability and subjective change.

The role of hypnotizability in the hypnotic response of asthma patients has not been well established. Of three studies reporting positive correlation between therapeutic response and hypnotizability, two based their findings primarily on subjective improvement (Collison 1975, cited in DePiano 1979; Maher-Loughnan 1962) and only one on objective measurements (Ewer 1986). Wagaman et al found that almost twice as many asthma patients, regardless of hypnotizability, responded to a posthypnotic suggestion for ease of breathing as responded to a posthypnotic suggestion to touch their ankles in response to a sound (Item #11 on the Harvard Group Scale of Hypnotic Susceptibility) (Wagaman 1997a). Although numbers are too small to be conclusive, motivation may play a significant role in determining hypnotic response in the medical patient. The contribution of the medical patient's hypnotic ability, versus other factors in the therapeutic response to hypnosis, warrants further investigation.

Other Considerations

Asthma patients have been found to exceed the norms in denial and in state anxiety (Wagaman 1997b). Both state and trait anxiety can influence the actual or perceived severity of illness and, therefore, affect the outcome (Kinsman 1980a; Kinsman 1980b; Kinsman 1980c). Dirks et al found that the combination of high state anxiety and average trait anxiety was associated with exceptionally good medical outcome. *The combination of both high state and high trait anxiety, however, was associated with exceptionally poor medical outcome* (Dirks 1977b; Dirks 1979). In my mind, however, although state anxiety serves a protective role in asthma, levels should be high enough for effective vigilance but not so high that they interfere with accurate assessment of symptoms or rational action. A study that appears to support my viewpoint was performed by Dahlem et al on patients who were matched for levels of pulmonary function. They found that those with low state anxiety scores were least likely to ask for medication to be prescribed on an "as needed" basis, regardless of the pulmonary function level. High scorers often requested medication at each level of pulmonary function. Only moderate scorers made more requests on days when pulmonary functions were lower (Dahlem 1977). Denial (repressive and defensive coping) can delay taking appropriate, lifesaving, action (Sibbald 1989; Steiner 1987; Yellowlees 1989).

THE CASE FOR HYPNOSIS

Hypnosis can help in the development of habits to ease an asthmatic attack. Breathing retraining, directed at restoring the ability to breathe diaphragmatically, and therefore more deeply and more slowly, can be very helpful for asthma patients. Retraining can be facilitated by a posthypnotic suggestion to utilize the diaphragmatic breathing in response to symptoms.

Asthmatic patients who are hypnotized must be informed that suggestions may alter perception but not necessarily actual physiological change (Isenberg et al 1992a and Rubenfield & Pain 1976, cited in Brown 1987). A portable peak expiratory flow meter enables patients to make this differentiation.

Methods

Although the extent to which hypnotizability determines therapeutic success in the medical patient remains controversial, I have found the administration of hypnotic susceptibility scales to be useful for two reasons: (1) It familiarizes patients with the hypnotic process prior to the therapeutic sessions; and (2) some of the hypnotic phenomena help to demonstrate the concept of mind/body interaction and to reinforce the patient's ability to respond to hypnosis.

Prior to initiating hypnotherapy, a thorough history should be taken. The patient should receive explanations of hypnosis, including myths and misconceptions, and the patient should have the opportunity to ask questions about asthma, too. Informed consent should then be obtained. If specific hypnotic procedures with the potential for increased risk or discomfort, such as symptom induction or regression, will be involved, these should also be explained and performed only with the knowledge and permission of the patient. These two procedures are of special concern in patients who have had very severe asthma attacks. The practitioner should be competent in both performing the selected techniques and in managing abreactions, if using regression. The practitioner should also be competent in the management of an asthma attack or have medical personnel who are readily available.

Light-to-medium trance depth is sufficient. The type of induction chosen should be one that neither focuses on breathing nor assumes the ability to breathe deeply or rhythmically. I have found eye fixation to be effective for most patients for several reasons: (1) It provides a focus other than their breathing, thereby providing distraction; (2) it does not require eye closure, and the patient may be too anxious to do so, yet this induction will almost always result in eye closure, anyway; (3) it is a method patients can adapt for use in many places and situations when brief intervals of focus are required for ease of symptoms, especially when reinforced by posthypnotic suggestion.

Suggestions during trance include ego strengthening and emphasizing the ability to do an appropriate assessment without overreacting or underreacting. Usually the asthma patient suffers from a feeling of loss of control. One of our goals during hypnosis is to re-establish a sense of control for them so they feel they are controlling the asthma rather than the asthma controlling them. Complete symptom removal is probably unrealistic and undesirable. Instead we are striving to reduce excessive physiologic and psychologic symptoms and achieve a balance resulting in appropriate levels of awareness, muscle tension, action, and control.

A frequently used method is symptom reduction, usually utilizing direct or indirect suggestions for diminished symptoms and increased comfort. Erickson (Rossi 1983) described the use of a fractional approach. He explained to the patient that some of his symptoms were caused by the asthma, some by fear, and some by muscle tension. He then suggested that the patient decrease his symptoms very gradually by small percentages, keeping just the percentage attributable to the organic asthma.

Imagery is helpful for many patients. They might visualize the muscles in their airways in their lungs relaxing and opening, with fresh air entering. They might visualize the inflammation in the walls of the airways changing from red, rough, and swollen to pink and smooth. Auditory and kinesthetic imagery can also be utilized to enhance some of the visual imagery, such as imagining tension in the neck, shoulder, and chest muscles being relieved by specific visualizations. Asthma patients are very sensitive to scents. It is prudent to avoid olfactory imagery. Do not mention a known triggering mechanism for that particular patient (e.g., cold temperature, cold air, meadow, hay, flowers, animals, and so on). The imagery of a ball, a swing, a pendulum, or waves and tides can establish rhythmic breathing.

Two closely related hypnotic techniques are hypnotic recall of easy breathing and hypnotic deconditioning. The latter involves retracing the steps of the initial incident so that the patient can reframe it (Rossi 1986).

A Controversial Method

Symptom challenge (symptom induction, symptom provocation) involves provoking symptoms, usually by hypnotic suggestion, and having the patient practice relieving them by using the self-regulatory measures he has learned. This technique remains controversial, even though, theoretically, symptoms induced by hypnotic suggestion should be able to be eliminated by hypnotic suggestion. Some practitioners have found this method to be very effective; others are not comfortable with it. In addition to the obvious concerns for the patient's comfort and safety, an experiment conducted by Thorne and Fisher involving both asthmatic and nonasthmatic subjects demonstrated that the physiologic response measured by pulmonary functions during a hypnotically suggested asthma experience, although different from presuggestion measures, differed in slope from a true asthmatic response. Additionally, response was related to hypnotizability and not to the presence or absence of asthma. Subjectively, however, the participants felt as if they were having a true asthma attack. This finding suggests that just as subjects can hallucinate feeling better without objective benefit, they can also hallucinate an attack without the actual physiologic changes (Thorne 1978). Therefore, we need to consider the possibility that we could be doing them a disservice by instilling a false sense of confidence in their ability to relieve a true attack if the symptoms during hypnosis are not authentic. Methacholine or exercise has also been used, although less frequently, to provoke true symptoms (Brown 1987). Symptom induction could result in a strong sense of mastery and control for the patient, if both the symptoms and the therapeutic response were documented objectively as well as subjectively. As usual, the risk–benefit ratio concerning the patient's safety and comfort must be considered. If utilized, I recommend restricting this technique initially to use under competent supervision rather than on a practice tape for home use and, as with other methods of hypnosis, instructing the patients to monitor

their peak expiratory flow. Rossi describes a related technique, "symptom scaling." The patient is asked to experience the problem and is also asked what percentage of the problem he or she is feeling, then to observe what changes occur spontaneously as he or she continues to focus on the symptom, and then to ratify the response by asking what percentage he or she feels in a little while. The therapeutic experience is completed when the patient reports some lowering of the original percentage. He cautions never to have a patient with a potentially life-threatening condition experience more than 25% to 30% of the worst previous episode, nor should symptom scaling exceed 50% of the type of response that could result in a medical emergency (Rossi 1993).

To Tape or Not to Tape?

Tapes can be very useful to patients for learning self-hypnosis and during episodes when they are too symptomatic or anxious to focus well. I prefer that they also learn to use self-hypnosis without a tape to avoid dependence on the tape and tape player. Self-hypnosis without a tape can be performed almost anywhere, almost anytime. If you make a tape for a patient, record on the tape that this tape was made for that individual (by name) only, and include the suggestion that he or she will be able to arouse and become alert and function well if and when necessary in an emergency. Caution the patient not to play the tape in the car, even if someone else is driving, because the driver could become hypnotized.

THE PATIENT WITH OTHER RESPIRATORY PROBLEMS

Chronic Obstructive Pulmonary Disease

Chronic obstructive pulmonary disease (COPD) is a nonspecific term that includes several specific disorders that may differ somewhat in clinical manifestations, pathologic findings, therapy, and prognosis. Patients have various degrees of cough, wheezing, expectoration, and bronchospasm. Dyspnea is frequently the predominant complaint. Unlike asthma, the symptoms are chronic, rather than intermittent, and the airway obstruction is not significantly reversible (Wyngaarden 1992).

Acosta-Austan has published a case report in which he utilized hypnotically induced relaxation with a 48-year-old woman hospitalized with severe COPD in an effort to decrease the intensity of dyspnea during periods of anxiety. Induction was performed by progressive relaxation after which suggestions were given for slow, deep breaths and further relaxation while breathing out gently through pursed lips. Respiratory rate, oxygen saturation (finger-pulse oximetry), and peak expiratory flow were evaluated before and after three hypnotic sessions to assess both results and safety of the procedure. All three parameters showed mild improvement after each session, as did the patient's subjective anxiety level. The patient was instructed in the use of a portable peak flow meter to guard against subjective improvement without corresponding objective benefit. The patient's hypnotizability was not specified (Acosta-Austan 1991). The same author (Acosta 1987) has reported using hypnotically induced relaxation with two anxious COPD patients on mechanical ventilators during prescribed "T piece" weaning periods. Both oximetry and anxiety scale measurements indicated that the patients were comfortable and secure during these periods.

Hyperventilation Syndrome

Hyperventilation occurs when ventilation increases out of proportion to carbon dioxide production, resulting in a decrease in the carbon dioxide pressure (Pco_2) of arterial blood. This result usually is caused by an increase in rate and depth of respirations (Wyngaarden 1992). The respiratory alkalosis and cerebral vasoconstriction cause the patient to feel lightheaded and possibly faint. Other symptoms may include a paradoxical sense of breathlessness, a feeling of impending doom, paresthesias, and carpopedal spasm (Crasilneck 1985; Kaplan 1994). Possible causes from medical disorders, psychiatric conditions, or drugs should be investigated, although hyperventilation can occur in normal persons during various emotional states, such as anxiety. Various hypnotherapeutic techniques (i.e., regression, ideomotor exploration, projective techniques, affect bridge, dream induction) may be useful in identifying covert sources of anxiety.

CHILDREN WITH RESPIRATORY PROBLEMS

Asthma

Asthma is the most common chronic illness involving children in the United States, affecting 6.9% of children between the ages of 3 and 17. It is the leading cause of absence from school because of chronic illness, accounting for 20% to 25% of absenteeism in the United States (Gevgen et al 1988, cited in Olness 1996).

The first controlled study of the use of hypnosis with asthma (Morrison et al 1960, cited in Maher-Loughnan 1962) failed to produce any improvement in response to hypnotic suggestion in 25 children. Treatment consisted of only two sessions, however, and patients were followed only 1 month. Diamond (cited in Wester 1984) reported that 40 of 55 children achieved complete symptom remission in response to hypnoanalytic techniques that included regression to the initial episode and insight-oriented approaches. Collison (cited in Watkins 1987) noted excellent or good responses in four out of six patients less than 10 years old and 32 out of 39 patients 11 to 20 years old, utilizing hypnotic relaxation, ego strengthening, suggestion for calmness, easy breathing, and exploration of related psychological factors. Diego (cited in Olness 1996) taught five adolescent boys to start and stop acute asthma attacks in hypnosis, followed by a posthypnotic suggestion of their ability to continue to be able to do this in the future; all reported subjective improvement. Smith and Burns (cited in Olness 1996) used direct suggestions for symptom relief with 25 children and adolescents 8 to 15 years of age; some reported subjective improvement but no objective improvement was demonstrated. Aronoff et al (cited in Olness 1996) used direct suggestion for easy breathing and decreased wheezing in an effort to abort acute attacks in 17 children and adolescents, 6 to 17 years of age. Most showed immediate improvement, both subjectively and objectively. Kohen noted an improvement in pulmonary function after 1 to 2 years of self-hypnosis (Kohen 1995). Self-hypnosis utilizing relaxation and mental imagery also resulted in decreased duration and severity of wheezing by subjective evaluation, reduced emergency room visits, and decreased number of days missed from school.

Anxiety, fearfulness, and feeling controlled by the disease are accompanying problems for children (Baron 1994; Bussing 1996; Wester 1991). Hypnosis may help the child cope with these feelings.

A simple explanation of asthma appropriate to the age of the child should be provided to the child and parents prior to hypnotherapy. Pictures are very helpful and do not need to be anatomically correct. Airways can be depicted as an upside down tree; the concept of bronchoconstriction versus bronchodilation can be illustrated by a tube of toothpaste with some areas in the original shape and some areas having been squeezed shut.

Induction should be performed by method(s) appropriate for age (see Chapter 8). Direct suggestions for calmness, easy breathing, and relaxation of the chest muscles and the muscles around the air tubes (the "inside" and the "outside" muscles) work well. Some children respond well to age progression, seeing themselves free of asthma and perhaps playing a sport. Some children do well with the posthypnotic suggestion to notice the very first early signs of respiratory difficulty and immediately take action. Imagery works well and can be tailored to the child's interests.

Cystic Fibrosis

Cystic fibrosis (CF) is an inherited multisystem disorder that is the major cause of severe chronic lung disease in children. Dysfunction of the exocrine glands causes a complex array of problems, particularly chronic obstruction and infection of the airways and maldigestion (Behrman 1992).

A pilot study (Belsky and Khanna 1994, cited in Olness 1996) assessed self-hypnosis as a coping strategy for 12 children and adolescents with CF. Hypnotic imagery was directed toward mastery of chronic illness and functional improvement with direct suggestions for thinner mucus, clearer lungs, easier breathing, and better absorption of medication. The experimental group demonstrated significant improvements in health locus of control, self-concept, and trait anxiety. They also showed improvements in peak expiratory flow. Kohen (conference abstract, 1994) has reported using various methods of hypnotherapy with CF patients for multiple problems. These include distraction, dissociation, imagery (such as switches to turn pain off or down or to regulate taste), and amnesia for painful experiences, relaxation, positive or negative hallucinations in an effort to control pain, anxiety, taste, and nausea.

Children with pulmonary problems, just like their adult counterparts, can benefit from hypnosis.

REFERENCES

Ackerman SJ: The new gestalt: Asthma as a chronic inflammatory disease [editorial]. J Asthma 20(6):331–333, 1989

Acosta F: Weaning the anxious ventilator patient using hypnotic fixation: Case reports. Am J Clin Hypn 29(4):272–280, 1987

Acosta-Austan F: Tolerance of chronic dyspnea using a hypnoeducational approach: A case report. Am J Clin Hypn 33(4):272–277, 1991

Ader R, Felten DL, Cohen N: Psychoneuro-Immunology, 2nd ed. San Diego, Academia Press, 1991

Alexander F: Psychosomatic medicine: Its Principles and Applications. New York, Norton, 1987

Barnes PJ: Effect of corticosteroid on airway hyper-responsiveness. American Review Respiratory Disease 141:570–576, 1990

Barnes PJ: New concepts in the pathogenesis of bronchial hyper-responsiveness in asthma. J Allergy Clin Immunol 83:1013–1026, 1989a

Barnes PJ: Our changing understanding of asthma. Respir Med 83(suppl):17–23, 1989b

Barnes PJ: The third nervous system in the lung: Physiology and clinical perspectives [editorial]. Thorax 39:5661–5667, 1984

Baron C, Marcotte JE: Role of panic attacks in the intractability of asthma in children. Pediatrics 94(1):108–110, 1994

Behrman RE, Cliegman RM, Nelson WE, et al: Nelson's Textbook of Pediatrics, 14th ed. Philadelphia, WB Saunders Company, 1992

Ben-Zvi Z, Spohn WA, Young SH, et al: Hypnosis for exercise induced asthma. American Review Respiratory Disease 125:392–395, 1982

Benson H, Arns PA, Hoffman JW: The relaxation response and hypnosis. Int J Clin Exp Hypn 29(3):259–270, 1981

Bowers KS: Hypnosis for the seriously curious. New York, Norton, 1976

Brown DP, Fromm E: Hypnosis and Behavioral Medicine. Hillsdale, New Jersey, Lawrence Erlbaum, 1987

Brown EA: The treatment of bronchial asthma by means of hypnosis as viewed by the allergist. Journal of the American Society of Psychosomatic Dentistry and Medicine 13:128–142, 1965

Brown EL, Kinsman RA, Johnson FA: Resolving intractable medical problems through psychological intervention: A clinical report. Psychotherapy 21(4):452–455, 1984

Bussing R, Burket RC, Kelleher ET: Prevalance of anxiety disorders in a clinic based sample of pediatric asthma patients. Psychosomatics 37(2):108–115, 1996

Butler C, Steptoe A: Placebo responses: An experimental study of psychophysiological processes in asthmatic volunteers. Br J Clin Psychol 25:173–183, 1986

Cheek DB, LeCron LM: Clinical Hypnotherapy. New York, Grune & Stratton, 1968

Chin TW, Nussbaum E: Detrimental effect of hypotonic cromolyn sodium. J Pediatr 120(4):641–643, 1992

Clark TJH, Godfrey S: Asthma, 2nd ed. London, Chapman and Hall, 1983

Cluss PA, Fireman P: Recent trends in asthma research. Annals of Behavioral Medicine 7(4):11–16, 1985

Crasilneck HB, Hall JA: Clinical hypnosis: Principles and Applications, 2nd ed. Orlando, Grune & Stratton, 1985

Crowne DP, Marlowe D: A new scale of social desirability independent of psychopathology. J Consult Psychol 24(4):349–354, 1960

Dahlem NW, Kinsman RA, Horton DJ: Panic-fear in asthma: Requests for as needed medications in relation to pulmonary function measurement. J Allergy Clin Immunol 60(5):295–300, 1977

Dekker E, Groen J: Reproducible psychogenic attacks of asthma. J Psychosom Res 1:58–67, 1956

DePiano FA, Salzberg HC: Clinical applications of hypnosis to three psychosomatic disorders. Psychol Bull 86(6):1223–1235, 1979

Dirks JF, Deiv M, Jones NF, et al: Panic-fear: A personality dimension related to intractability in asthma. Psychosom Med 39(2):120–126, 1977a

Dirks JF, Deiv M, Kinsman RA, et al: Panic-fear: A personality dimension related to length of hospitalization in respiratory illness. J Asthma Res 14(2):61–71, 1977b

Dirks JF, Fross KH, Evans NW: Panic-fear in asthma: Generalized personality trait versus specific situational state. J Asthma Res 14(4):161–167, 1977c

Dirks JF, Kinsman RA, Staudenmayer H, et al: Panic-fear in asthma: Symptomatology as an index of signal anxiety and personality as an index of ego resources. J Nerv Ment Dis 167(10):615–619, 1979

Dirks JF, Robinson SK, Moore PN: The prediction of psychomaintenance in chronic asthma. Psychother Psychosom 36(2):105–115, 1981

Djukanovic R, Rosche WR, Wilson JW, et al: Mucosal inflammation in asthma. American Review of Respiratory Disease 142:434–457, 1990

Edwards G: Hypnotic treatment of asthma: Real and illusory results. BMJ 2:492–497, 1960

Erskine-Milliss J, Schonell M: Relaxation therapy in bronchial asthma. J Psychosom Res 23:131–139, 1979

Erskine-Milliss J, Schonell M: Relaxation therapy in asthma: A critical review. Psychosom Med 43(4):365–371, 1981

Ewer TC, Stewart DE: Improvement in bronchial hyper-responsiveness in patients with moderate asthma after treatment with a hypnotic technique: A randomized controlled trial. BMJ 293:1129–1132, 1986

Ford FM, Hunter M, Hensley MJ, et al: Hypertension and asthma: Psychological aspects. Soc Sc Med 29(1):79–84, 1989

Goreczny AJ, Brantley PJ, Buss RR, et al: Daily stress and anxiety in the relation to daily fluctuation of symptoms in asthma and chronic obstructive pulmonary disease patients. Journal of Psychopathology and Behavioral Assessment 10(3):259–267, 1989

Gustafsson PA, Bjorksten B, Kjellman NIM: Family dysfunction in asthma: A prospective study of illness development. J Pediatr 125(33):493–498, 1994

Hall HR: Hypnosis and the immune system: A review with implications for cancer and the psychology of healing. Am J Clin Hypn 25(2–3):92–103, 1983

Hall HR: Research in the area of voluntary immunomodulation: Complexities, consistencies and future research consideration. Int J Neurosci 47:81–89, 1989

Hanley FW: Individualized hypnotherapy of asthma. Am J Clin Hypn 16(4):275–279, 1974

Hogg JC: Mucosal permeability and smooth muscle function in asthma. Med Clin North Am 74(3):731–740, 1990

Horton DJ, Suda WL, Kinsman RA, et al: Bronchoconstrictive suggestion in asthma: A role for airway hyper-reactivity and emotions. American Review of Respiratory Disease 117:1029–1038, 1978

Hudgel DW, Cooperson DM, Kinsman RA: Recognition of added resistive loads in asthma: The importance of behavior styles. American Review Respiratory Disease 126(1):121–125, 1982

Isenberg SA, Lehrer PM, Hockron S: The effects of suggestion and emotional arousal on pulmonary function in asthma: A review and hypothesis regarding vagal mediation. Psychosom Med 54:192–216, 1992a

Isenberg SA, Lehrer PM, Hockron S: The effects of suggestion on airways of asthmatic subjects breathing room air as a suggested bronchoconstrictor and bronchodilator. J Psychosom Res 36(8):769–776, 1992b

James AL, Pare PD, Hogg JC: The mechanics of airway narrowing in asthma. American Review Respiratory Disease 139:242–248, 1989

Janson-Bjerklie S, Boushey HA, Carrieri VK, et al: Emotionally triggered asthma as a predictor of airway response to suggestion. Res Nurs Health 9:163–170, 1986

Janson-Bjerklie S, Shnell S: Effects of peak flow information on patterns of self-care in adult asthma. Heart Lung 17(5):543–549, 1988

Jencks B: Your Body: Biofeedback at Its Best. Chicago, Nelson Hall, 1977

Jones MF, Kinsman RA, Schum R, et al: Personality profiles in asthma. J Clin Psychol 32(2):285–291, 1970

Kaplan HI, Sadock BJ, Grebb JA: Kaplan and Sadock's Synopsis of Psychiatry, 7th ed. Baltimore, Williams & Wilkins, 1994

Kikuchi Y, et al: Chemosensitivity and perception of dyspnea in patients with a history of near fatal asthma. New Engl J Med 330(19):1329–1334, 1994

King NJ: The behavioral management of asthma and asthma related problems in children: A critical review of the literature. J Behav Med 3(2):169–189, 1980

Kinsman RA, Dirks JF, Dahlem NW, et al: Anxiety in asthma: Panic-fear symptomatology and personality in relation to manifest anxiety. Psychol Rep 46:196–198, 1980a

Kinsman RA, Dirks JF, Jones NF, et al: Anxiety reduction in asthma: Four catches to general application. Psychosom Med 42(4):397–405, 1980b

Kinsman RA, Dirks JF, Jones NF: Levels of psychological experience in asthma: General and illness specific concomitants of panic-fear personality. J Clin Psychol 36(2):552–561, 1980c

Kohen DP: Relaxation/mental imagery (self hypnosis) for childhood asthma: Behavioral outcomes in a prospective, controlled study. Hypnos 22(3):132–144, 1995

Kohen DP: Self-regulation by children and adolescents with cystic fibrosis: Applications of relaxation/mental imagery (self-hypnosis). Paper presented to 36th annual scientific meeting of the American Society of Clinical Hypnosis, Philadelphia, 1994

Kroger WS, Fezler WD: Hypnosis and Behavior Modification: Imagery Conditioning. Philadelphia, Lippincott-Raven, 1976

LeBaron S, Zeltzer L: The treatment of asthma with behavioral intervention: Does it work? Tex Med 79:40–42, 1983

Lehrer TM: Psychological processes in asthma. Presented at the annual meeting of the Association for Applied Psychophysiology and Biofeedback, Los Angeles, 1993

Lehrer PM: Health, homeostatis, and healing: Promises and paradoxes in the applied psychophysiology of asthma. Biofeedback 25(2):4–7, 1997

Lewis RA, Lewis MN, Tattersfield AE: Asthma induced by suggestion: Is it due to airway cooling? American Review of Respiratory Disease 129:691–695, 1984

Liu MC, Bleecker ER, Lichtenstein LM, et al: Evidence for elevated levels of histamine, prostaglandin D$_2$, and other bronchoconstricting prostaglandins in the airway of subjects with mild asthma. American Review of Respiratory Disease 142:126–132, 1990

Luparello TJ, Lyons HA, Bleecker ER, et al: Influences of suggestion on airway reactivity in asthmatic subjects. Psychosom Med 30:819–825, 1968

Luparello TJ, Leist N, Lourie CH, et al: The interaction of psychologic stimuli and pharmacologic agents on airway reactivity in asthmatic subjects. Psychosom Med 32(5):509–513, 1970

McFadden Jr ER, Gilbert IA: Asthma. New Engl J Med 327(27):1928–1937, 1992

McFadden Jr ER, Luparello T, Lyons AJ, et al: The mechanism of action of suggestion in the induction of acute asthma attacks. Psychosom Med 31(2):134–143, 1969

Mackenzie JN: The production of the so called "rose cold" by means of an artificial rose. Am J Med Sci 91:45–57, 1886

Madrid AD, Barnes S: A hypnotic protocol for eliciting physical changes through suggestions of biochemical responses. Am J Clin Hypn 34(2):122–128, 1991

Maes S, Schlosser M: Changing health behavior outcomes in asthmatic patients: A pilot intervention study. Soc Sci Med 26(3):359–364, 1988

Maher-Loughnan GP: Hypnosis and auto-hypnosis for the treatment of asthma. Int J Clin Exp Hypn 18(1):1–14, 1970

Maher-Loughnan GP, Kinsley BJ: Hypnosis for asthma—a controlled trial. BMJ 4:71–76, 1968

Maher-Loughnan GP, Mason AA, MacDonald N, et al: A controlled trial of hypnosis in the symptomatic treatment of asthma. BMJ 11:371–376, 1962

Mather MD, Degun GS: A comparative study of hypnosis and relaxation. Br J Med Psychol 48:55–63, 1975

Matus I, Bush D: Asthma attack frequency in a pediatric population. Psychosom Med 1(8):629–636, 1979

Moorefield CW: The use of hypnosis and behavior therapy in asthma. Am J Clin Hypn 13(3):162–168, 1971

Morley J: Prostaglandins and the lung. Postgrad Med 53:652–653, 1977

Morrison JB: Report on 33 asthmatic patients whose treatment was modified by hypnotherapy. North Wales, Abergele Hospital, 1976

Murphy AI, Lehrer PM, Karlin R, et al: Hypnotic susceptibility and its relationship to outcome in the behavioral treatment of asthma: Some preliminary data. Psychol Rep 65:691–698, 1989

National Institutes of Health: Guidelines for the diagnosis and management of asthma. Publication No. 91-3042, U.S. Department of Health and Human Services, Bethesda, 1991

Neijens HJ: Determinants and regulating processes in bronchial hyper-reactivity. Lung (suppl) 168:268–277, 1990

Neild JE, Cameron IR: Bronchoconstriction in response to suggestion: Its prevention by an inhaled anticholinergic agent. BMJ 290:674, 1985

Neinstein LS, Dash J: Hypnosis as an adjunct therapy for asthma: Case report. Journal of Adolescent Health Care 3:45–48, 1982

Nijkamp FP, Sitsen JMA: Leukotrienes, allergy and inflammation. Pharmaceutisch Weekblad Scientific Edition 4:165–171, 1982

Nowak J: Anatomopathologic changes in the bronchial walls in chronic inflammation, with special reference to the basement membrane, in the course of bronchial asthma. ACTA Medica Polona 10(2):11–172, 1969

Olness K, Kohen DP: Hypnosis and Hypnotherapy with Children, 3rd ed. New York, Guilford, 1996

Philipp RL, Wilde GJS, Day JH: Suggestion and relaxation in asthmatics. J Psychosom Res 16:193–204, 1972

Randall T: International consensus report urges sweeping reform in asthma treatment. JAMA 267(16):2153–2154, 1992

Richter R, Dahme B: Bronchial asthma in adults: There is little evidence of the effectiveness of behavioral therapy and relaxation. J Psychosom Res 26(5):533–540, 1982

Rossi EL: The Psychobiology of Mind-Body Healing, revised ed. New York, Norton, 1993

Rossi EL, Ryan MO: Mind Body Communication in Hypnosis: The Seminars, Workshops, and Lectures of Milton H. Erickson, vol. 3. New York, Irvington, 1986

Rossi EL, Ryan MO, Sharp FA: Healing in Hypnosis: The Seminars, Workshops, and Lectures of Milton H. Erickson, vol 1. New York, Irvington, 1983

Sachar EJ, Fishman JR, Mason JW: Influence of the hypnotic trance of plasma 17-hydroxycorticosteroid concentration. Psychosom Med 27(4):330–341, 1965

Schleimer RP: Effects of glucocorticosteroids on inflammatory cells relevant to the therapeutic applications in asthma. American Review Respiratory Disease 141:S59–S69, 1990

Sibbald B: Patient self-care in acute asthma. Thorax 44(2):97–101, 1989

Simonsson BG, Jacobs FM, Nadel JA: Role of the autonomic nervous system in the cough reflex in the increased responsiveness of airways in patients with obstructive airway disease. J Clin Invest 46(11):1812–1818, 1967

Sinclair-Gieben AHC: Treatment of status asthmaticus by hypnosis. BMJ 2:1651–1652, 1960

Smith MM, Colebatch HJH, Clarke PS: Increase and decrease in pulmonary resistance with hypnotic suggestion in asthma. American Review of Respiratory Disease 102:236–242, 1970

Spector S, Luparello TJ, Kopetzky MT, et al: Response of asthmatics to methacholine suggestion. American Review of Respiratory Disease 113:43–50, 1976

Spittle BJ, Sears MR: Bronchial asthma: Lack of relationships between allergic factors, illness severity and psychosocial variables in adult patients attending an asthma clinic. Psychol Med 14(4):847–852, 1984

Steiner H, Higgs CM, Fritz GK, et al: Defense style and the perception of asthma. Psychosom Med 49(1):35–44, 1987

Sterling GM: The mechanism of bronchoconstriction due to hypocapnia in man. Clin Sci (Colch) 34:277–285, 1968

Strupp HH, Levenson RW, Manuck SB, et al: Effects of suggestion on total respiratory resistance in mild asthmatics. J Psychosom Res 18:337–346, 1974

Thorne DE, Fisher AG: Hypnotically suggested asthma. Int J Clin Exp Hypn 26(2):92–103, 1978

Wagaman MJ, Doyle RP, Robbins N: Motivation and hypnotic response in asthma patients. Scientific Presentation Abstracts of 14th International Congress of Hypnosis, San Diego, 1997a

Wagaman MJ, Doyle RP, Cella JP, et al: Physical and psychological effects of hypnosis with asthma patients. Scientific Presentation Abstracts 14th International Congress of Hypnosis, San Diego, 1997b

Watkins JG: Hypnotherapeutic Techniques: The Practice of Clinical Hypnosis, vol. 1. New York, Irvington, 1987

Waxman D: Hartland's Medical and Dental Hypnosis, 3rd ed. London, Bailliere Tindall, 1989

Weiner HM: Stress, relaxation and asthma. Int J Psychosom 34(1):21–24, 1987

Wester WC, O'Grady DJ: Clinical Hypnosis with Children. New York, Brunner/Mazel, 1991

Wester WC, Smith AH: Clinical Hypnosis: A Multidisciplinary Approach. Philadelphia, Lippincott-Raven, 1984

White HC: Hypnosis in bronchial asthma. J Psychosom Res 5:272–279, 1961

Wickramasekera I: A conditioned response model of the placebo effect. Biofeedback and Self-Regulation 5(1):5–18, 1980

Wickramasekera IE: Clinical Behavioral Medicine. New York, Plenum Publishing Corp, 1988

Wistuba F: Significance of allergy in asthma from a behavioral medicine viewpoint. Psychother Psychosom 45:186–194, 1986

Wong-Chung D, Mateijsen N, West R, et al: Assessing the functional status during an asthma attack with Dartmouth COOP charts: Validity with respect to the change in asthma. Family Practice 8(4):404–408, 1991

Wyngaarden JB, Smith LH, Bennett JC: Cecil Textbook of Medicine, 19th ed. Philadelphia, WB Saunders, 1992

Yellowlees PM, Ruffin RE: Psychological defenses and coping styles in patients following a life threatening attack of asthma. Chest 95(6):1298–1303, 1989

part three

Hypnosis and Other Health Care Professions

12

Dentistry

Samuel Perlman

INTRODUCTION

Hypnosis is a tool used in dentistry and is a source of unexpected pleasure both for the dentist and patient. Many patients search for more than just a good filling or a fast cleaning; they seek personal attention and thrive in an atmosphere in which personal care is provided. Hypnosis helps the dentist alleviate patient anxiety yet still use time effectively. When the patient is in trance he is more amenable to treatment, more cooperative, and thus the dentist can work more efficiently. Rapid methods of induction are available, and after the initial encounter with trance, returning to trance during subsequent visits is even faster. The use of language and stories leads to conversational trance. Posthypnotic suggestions give more comfort to the patient between dental visits and enable the patient to approach the next dental encounter calmly.

ANXIETY AND HYPNOSIS

Some patients think about dental treatment and feel impending doom. Such anxiety is the primary cause of why more than 10 million people do not receive appropriate dental care (Reilly 1990).

Hypnosis can be used for patients who are reluctant to seek dental treatment because of anxiety or phobia. A meditative hypnotic induction is especially useful in reducing anxiety prior to dental procedures (Fabian 1995).

The cause of dental anxiety is most commonly a single or multiple traumatic event from childhood. Some parents may inadvertently portray dentistry as an area to be feared because of their own memories of pain or feelings of helplessness. Fear of the unknown, separation from primary caregivers, stories from significant others, and media stereotypes create personal myths for the patient. They enhance the individual's sense of vulnerability and inadequacy in coping effectively when receiving dental care. Avoiding treatment permits the patient to avoid feeling helpless or embarrassed. The stronger the misperceptions, the greater the anxiety. As this anxiety increases, it is likely to produce phobia. A patient may be anxious or phobic about the dentist and have no fears in other areas of life. Alleviating anxiety by rational explanation may not be sufficient in all phobic patients (Katz 1996). Greater success is achieved by other modalities such as behavioral relaxation techniques and hypnotism. As the patient avoids the dentist, he feels more able to cope. When treatment is started, it is often terminated before completion (Katz 1996).

The American Dental Association's *Dental Newsline* on the Internet, in a section titled "Overcoming Dental Anxiety," states that "good old-fashioned daydreaming or relaxing takes place courtesy of your imagination." This suggestion is actually a hypnotic modality.

A possible consequence of anxiety is the disturbance of cognitive functioning, making it difficult to think clearly, use proper judgment, learn efficiently, or remember accurately. Hypnosis can alter some psychophysiological functions, and thus we can use hypnotic techniques to overcome anxiety associated with a visit to the dentist. Hypnosis can also increase coping skills and bolster feelings of self-worth, which are important factors in reducing anxiety (Finkelstein 1991).

Hypnotism may be defined as suggestion and repetition, suggesting being the process by which an individual accepts a proposition put to him by another person, without having the slightest logical reason for doing so (Peretz 1996b).

HYPNOTIC METHODS

The preparation of the patient for hypnosis, and the success of this modality, depend upon the motivation of the patient. *The patient manages his own trance.* Factors such as the length and severity of the dental procedure, the patient's perception of the skill of the dentist, the patient's perception of the outcome, and the attitude of family members, are influential. Coping with anxiety varies with one's physical condition. When tired, ill, or injured, people are more easily threatened (Finkelstein 1991).

Hypnosis encourages the patient to enter into an analgesic state. This feeling of well-being is one of the primary uses for hypnotism in dentistry. Anxiety is replaced, in trance, by something pleasant, something that is easy for the patient to control. A deep trance isn't always needed. Merely occupying the mind by experiencing something safe and pleasant may be all that is required. When the patient is in trance and relaxed there is moderate pain relief and suppression of the gag reflex. When the patient is in trance, the dentist can treat more efficiently, and have less of his own tensions concerning patient comfort. Without formal trance, indirect hypnotic techniques using everyday communication patterns, both verbal and nonverbal, can be used by the dentist to induce deep relaxation for patients. Three components are used: (1) "pacing," which is the monitoring and feeding back to the patient his observable and reactive behavior; (2) "leading," which is suggesting positive behavior modification; and (3) "utilization," which is using all that is known about the patient to strengthen the dentist–patient relationship (Dinninger, Heinz and Kunzellman 1998).

There is sometimes a fear of losing control with hypnosis, so it is suggested that in the induction the patient be told that he may terminate the hypnotic procedure at any time and that he will feel that he is always in control (Eli 1991). This suggestion minimizes the threat of losing autonomy.

HYPNOSIS AS DENTAL ANESTHESIA

Hypnosis may be used to obtain anesthesia for dental treatment without chemical agents. Hypnosis can reduce the amount of sedative drugs needed (Lu and Lu 1996), which is particularly beneficial to medically compromised patients, such as geriatric patients, patients with cardiac, kidney, or liver diseases, or patients with other severe systemic conditions. Hypnosis effectively allows for a reduction in the sedative dose and still provides successful and comfortable dental treatment.

Hypnosis can be used in conjunction with nitrous oxide sedation as in the case of the patient who presents with a history of fainting whenever local anesthetics are used for dentistry. In this case, hypnotism is used mainly to facilitate the anxiety of treatment, and the inhalation is used for sedation for pain relief (Shelagh 1994).

Conscious sedation in patients who are physically dependent on central-acting drugs is problematic for the dental anesthesiologist because of the development of tolerance to standard sedative agents (Lu and Lu 1995). Those patients require higher doses than recommended and have an increased risk of drug overdose; however, hypnosis combined with lower and safer doses of chemicals produces good to excellent outcomes. Hypnosis can augment the effects of drugs in this patient population.

Also, patients with multiple allergies to local anesthetics who require extraction or other surgical or potentially painful procedures can use hypnosis to mobilize their own psychophysical capacities to control pain and anxiety (Herod 1995).

RAPID INDUCTIONS

Because dentistry is a time-sensitive profession, the ability to induce a trance rapidly is important. One reason that hypnosis is not more widely used in dentistry is because of the perceived loss of time. Rapid induction to trance can easily be accomplished with practice. Methods for this rapid induction include the handshake induction, the coin drop induction, the arm rub induction, and the arms together induction. The upcoming procedures are efficient and lead to more rapid deepening procedures.

Handshake Induction (Erickson 1990)

The patient, seated in the dental chair expecting hypnosis, is asked to shake hands with the dentist. When the dentist grasps the patient's hand, instead of the usual grasp and shake, the dentist takes the patient's hand as usual, but then presses his index finger lightly on the patient's wrist, presses his middle finger on the side of the patient's hand, and then his thumb on the bottom of his clasp (top of the patient's hand), all the while extending the patient's arm slightly. The dentist then says, while looking directly at the patient, "that feels comfortable, doesn't it?" This takes the patient by surprise and he will most often respond "yes." The dentist then places his left hand on the patient's arm slightly above the elbow and starts bending the arm upward, while his right hand continues to extend it slightly. During this time the dentist maintains steady eye contact with the patient. He then slowly moves his right hand away from the patient's hand, but keeps his left hand gently under the patient's right arm. Soon the patient's arm will begin levitating. The dentist then moves away his left hand. If the arm doesn't start levitating, the dentist can suggest that balloons filled with helium are attached to the wrist and causing the arm to float. The benefit of this induction is not only its speed but also the ratification of trance by the patient watching or feeling the arm rise or become weightless, floating in air. Any deepening procedure may be used here, and if glove anesthesia is indicated, the dentist is well on his way to achieving it (Erickson 1990).

Case study 12–1

Dolly, a 66-year-old woman who has been a patient of mine for over 20 years, has had all dentistry done without anesthesia because she cannot bear the thought of an injection. When Dolly presented with a tooth that needed extraction she announced that of course she "couldn't have a needle." She didn't want anything else either but didn't know if she could endure the pain of surgery. I told her that I would use a "special way." She agreed and when she presented for her next appointment I used a handshake induction followed by arm levitation with the suggestion that a rubber band was stretched between her hand and her face. I suggested that as her hand moved closer to her face, she would become more and more relaxed and finally when it touched her face, she could allow it to drop to her side. I then used glove anesthesia. To accomplish this anesthesia, I utilized the arm that was in an elevated state and suggested to her that as I moved my hand down her hand from the wrist to her fingers, with her permission, her hand would gradually become numb. I indicated that the feeling she would achieve would be unusual, and gradually would become more and more numb. The sensation could be warm, cold, or tingling and I left it to her to make the choice. Slowly, she reported that her entire hand became numb. Glove anesthesia partially derives its name from the fact that the hypnotist can indicate that the hand might feel as if it were in a glove and the area covered by the glove becomes numb. After the glove anesthesia I again used arm levitation to have that hand move slowly to her face and transfer the numbness from the hand first to her lips, then her gums and finally to her tooth. During this entire inducton, Dolly was communicating verbally, and her eyes were open. We periodically joked about how things were "just happening." She was amazed and delighted. After she was numb, through hypnosis only, I removed the tooth. She had no discomfort, no pain at all. She couldn't believe it. I reoriented her, and then she said that she felt pain.

I had given her no posthypnotic suggestion about comfort. I quickly shook her hand again and returned her to trance, this time telling her that as her arm moved up and touched her face she would be completely comfortable and remain that way. The patient left the office thrilled and unable to believe that she had been hypnotized, and the extraction painlessly accomplished.

Arm Rub Induction

This method is similar to the handshake induction. First, permission is requested from the patient for the dentist to rub the patient's arm lightly, from the elbow to the wrist, to the tip of the fingers. The patient is told that after several passes along that arm, he will be very relaxed and comfortable, and that the hand will start feeling unusual below the wrist. The dentist then moves his finger across the wrist, drawing a line. The dentist says that he doesn't know if the hand is warmer or cooler, or maybe tingly, or maybe lighter, or heavier, or maybe even numb, but he does know it is feeling different than usual. An alternative is to continue stroking the arm while speaking. Then suggest that as the patient feels comfortable and relaxed, he can close his eyes if he wants. Soon the patient's eyes close, and then the dentist can continue with glove anesthesia (Finklestein S, personal communication).

Coin Drop Induction

The patient is seated in the dental chair, and with the chair moderately reclined is given a coin to hold between his right thumb and forefinger. He is asked to hold his wrist higher than his fingers so that gravity takes over. The patient is told to pay careful attention to the thumb nail on that hand, noticing lines and crevices that may never have been noticed before. He is instructed not to take his eyes off that thumb nail. The dentist continues to talk, explaining that as the fingers holding the coin get more and more relaxed, the coin is going to drop, all by itself, from between the fingers. When the coin drops the patient will know that this is a signal to close his eyes, drop his arm to his lap, and allow himself to become very relaxed and comfortable, sinking into the dental chair. He is told that when the coin drops, the dentist will catch it. He is told that his eyelids may become very tired and heavy. The dentist continues to speak, telling the patient how relaxed his fingers are, and how tired his eyes are becoming. When the coin is finally dropped it signals the end of the induction part of trance, and the patient is ready for deepening.

Hands Together Induction

The hands together induction is useful because it is rapid and because it is visual, ratifying the trance. The patient, seated in the dental chair, is asked to hold his arms extended in front of him with the palms of his hands facing each other. He is told to allow the arms to come together at their own speed while watching them, and when they do come together and the hands touch, he will become very deeply comfortable. His hands will lower into his lap and he will wish to close his eyes, becoming increasingly more comfortable. And as he watches his hands, and they start coming together, he can notice the relaxation and comfort starting, ever so gradually, yet rapidly, as the hands come together all by themselves, at their own rate. The hands ultimately come together and trance ensues. Throughout this induction the dentist speaks in a slow, soothing voice, encouraging relaxation.

DIRECT TECHNIQUES

Hypnotic techniques that are more direct include the substitution of a pleasant experience for the fear of a negative one. During trance the patient can travel to a safe and comfortable place, concentrating on sights, sounds, touch, and smells in that place and associations that are pleasant and not threatening. The hypnotist directs the patient to select a place that is comfortable and safe. This permisive induction allows the patient to choose the content of the trance. The hypnotist may mention experiences that the patient could observe in that place but generally leaves room for the patient to embellish the experience himself.

Another hypnotic approach is the use of guided imagery, such as story telling. In this technique the hypnotist guides the patient on an excursion to a place selected by the hypnotist. The details are supplied in the story, utilizing, as above, as many sensory inputs as is feasible. One format that is often used is to let patients know that you're going to tell a story, and that they can allow themselves to concentrate on what is being said. For example, the dentist may begin by guiding the patient through a field of flowers of various colors, having him observe the pink ones, the white ones, and the yellow ones, while walking along a safe, wide path, sort of like a yellow brick road. As the patient continues along this path he comes to a stream with a very solid, safe stone bridge that passes over it. In the middle of the bridge is a comfortable seat to overlook the calm water of the stream and perhaps watch a leaf floating slowly down the stream, moving ever so slowly, at its own pace, with the flow. Throughout this experience, the patient is encouraged to give the dentist feedback that acknowledges the trance. The dentist tells the patient to pass over the bridge, follow the path, and notice the specimen trees and plants and the lush lawn. The patient passes the caretaker's cottage where the caretaker and his mate wave to him. It is suggested that the patient notice what the caretaker looks like. He then comes upon a large and beautiful castle with an ornately carved wooden door. The patient is encouraged to carefully look at this door and notice the carving. The carving, he is told, may mean something special to him. Upon opening the door he comes into a special lobby containing a large marble staircase with a red carpet and firm handrails on either side, an elevator with a safe wide seat, and an escalator. He is encouraged to carefully go downward in the manner most comfortable for him, taking note of the statues and paintings. The sights and sounds within the castle or on the grounds enhance separation from the present. The tour continues until the dentistry is completed. At that time the patient retraces his steps, returns to the fields and ultimately back to the path where he waves goodbye to the caretaker, again crosses the bridge and returns to the present. The embedded suggestions here deepen the trance and enhance feelings of safety and well being.

HYPNOSIS FOR BRUXISM

Bruxism, the clenching or grinding of teeth, can occur either at night during sleep, or while awake during the day. Often the patient is unaware that he has a problem. Use of a hand mirror to show him the actual wear that has taken place on tooth structure gives a visual stimulus for compliance to treatment suggestions. It is important to determine whether the clenching or grinding is done during the day or at night, or both. If it is at night it often is heard by another person. If there is no one to hear the sound, querying the patient about whether his jaw feels tired in the morning or if he feels as though he chewed gum in his sleep is useful (Clark 1991). Hypnosis can provide long-term relief from bruxing (Felicity 1994).

Case Example

Bruxism at night may be treated by placing the patient in a moderately deep trance. During the trance the sensations of the feeling of grinding may be elicited. The posthypnotic suggestion is made that every time his teeth touch he will be awakened and angry that the teeth woke him, be happy that he was able to notice it, and then be able to go right back to sleep. This suggestion allows the unpleasant stimulus of bruxing to awaken the patient, and the pleasant anchor of awareness of the problem to allow him to go calmly back to sleep.

Bruxism during the day is treated similarly, but the posthypnotic suggestion is modified to suggest that each time the teeth touch in a bruxing manner, a message is sent to the tongue to place it between the upper and lower teeth and remind the patient that he should stop. Also, in a conversational trance it may be suggested to the patient that he look for clenching during the day not only at times of tension or anxiety, but at times of relaxation, such as watching television, reading, driving, or commuting on the train.

HYPNOSIS AND THE GAG REFLEX

Hypnosis is extremely effective with patients who have a heightened gag reflex. Sedation is one of the measures that is used to deal with the hyperactive gag response, and hypnosis is a way to sedate (Crothers 1996). Hypnosis can provide a set of techniques that may be used to augment or facilitate a particular course of treatment. Principles using relaxation, anxiety control, conditioning/desensitization, and confidence boosting technique help to control the gag reflex (Barsby 1994).

Case study 12–2

One patient, Marc, had been abused by his father. When Marc misbehaved his father placed a pillow over his mouth or rags in his mouth when further punishment was needed. Marc had suffered mentally to the extent that he had to give up his job, was separated from his family, and had been hospitalized. Before hypnosis was considered, his therapist was consulted and permission received. Marc demanded that nitrous oxide be used during treatment, for he was sure that he would gag without it, and perhaps even with it. He was placed in a deep trance and sent to his favorite place in his mind. Nitrous oxide sedation was used concurrent with hypnosis. During the course of treatment he was not told that the nitrous oxide was being turned off, leaving only the hypnosis. No local anesthetic agent was used. Crown and bridge procedures that would normally have caused him great anxiety, gagging, and pain or discomfort were performed with ease and at rapid speed because of his comfort. Before reorienting, he was told that the nitrous oxide had been turned off early in the visit and that only hypnosis was used. He was given the posthypnotic suggestion that he would be extremely relaxed when he returned to the office for his next visit. At the time of the subsequent visit he said, "Hey Doc, do you pump that sweet air into the waiting room? I feel so comfortable when I come in here."

REDUCTION OF BLEEDING AND POSTHYPNOTIC SUGGESTIONS FOR HEALING

The reduction of bleeding can be useful in many dental procedures, including postsurgical healing, prosthetic impression taking, root canal therapy, and periodontal treatment. Also, hypnosis can be used for bleeding control in patients with hemophilia (Lucas 1985). Patients receiving preoperative suggestions exhibit a 30% reduction in blood loss (Bystedt, Enqvist, and von Konow 1995).

Case Example

A dialogue with patients, either in formal or conversational trance, may include "You know that we can control how our body helps with healing. It's accepted that people can reduce their blood pressure and heart rate using techniques such as biofeedback. You've heard about that, haven't you? (a yes set). Well, we can also reduce the amount of bleeding that occurs. Of course, we want just enough to allow fresh blood to come to the surgical site to bring nutrients and oxygen needed but we don't need too much (Larkin D, personal communication), just the right amount. So even if you think it is strange, just spend a few moments now talking or thinking to yourself, that just the right amount of bleeding can occur and then it can stop rapidly at just the right time. Your body has the resources within it to know when the time is right. So either with your eyes closed or with them remaining open, just tell yourself to have your body do what it knows it should do."

Enqvist and Fisher evaluated the use of preoperative hypnotic techniques used for patients planned for dental surgery (Enqvist 1997). Both a reduction of anxiety prior to surgery and the amount of postoperative analgesics needed were noted. The phrase, "usually when there is very little difficulty removing a tooth as we just noticed, the healing occurs very smoothly and comfortably," provides a posthypnotic suggestion. When medication is expected to be needed the phrase, "It's interesting to notice that exactly 20 minutes after you take this pill it starts to work and gives the comfort you expect."

When taking dental impressions it is important to have an operative field that is free of blood and fluids. We can control most saliva by use of devices such as cotton rolls or other evacuation aids. It is possible to control the seepage of fluids, including blood, merely asking the patients to just take a moment to tell their body to stop any seeping or bleeding so that we can take the needed impression. This same method can be used during endodontic treatment to stop bleeding if it occurs in the root canal.

Similar control of bleeding can be used in deep periodontal curettage. After the procedure, the posthypnotic suggestion that "following treatment you can remain remarkably comfortable with very rapid healing" usually ensures comfort.

Case study 12–3

A patient who was previously hypnotized, and therefore oriented to successfully use suggestions, needed a root canal. Treatment was started by anesthetizing the area to be treated, a maxillary right lateral incisor. The patient was aware of the procedure and was placed in a conversational trance discussing new changes to her workplace, an outpatient psychiatric center. When I had my turn in the conversation, holding her lip up as I was speaking, I injected, with no pause in conversation. She didn't feel the injection, and treatment continued. When instrumenting the canal there was a lot of bleeding. I told her about this and mentioned that it could impede treatment. She was asked to just tell this bleeding to stop. She spontaneously closed her eyes and after a moment opened them and the bleeding stopped.

HYPNOSIS IN PEDIATRIC DENTISTRY

Children in the dental office offer a challenge and a reward. They may be cooperative at one visit and impossibly difficult at the next. Hypnosis can be effectively used to treat the hesitant, scared, or reluctant child. If hypnosis were used more often, the number of children requiring general anesthesia would be lowered (Niven 1996). By giving the child an expectation of his visit, he will come to the dental office anticipating a pleasant diversion. This diversion is determined during a pretrance in which the dentist learns about the likes and dislikes of the child. Some children like sports, others like television cartoons, while others enjoy thinking about places the family has gone on trips. Dissociating from the place of treatment is the goal. Children enjoy placing themselves outside of the dental experience while treatment is accomplished. Some dentists have the children watch a television screen. The child is told that his mind has the ability to flip channels, enter the show he is watching, and if he wishes, become a performer, taking an active part in the script.

Peretz states that for some children, suggestions that

Case study 12–4

Mike, 7 years old, presented with a history of unhappy and unsuccessful attempts at dental care. One dentist was rushed and another was demanding and authoritative. Mike didn't cooperate with the second dentist, and that dentist became gruff, causing Mike to become more withdrawn and more reluctant to allow treatment. Mike's mother sought hypnotic treatment from a colleague to prepare Mike for dentistry. The hypnotist taught Mike what to expect in the dental office by using a series of treatment scenarios. I was contacted when Mike had a toothache. The mother, while talking to me on the phone, with Mike right there, used language that I thought might encourage fear in her son (e.g., statements such as, "he can't hurt you over the phone"). Mike talked to me and agreed to come to my office to let me look at his tooth and put on some "gray stuff" (medicated filling) to make him feel more comfortable. He arrived with his stuffed animal, named "Brother Dog." Classic induction methods did not succeed and often caused tears. A conversational trance approach was then used. My continued talking gradually drew Mike into the conversation. He told me how upset he was with x-rays, and we made a "deal" that none would be taken at this visit. I continued to tell Mike about our neat things, showed him how I could squirt his mother with air, and how I could spray the plants. Gradually, I introduced new dental equipment to him. I vacuumed his arm and talked as a make believe filling was placed in "Brother Dog's" mouth. Soon Mike allowed me to spray his mouth with the whistling squirter, my high speed handpiece, and to

place a temporary filling, the gray stuff, in the tooth that needed restoration. Mike agreed that when he returned for treatment, I could tickle his tooth.

When he presented at the next visit he presented without "Brother Dog." Because he was much more comfortable, a more classic induction involving glove anesthesia was considered. I told Mike that as I moved my hand gradually down his arm from his elbow to his wrist and across his fingers, his hand would start feeling different, either warmer or colder or tingly or just different. Soon he agreed that it did feel different. His cooperation indicated trance, even though he was squirming and wriggling (children in trance often move about). I then had him try to levitate his arm to bring his hand to the tooth that needed treatment. I wanted him to transfer the anesthesia he felt in his hand to the tooth. He couldn't make the arm move by itself, so I suggested that he himself make it lift. He did it while paying attention to me, and as the hand touched the tooth, I suggested that the tooth would also feel different. He agreed that it did. I then suggested that he press that tooth very firmly to make sure that it felt funny and was numb. He allowed the use of the high speed drill, evacuation of fluids with a suction tip, the use of a spoon excavator and placement of an amalgam restoration. With a great deal of praise, he proudly inspected his new silver tooth. Before dismissing Mike, the subject of x-rays was again discussed. Although none were taken at that visit, a promise was made to take them next time.

---

are made in trance are not only more readily accepted but also are more powerfully acted upon than in normal situations (Peretz 1996).

Shaw and Welbury state that hypnosis is a useful adjunct in children who are unable to accept dental extractions using inhalation sedation and local anesthesia. When these latter techniques were unsuccessful, hypnotic imagery was used. Sixteen of twenty formerly untreatable patients were able to be treated. Parents indicated in a written evaluation of the procedure that they were happy with their child's treatment. Hypnotic imagery can be used as an adjunct to inhalation sedation and conventional management tools for dental extractions in children (Shaw 1996).

TIME DISTORTION

Hypnotism can be used to perceive either a shortened or a lengthened dental office visit. Fabian found that

time distortion occurred in dental treatment carried out under hypnosis in 64% of the patients sampled. Of course, most patients wish that "time flies" when they are in the dentist's chair (Fabian 1996).

ABNORMAL REACTIONS

There are very few contraindications for the use of hypnosis in dentistry. Attention, however, must be paid to the patient who is undergoing psychotherapy for an unusually traumatic or threatening issue, or who is in unstable mental health.

CONCLUSION

Millions of people receive incomplete dental care or no dental care at all because of dental anxiety and dental

---

Case study 12–5

Ellen presented at my office for an extraction. She is a 55-year-old woman in good physical health, a patient of record for many years, and the wife of a psychologist. Previous dental treatment, whether extensive or minor, was accompanied by moderate anxiety, but with self-control by the patient. Ellen had been seeing a psychiatrist for many years and told me that she was in stable mental health. She was apprehensive about the surgery, but more anxious about the actual loss of the tooth than of the procedure itself. We had discussed my use of hypnosis at previous visits, and she asked if I would hypnotize her for this procedure to reduce anxiety. She requested local anesthetic for pain control. I agreed. All went fine. The tooth was removed and she was very relaxed and comfortable. When I reoriented her, she stood up, sank to her knees and started moaning incoherently about her daughter. She started crying hysterically and would not allow anyone to talk to her except me. I escorted her to the business area of my office. She was totally incoherent. I tried to further reorient her by counting back from ten to one and having her follow me. She could get from ten to seven and then would start flailing and screaming about her daughter. She would not allow my staff to help, and in fact was abusive to them. When I suggested that she might be more comfortable in my private office

she responded with a primal scream. During this time she was able to give me the name of her psychiatrist. Several telephone calls with clear messages of an emergency situation did not elicit a return call. I called her husband, but he said that he was unable to cancel his day and could not leave his office. Only after the psychiatrist finally returned the call and increased her medication, which was in her purse all the time, did Ellen become slightly less agitated. Her husband finally came to pick her up. He then told me that she had been despondent during the past week and was losing touch with reality. He said that he should have told me but just didn't think about it before her appointment. Her psychiatrist also knew that she was coming to the dentist for an extraction and admitted that she should have contacted me because of the patient's deteriorating psychiatric condition; she just didn't think to do so. The next day Ellen called to apologize, not remembering much of what took place, except that she was embarrassed by her actions. I had taken a thorough medical history, but not a thorough mental history. It is mandatory to do so and confer with the therapist prior to use of hypnosis to be certain the patient is not in the midst of a psychotic break or other decompensating condition. Hypnosis is contraindicated for psychotic patients.

---

phobia (Feldman 1958). Dentists report that patients with anxiety disorders are likely to begin treatment and then terminate before completion of the necessary work. Hypnotherapy can reduce the fear and the tension associated with going to the dentist and reduce, if not eliminate, dental phobia (Baker 1983). Teaching self-hypnosis to the patients is valuable, too. The patient appreciates the increased sense of control that reduces feelings of vulnerability. Hypnosis is effective for children as well as adults.

REFERENCES

American Dental Association: Overcoming Dental Anxiety. ADA Dental Newsline, 1977

Baker R, Boaz D: The partial reformulation of a traumatic memory of a dental phobia during trance. Int J Clin Exp Hypn 31:14–18, 1983

Barsby MJ: The use of hypnois in the management of gagging and intolerance to dentures. Br Dent J 176(3):97–102, 1994

Bystedt H, Enqvist B, von Konow L: Pre- and perioperative suggestions in maxillofacial surgery: Effects on blood loss and recovery. Int J Clin Exp Hypn 43(3):284–294, 1995

Clarke HJ, Reynolds PJ: Suggestive hypnotherapy for nocturnal bruxism: A pilot study. Am J Clin Hypn 33(4):248–253, 1991

Crothers AJ, Robb ND: Sedation in dentistry, part 2: Management of the gagging patient. Dental update 23(5):182–186, 1996

Dubin L, Shapiro S: Use of hypnosis to facilitate dental extraction and hemostatis in a classic hemophiliac with a high antibody titer to Factor VII. Am J Clin Hypn 17(2):79–83, 1974

Eli I, Kleinhauz M: Hypnotic induction in dentistry: Coping with fear of losing control (autonomy). Int J Clin Exp Hypn 39(3):July 125–128, 1991

Enqvist B, Fisher K: Preoperative hypnotic techniques reduce consumption of analgesics after removal of third molars: A brief communication. Int J Clin Exp Hypn 45(2):102–108, 1997

Erickson MH: Collected Papers of Milton H Erickson on Hypnosis. New York, Irvington Publishers, 1990

Fabian TK: Hypnosis in dentistry: Comparative evaluation of 45 cases of hypnosis. Forgorv Sz 88(3):111–115, 1995

Fabian TK: Hypnosis in dentistry 2 amnesia, loss of time perception: Spontaneous manifestations during use of hypnosis in dentistry. FOGORV SZ, 88(3):111–115, 1995

Feldman J, Freidson E: The public looks at dental care. J Am Dent Assoc 57:325–335, 1958

Felicity W: Hypnosis in the treatment of bruxism. Australian Journal of Clinical and Experimental Hypnosis 22(2):97–107, 1994

Finkelstein, Selig: Hypnotically assisted preparation of the anxious patient for medical and dental treatment. Am J Clin Hypn 33(3):187–191, 1991

Herod EL: Psychological pain control during tooth extraction. General Dentistry 43(3):267–269, 1995

Katz J, Peretz B, Shemer J, et al: Treating dental phobia patients in the Israeli Defense Force. International Journal of Dentistry 46(2):108–112, 1996

Lu DP, Lu GP, Hersh EV: Augmenting sedation with hypnosis in drug dependent patients. Anesthesia Progress 42(3–4):139–143, 1995

Lu DP, Lu GP: Hypnosis and pharmacological sedation for medically compromised patients. Compendium of Continuing Education in Dentistry 17:1, 32, 34–40, 1996

Lucas O: Dental extractions in the hemophiliac: Control of the emotional factors for hypnosis. Am J Clin Hypn VII:301–307, 1985

Niven N, Shaw AJ: Theoretical concepts and practical applications of hypnosis in the treatment of children and adolescents with dental fear and anxiety. Br J Dent 180(1):11–16, 1996

Peretz B: Confusion as a technique to induce hypnosis in a severely anxious pediatric patient. Journal of Pediatric Dentistry 21(1):27–30, 1996a

Pertez B: Relaxation and hypnosis in pediatric dental patients. Journal for Clinical Pediatric Dentistry 20(3):205–207, 1996b

Reilley RR, Rodolfa ER: Etiology and treatment of dental anxiety and phobia. Am J Clin Hypn 33(1):22–28, 1990

Shaw AJ, Welbury RR: The use of hypnosis in a sedation clinic for dental extractions in children: Report of 20 cases. Journal of Dentistry for Children 63(6):413–420, 1996

Thompson S: The use of hypnosis as an adjunct to nitrous oxide sedation in the treatment of anxiety. Contemporary Hypnosis 11(2):77–83, 1994

13

Nursing
Dorothy Larkin

INTRODUCTION

There are extensive opportunities for a nurse to use hypnosis. Hypnosis can help alleviate the suffering associated with burns, cancer, labor and delivery, emergency care, surgical preparation, recovery from surgery, and cardiac procedures. Patients with chronic diseases and with life-threatening illnesses, too, can benefit from hypnosis. Also, hypnosis can be used for health promotion for children and adults by fostering active participation and cooperation with medical regimens.

Nurses can easily integrate the principles of therapeutic suggestion into daily conversations with patients, families, and groups. Additionally, hypnosis can facilitate staff cohesiveness, stress management, and conflict resolution.

The subjective experience of hypnosis is ". . . a form of self-induced, focused attention" (Olness 1993). Milton Erickson said that providing hypnosis is providing therapeutic communication. He said, "Hypnosis is essentially a communication of ideas to a patient in such a fashion that he will be most receptive to the presented ideas and thereby motivated to explore his own body potentials for the control of his psychological and physiological responses and behavior" (Erickson & Rossi 1980).

Erickson claimed that during trance, "learning and openness to change are most likely to occur" (Rosen 1982). Facilitators help patients enter a hypnotic trance by capturing their attention and directing it inward, leading them to an inner search in which they are more responsive to discovering and utilizing unconscious learnings and inner resources (Rosen 1982).

When I teach nurses about hypnosis, I emphasize the Ericksonian strategy of utilization. Utilization is the technique of catering inductions to the unique responsiveness of each patient. Word choices and subject choice are most important. Nurses using hypnosis have as their first goal the establishment of an intense therapeutic rapport with their patients. Nurses need to be aware of the ways in which their patients will best respond. Some patients respond well to autocratic, directive suggestions, whereas others respond better to indirect, permissive suggestions, analogies, metaphors, or therapeutic storytelling (Erickson 1976; Larkin 1988; Larkin 1990).

INDUCTIONS AND STYLES

Nurses utilizing therapeutic hypnosis should know the following hypnotic principles and induction styles and then cater all inductions to the unique needs of each patient.

Progressive Muscle Relaxation. A typical induction might include some of the following suggestions. "You can imagine softening of muscle fibers, beginning to relax the muscles in your head, face, and neck like a tight rubber band loosening, releasing any unnecessary tension, with each breath deepening your sense of relaxation and comfort."

Imagery of a Peaceful Place in Nature. The nurse should explore and then utilize each patient's preference regarding a peaceful, comfortable place in nature. The imagery should include encouragement to explore that place using all senses and to memorize the experience of replenishment, so it can be retrieved whenever wanted or needed.

Pacing and Leading. The nurse aligns with the patterns, rhythms, or perceptions of the patient. Leading involves therapeutically and suggestively guiding the patient toward discovery of healthful possibilities.

The Interspersal Approach. The nurse purposely intersperses direct suggestions for enhancing comfort, within the context of a larger conversation. This approach is illustrated by Erickson's famous "Joe" story, in which a terminally ill gardener hospitalized in intensive care, on a respirator and in intractable pain, listened to Ericksonian hypnotically drone on with emphasized interspersed suggestions how "tomato plants can [*feel comfortable, Joe, rest comfortably, enjoy food and fluids, live the fullness of each day, Joe*] . . . " (Erickson 1966).

Therapeutic Storytelling and Metaphors. (Crowley and Mills 1986; Larkin 1988.) The nurse develops a metaphor or story that is isomorphic or similar in some way to the patient's experience. It may be a story about another person with a similar problem and how he or she resolved that problem. This method is an indirect way to suggest to your patient a possible strategy for resolving the problem. Erickson often spoke about how a young child is challenged in learning the alphabet, and although it may feel like a seemingly insurmountable task, gradually the letters are learned, and then the child learns to create words, sentences, and paragraphs. The alphabet creates a foundation for a lifetime of learning. This story can metaphorically parallel the challenges a person may experience in working to successfully resolve a problem.

Reframing. This technique changes the meaning of an experience or situation into a perception that is more favorable or conducive to health promotion. An example of reframing was provided by Jennifer White, BSN, RN, who worked in an ambulatory care unit in Maine: A 19-year-old woman required catheterization of the bladder. The patient was tense and fearful. Before the procedure was explained to her, she asked, "Are you going to shove that thing into my bladder?" Ms. White replied, "Oh no, I'm going to gently slide the tube in." The patient relaxed and the tube slid in, uneventfully (cited in Larkin 1988).

Patients who learn self-hypnosis become self-sufficient in evoking comfort. Because hypnosis is a learned ability that improves with practice, patients often benefit from a series of educational sessions.

HEALTH PROMOTION

I teach nursing hypnosis within the context of the theoretical framework of Rogers' Science of Unitary Human Beings (Rogers 1992). Rogers described the purpose of nursing as promoting multidimensional patterns of health and well being for all people. Hypnosis facilitates health by (1) countering Selyes' generalized adaptation syndrome that depicts the maladaptive physiological response to distress: (2) augmenting Benson's relaxation response that counters the maladaptive stress response (Benson 1975; Benson 1984); and (3) evoking or enhancing active patient participation that may augment immunological functions as suggested by psychoneuroimmunological research.

The growing field of psychoneuroimmunology suggests multiple benefits of hypnosis (Hall 1982; Levitan 1991). Levy reviewed studies on the psychoneuroimmunological implications of emotions and cancer progression and reported that helplessness and poor coping are associated with lower survival rates from cancer. Relaxation techniques and hypnosis are health-promoting strategies that can counter the experience of helplessness, enhance patients' active participation in care, and potentially augment immunological strength (Levy 1981).

I emphasize to nursing students and patients that even such a simple intervention as progressive relaxation can have profound health-promoting benefits. Kiecolt-Glaser et al studied 45 geriatric residents in an independent living center. They showed a significant increase in the activity of their natural killer cells after a month's training in relaxation techniques (Kiecolt-Glaser J 1985).

SYMPTOM MANAGEMENT

Hypnosis can ease symptomology associated with disease. Erickson describes pain as a "subjective experience" and ". . . a complex, a construct, composed of past remembered pain, of present pain experience, and of anticipated pain in the future. Thus, immediate pain is augmented by past pain and is enhanced by the future possibilities of pain" (Erickson 1980). Erickson illustrates how hypnosis may benefit pain management: ". . . any hypnotic alteration of any single interpretive quality of the pain sensation serves to effect an alteration of the total pain complex" (Erickson 1980). For example, if a patient describes his pain as red hot, suggestions to shift the image by adding drops of cooling yellow to dilute the intensity can change a patient's experience of pain. This simple imagery exercise illustrates to patients the possibilities of shifting their perception of their symptoms.

A young burn patient needed to do frequent exercises to prevent muscle contractures. One day as her arm was being flexed, she screamed in pain, "It's pulsing. I can feel it pulsing." I utilized her perception and said, "Yes. I'll take your pulse now and let's see if your count of those beats will be the same as mine." The patient immediately became absorbed in the task of counting; she was no longer panic stricken. The counting task distracted her. She was then in a suggestible state and was easily hypnotized, while she continued to permit her arms to be exercised.

PAIN MANAGEMENT

When I work as a nurse pain management consultant, I often offer patients a permissive induction that may consist of progressive relaxation and imagery of being in a peaceful, replenishing place in nature. Within this conversation I intersperse therapeutic suggestions for healthful living. I discuss with patients the natural capacity to shift and reframe perceptions and teach them that this flexibility of awareness as a natural capacity can be augmented with hypnosis. With interspersed suggestions and therapeutic stories, I fuse awareness of living in the present with an appreciation of the learnings of the past, which is then coupled with an expectant

anticipation of the therapeutic possibilities in the future. For example, a person with chronic pain can be taught how to enhance selective awareness. That patient can be taught, with hypnosis, to delete or diminish awareness of pain, while at the same time to notice an increased sense of relaxation, comfort, love, and connection with family and friends.

After learning hypnosis, pain patients often say they still have their pain, but they no longer feel bothered by it. This dichotomy of perception is understood as *dissociation* in hypnosis, described by Pierre Janet in 1889 as a "division of consciousness" (cited in Hilgard 1983) and by Hilgard (1977) as the "hidden observer." Hilgard and LeBaron describe trance as an altered state of consciousness, in terms of "degrees of dissociation." They depict the ambiguity of this experience in their claim:

An altered state of consciousness is characterized by a shift in subject experience or in psychological functioning that one perceives as distinctly different from the usual alert, waking consciousness. It is not possible to draw a fine line between a minor dissociation and an altered state of consciousness because they often shade gradually from one to the other, much like the transition periods of such ambiguous states as dawn and dusk (Hilgard 1984).

Redd et al describe helping six patients control chemotherapy side effects. They suggest it is the dissociative nature of hypnosis that enables subjects to "experience pain at a physiological level while hypnotized, but the discomfort is no longer bothersome at the psychological level" (Redd 1982). Their description of the hypnotic induction process involves the following three steps:

First, the patient was asked to focus on a fixed point on the wall or ceiling and then concentrate on the psychologist's voice and suggestions. Then, deep muscle relaxation was induced by suggesting comfortable sensations in different muscle groups, while progressing from the feet to the head and back two times. Next, relaxing imagery was introduced by the therapist describing various pleasant scenes. Interwoven with the imagery were suggestions of comfort. After 30 minutes, the patient was aroused by the therapist counting from 1 to 20. This training session was audiotape recorded and the patient was instructed to listen to the tape daily in order to increase her responsiveness to hypnosis (Redd 1982).

One week later, patients received a second training session that included the former induction and a "description of the sequence of events leading to the chemotherapy, including being carried by wheelchair to and from the chemotherapy room." The third session occurred the day of the chemotherapy treatment, and subjects then completed a visual analogue scale rating their experience of nausea. All subjects reported no anticipatory emesis and little nausea following chemotherapy. The researchers speculated that the deep relaxation associated with hypnosis may have inhibited the muscle activity in the upper small bowel, esophagus, and stomach, and that reduced the patients' nausea and emesis.

Margolis presented a clinical report of personalized hypnotic interventions with six cancer patients (Margolis 1982). She claims, "Deep relaxation, ego strengthening, imagery and suggestions for changes in perception and awareness are the principal techniques used to reduce suffering and to promote a sense of well being among cancer patients. . . ." She emphasizes the need to individualize hypnotic inductions and utilize "a patient's distinctive experiences, feelings, convictions, or resources in order to effectively offer comfort, distraction, shifts of psychological mood or state, insight, even resolutions of unfinished business, as well as relief from pain." For example, a 27-year-old man diagnosed with lymphoma created his own hypnotic images to ease his nausea and vomiting after chemotherapy, in which he would "remove himself from the procedures by putting himself in trance, visiting (in trance) a comfortable place where he had always enjoyed good health and a sense of well-being. He chose a lush green mountain resort where he sat on a stone terrace overlooking a woods below. He would feel himself blending into the wide expanse of blue sky, he could see the full green trees, and feel the cool breeze. He was able to recreate the strength and euphoria . . . (and) . . . managed to substantially reduce his feelings of nausea and vomiting" (Margolis 1982).

This kind of multisensory imaging process is a common experience reported by hypnotized patients and illustrates the therapeutic benefits of distraction techniques. Redd et al describes the contribution of distraction: "The monotonous stimulation of the therapist's voice and the narrow focus of attention upon the experience of relaxation or pleasant imagery may prevent the patient from attending to internal cues of nausea or nausea-eliciting conditioned stimuli" (Redd 1982).

PREOPERATIVE CARE

Preoperative hypnotic education offers many opportunities for utilizing therapeutic suggestions. Merely educating the patient as to what to expect postoperatively is an implication that the patient will survive surgery. Suggestions made to the patient preoperatively can greatly facilitate postoperative comfort, voiding coughing, reorientation, and ultimately lead to earlier discharges from the hospital. Suggestive preoperative education helps patients relax prior to surgery because some of their fear of the unknown has been alleviated by specific information of what to expect postoperatively (Larkin 1988). Positive

suggestions during the preoperative education phase are easy to incorporate and will help lower the patient's anxiety. Typical suggestions include, "Blood works to nourish cells and cleanse wounds as they heal properly and comfortably," or "Deep breaths will replenish the oxygen in the blood that will feed those healing cells and help them grow stronger."

To teach preoperative patients how to splint abdominal muscles for coughing, a positive suggestion could be, "This will give you support, so when you cough and clean out your lungs, it can be more comfortable and more oxygen can get to the cells to speed your healing."

Rapkin et al used brief preoperative hypnosis with a sample of 36 head and neck cancer surgery patients. One to three days preoperatively, patients in the hypnotic group (n = 15) were administered a consent procedure, personality questionnaires, and a 20-minute imagery–hypnosis script. The induction was described as "indirect and permissive because, although high hypnotizable individuals may respond to direct suggestions, low hypnotizables may be more responsive to indirect suggestions" (Rapkin 1991). According to Rapkin "patients were invited, through suggestions, to develop their own images because (1) pleasurable, comforting images are to some extent idiosyncratic, and (2) self-generated images would be expected to involve internal enactment rather than to be passively received." A portion of the script was published and described permissive imagery of relaxing in a soothing, healing tub of water (i.e., "you might notice that you find yourself gently lowering yourself into the tub. . . ."), as well as a future orientation suggestion to "allow your imagination to take you ahead to the future . . . to some time after your surgery when your body has healed." Postoperative hospitalizations for the hypnotic group (mean stay of 8.7 days) were reported as significantly shorter than the group who received usual care (mean stay of 13.9 days). Further research with a larger sample size for randomization intervention study was recommended. Such encouraging findings will likely attract attention and support for adjunctive hypnotherapy because cost effectiveness is of paramount concern in our health care system today.

HYPNOSIS IN GROUPS

Spiegel reported that he used hypnosis in support groups for women with breast cancer. His research began in 1976 with 86 women with breast cancer. Fifty were randomly assigned to support groups, and 36 did not attend groups. He conveyed his deep surprise when the results indicated the women in the support groups "lived an average of 18 months longer than did women with comparable breast cancer and medical care who did not go to such groups" (Spiegel 1993). Although he attributes these findings to social support, the women in the groups also received training in self-hypnosis. These group patients who "were trained in self-hypnosis to combat pain also reported half as much pain as the control patients." This preliminary work suggests life-saving potentials and the need for more research on the use of hypnotherapy in groups.

CONVERSATIONAL INDUCTIONS

While working in an active New York City emergency room, I enjoyed overhearing another nurse complain that, "Dorothy always gets the easy patients." My perspective was that the hypnotic suggestions I interspersed into daily conversations with emergency room patients facilitated their cooperation, and this, in turn, eased my delivery of care.

The following examples illustrate conversational inductions and nursing hypnosis.

Therapeutic Nursing Suggestions in an Emergency Room Setting

The wide variety of patients seen in emergency rooms provides a multitude of opportunities for utilizing therapeutic suggestions. When the concepts of direct and indirect suggestions are understood by the nurse, every interaction with these patients can include therapeutic suggestions. Patients usually come to the emergency room with some level of fear and anxiety. The triage nurse can begin to make therapeutic suggestions while taking their vital signs, telling them something about their body that is properly functioning: "Your pulse is a good rate, nice and steady"; "you've got a good, healthy blood pressure"; "that bleeding has been cleaning out that wound properly, so it can heal better." The rationale for these comments is consistent with Milton Erickson's utilization technique. This approach implies accepting and utilizing something the patient is doing appropriately and then leading the patient with a conjunctive clause, such as "and when you have this gown on with the opening to the back, you can sit here and be comfortable and the doctor will be right with you." This suggestion includes the implied directive: "when you put this gown on," the permissive "you can," and an interspersed direct suggestion, "sit here and be comfortable." Patients who receive this simple type of introduction generally are more compliant and patient while they wait in the emergency room.

Any drugs given can be linked with therapeutic suggestions for their effective therapeutic action. For example, "Mr. Smith, this medication will help open up the blood vessels in your heart so more oxygen will nourish the area and you should begin to feel more comfortable very soon." Therapeutic interventions should also be offered with suggestions. For example, "This neck brace will help remind you to keep your muscles relaxed and comfortable while they heal properly."

When performing invasive procedures, the nurse can explain the rationale for the process with suggestions for a healthful outcome. Suggestions for relaxation or imagery can easily be interspersed. For example, "George, I'm going to gently clean these burns so the area can heal more quickly." An isomorphic metaphor with implied suggestions for healing is as follows: "It's like tending a garden and weeding out anything that might interfere with the healthy growth of your vegetables. This cleansing will help make the area fertile for new cells to grow, just like the flowers and vegetables need to be tended, and as they grow and heal properly, nourished by the oxygen in the blood, it's like the garden needs the rain; those cells can grow comfortably. . . ."

Asthmatic patients present to the emergency room in acute physiological and psychological distress. As an adjunct to the traditional medical treatment of oxygen and inhalation treatments, patients can be taught how to perform diaphragmatic breathing. The nurse can utilize therapeutic suggestions while teaching and thus reduce anxiety and the severity of the attack. For example: "I want you to breathe with your diaphragm (demonstrate with hand on stomach, pushing out abdomen with each inhalation) and then those tubes in your lungs can open up and bring you more air." (Form tube with hand and enlarge for visual demonstration. The patient should join the nurse in this breathing. Patient's hands are on his stomach.) The nurse can diaphragmatically breathe with the patient, observing and commenting about what he is doing correctly, praising him when correct technique is shown. The patient is then asked to practice and demonstrate to the nurse to show "how well you can do it," and "to notice the feelings as your tubes in your windpipe relax and open up." He is left with the therapeutic suggestion that asthmatics who breathe this way find it relaxing and mediative. When the patient repeats the demonstration correctly, the nurse can offer a double-bind, future-oriented suggestion of "I don't know whether your stomach will tell, or show, your mind when to breathe this way, but you can help open those tubes. It probably does not matter how you choose to breathe this way because you know how to do it, and you can do it whenever you need to without even thinking about it." Variations of this basic conversation can be utilized with all patients, from pediatric to geriatric (Larkin 1988).

Therapeutic Nursing Suggestions and Imagery for the Control of Bleeding

A 4-year-old girl with leukemia was admitted to the pediatric oncology unit with an uncontrollable nosebleed. Her initial emergency medical treatment consisted of nasal packing and platelet transfusion. The following night she suddenly developed another nosebleed. As charge nurse, I responded when her mother came to the nursing station, frantically exclaiming, "It started again!"

I entered the patient's room, got down to her eye level and told her I would apply pressure on her nose to help *stop the bleeding*. I then began to gently stroke her cheek to match the rhythm of her breathing. This technique is known as "pacing," which is implicit in Erickson's utilization approach. The utilization approach accepts and utilizes the patient's rhythms and then therapeutically guides the patient. When the patient and facilitator's rhythms are matched, the facilitator (here, the nurse) can then "lead" the patient. I did this by slowing down the stroking of her cheek to help her relax and slow down her respiratory rate. At the same time, I suggested to her "Some children I know like to go inside their mind and see cartoons. Now, I don't know if when you look inside your mind you see Bugs Bunny or Donald Duck." (This is a therapeutic double-bind.) Her eyes were closed for a moment while I continued to pace and lead my stroking with her breathing, and she whispered, "Bugs Bunny."

I utilized her response by saying, "That's right, and Bugs Bunny looks like he's exploring all around the corners in there, and I don't know if you can see what he's hiding behind his back, so I'll tell you. He's got some Krazy Glue. . . . Can you see it now?" She nodded her head and I responded with, "Maybe you can tell me when Bugs Bunny finds that little hole and patches it up with the Krazy Glue so it doesn't leak anymore. . . . Has he found it yet?" She nodded, and I said, "OK, and now you can just watch him put that strong glue in and watch it dry, but I'm not going to take my finger off your nose until you know it's absolutely dry. . . . Is it dry yet?" She slowly shook her head. I reassured her, "OK, you can let me know when it's strong and dry; I know that stuff works fast. . . . Is it dry now?" She nodded. I released the pressure and her bleeding had stopped. As she opened her eyes to meet mine, I continued to pace and stroke her cheek, offering a future-oriented suggestion: "You can do that whenever you need to. Bugs Bunny will always be there with the Krazy Glue."

A direct and active approach characterized the interaction during this crisis. This approach captured the attention and cooperation of the patient and subsequently reduced both her anxiety and that of her mother. The interspersed suggestions were emphasized by a change in my voice modulation, prefaced by permissive or qualifying comments, such as, "you can" and "when." These comments encourage active participation of the patient and help avoid resistance to the therapeutic suggestions. A consistent direct and implied message continued to be that she could control and stop the bleeding. Her mother listened to this interaction and discovered strategies that could be useful to her daughter; strategies that went beyond traditional medical care. In hypnotic education it is important to include a suggestion about future learning and future applicability of the current suggestion.

Therapeutic Distraction

It is theorized that when patients are confused they change their perceptual attention, and that change closes the "sensory gate" to incoming painful stimuli (Melzack and Wall). Tina, a 6-year-old girl who was fighting with the nurses as they attempted to change the dressing on her wounded leg, was able to distract herself from feeling severe pain when I intervened as follows:

Nurse #1: Tina, have you met Dorothy?

D: (Tina looked at me. I captured her gaze, and spoke in a slow, deep voice.) May I call you Fred?
Tina: (Appeared shocked.) NO!

D: Oh, well. How about George?
Tina: (A momentary pause and then an indignant shake of the head.) I'm a GIRL!

D: I'm a girl, too, and it's all right if you call me Fred. (This shows Tina that even if something is unquestionably what it is, it is okay to pretend that it can seem different. I wanted her experience of pain to be included in this generalization.)

I then sat behind Tina while the other nurses began to cut away her dressing. I whispered secret challenges into her ear. For example, "Bet you don't know how many muscles you use when you lift that leg." The words "that leg" were to help her dissociate, and "lift that leg" was an interspersed direct suggestion.

The minimal time required for these interventions suggests benefits for educating bedside nurses in hypnotherapeutic approaches. These examples are presented in greater detail in Zahourek's books on relaxation and imagery (Larkin 1988; Zahourek 1990).

Suggestions Go Everywhere

Therapeutic suggestions communicated to one individual can also evoke beneficial responses from persons overhearing the conversation. Such suggestions can actually be intended for present persons to whom the nurse is not overtly speaking. The following is an example from my work with a 12-year-old girl with chronic renal problems and an intravenous technician.

The highly competent technician distressingly reported that Julie's intravenous needle needed to be restarted. The technician said that she had trouble starting the intravenous drip last time because Julie has terrible veins. She then emphatically stated that she would try only three times and then the doctors would have to start it.

I entered Julie's room on morning rounds while the IV technician was setting up the necessary equipment. I had not met Julie before and walked up to her bed to introduce myself. To establish rapport, I lowered to her eye level and gently squeezed her arm where the intravenous needle would likely be inserted. The following conversation occurred:

"Hi Julie. My name is Dorothy and I hear you need a new IV. Why don't you make those veins big so she can get it in on the first try? I bet you didn't know you could do that, did you? You can tell me later how well you did it."

Julie looked a bit surprised and then nodded. The IV technician overheard our conversation with the interspersed suggestion "she can get it in on the first try." The interspersed direct suggestion for Julie to "make those veins big" was prefaced by my permissive comment of wondering if she already knows how to do it. This implication that it can be done is followed by the interspersed suggestion, "you could do that." The final comment implies future satisfaction for a job well done.

Ten minutes later the IV technician rushed up to me and joyfully announced that she got it on the first try! I congratulated her and then returned to Julie's room to extend further congratulations. When I greeted the beaming Julie with my thumbs up, I offered the future-oriented suggestion, "And now that you know how to do it, you can think those veins big anytime you need to, and isn't that good news?"

Jennifer White, BSN, RN, reports her experience with a 16-year-old girl who had eye surgery under general anesthesia. The patient returned to the day surgery unit very groggy, but arousable. She remained stable throughout the postoperative course but maintained a state of grogginess or sleep for the next 4 hours. The patient's mother was at the bedside during the patient's recovery period. She verbalized concern over her daughter's "slow" recovery; she had observed many other patients in the unit who recovered more rapidly and were already discharged. She felt her daughter

should be admitted for an overnight stay. Discussing the situation with the patient's mother, I reassured her that an overnight stay was a possibility, but we would continue to monitor the patient's recovery for at least 1 more hour before making such a decision. Still within the patient's hearing range, I discussed the individuality of a patient's recovery from anesthesia (suggestions go everywhere). We reviewed the range of possibilities from a very gradual recovery to a sudden coming to alertness after a long period of sleeping (this double bind implies that the question is not "if" the patient will recover today but "how" the patient will recover today). Fifty minutes later the patient sat upright in bed and was totally alert. She announced she felt "much better," was hungry, and was ready to be discharged.

NONTHERAPEUTIC SUGGESTIONS AND COUNTERING MEASURES

Practitioners may need to counter nontherapeutic suggestions made by other health care providers and family members. Well meaning people may be unaware of their statements' potential maladaptive impact upon the patient. A professional's benevolent intent of truthfully conveying to patients probable perceptions of medical procedures is legally warranted and ethically appropriate, but too often it is the negative potential response that is emphasized at the expense of positive or neutral responses. In working with burn patients, it is necessary to dress the wounds with an antibiotic that is frequently perceived as uncomfortably hot. Other nurses often warn patients with the negative suggestion, "Get ready, this dressing is going to burn." Naturally, the patients apprehensively pay attention to the predicted burning sensation and subsequently complain or grimace when the heat is felt. A therapeutic approach to the same situation is to advise the patient that the dressing is going to feel wet and warm (a simultaneous perceptual experience). The occasional patient who reports discomfort from excessive warmth would have that experience accepted and acknowledged. Her attention could be redirected to another experience that was a simultaneous truthful perception, such as the concept of time: "Yes, but most patients say the heat lasts only a short time and I wonder how soon yours will quit?" (This is an example of an interspersed suggestion for brevity of discomfort.)

On another occasion, I was assisting a patient for his first postoperative burn cleansing tank immersion procedure. The attending physician loudly announced, within the patient's hearing range, "Get the thrombin ready, he was just debrided and he's going to lose a lot of blood." To counter this nontherapeutic suggestion,

I calmly and emphatically stated at the patient's ear level, "Although I wonder how interesting it might be to notice how little you need to bleed, perhaps just the amount needed to cleanse the burns properly, so they can heal even quicker. After all, you have been stopping the bleeding all your life and even if you don't fully know how you do it, maybe you could just watch to see how it's done properly this time." These suggestions were subtly re-emphasized throughout the tanking procedure and were interspersed with suggestions for relaxation, deep breathing, and enhanced comfort. The patient was compliant, relaxed, and required very little thrombin.

Another example of countering nontherapeutic suggestions was when a 9-year-old boy with terminal leukemia needed to be logrolled and weighed. The process was complicated by the Swan, arterial and intravenous lines, ventilator tubing, and chest tubes. The primary attending nurse told the boy she was sorry, but this was going to hurt him. The patient responded with a grimace and a moan. I then commented, "Sometimes it can be more comfortable if we move very slowly, carefully and gently, and maybe if you take a few slow, deep breaths, that can really help." The patient's furrowed brow relaxed; he took a deep breath and began to assist us by slowly moving one arm and leg. The other nurse responded with, "Oh no, there's no way you can be comfortable logrolling with chest tubes. Chest tubes always make you hurt." The boy's frown and grimace returned. I countered with, "I'm not so sure about that, but it might be really interesting to find out how comfortable it could be . . . with deep breaths, and slow, careful movements, right now . . . so maybe the hurt won't even need to bother him." The patient's forehead again relaxed and he proceeded to assist us further. The other nurse was verbally persistent in maintaining her position that comfort could not exist and the conversation continued to offer the patient opposing suggestions (to which the patient correspondingly alternated relaxed and furrowed brow) until I chose to monopolize the conversation. The procedure was completed with willing patient participation and minimal nonverbal indications of discomfort.

COST EFFECTIVENESS OF HYPNOSIS

Cost effectiveness is a primary issue and concern in the current climate of managed care. A recent example from my practice illustrates the encouraging cost effectiveness of utilizing hypnotherapeutic approaches in nursing practice. A 4-year-old boy was seen with multiple warts (over 30) throughout his body. A colleague had requested a hypnotherapeutic consultation prior to the medically recommended surgical excisions. I met with the child and parents once and utilized a conversational induction to induce rapport. As in all utilization approaches (Erickson and Rossi 1980), I tailored the induction to the unique awareness, responsiveness, and experience of the patient. Therapeutic suggestions woven into daily conversations are particularly effective in facilitating patients' active participation and cooperation with therapeutic regimes. With this little boy, I conversationally and with vocal emphasis introduced the idea that dinosaurs are now extinct, but we know what they looked like (he had a toy dinosaur in his bag). I suggested he should go home and memorize what his warts looked like so he could remember them after they cleared. I then blew bubbles and commented, "Now you see them; now you don't," and I asked him to feel tingles at each wart "so you know your body is clearing them up." One month later the warts had "spontaneously" cleared; surgical removal was not required.

Another example of the cost effectiveness of hypnosis in nursing was with an 87-year-old woman hospitalized after gynecological surgery for 3 weeks beyond her expected discharge date. I met her on rounds and introduced myself as her per diem nurse. When asked how she was, she emphatically stated, while surrounded by visitors, that her extended stay was because "I can't pee." I accepted and utilized her perspective and then reframed it as appropriate behavior with an exuberant comment, "Of course not, certainly not while you're in bed and your friends are here!" She looked surprised, and I said I would come back soon and we could talk about it. When I returned at her required routine catheterization time, I brought her into the bathroom and conversationally and hypnotically talked about how muscles can tighten and relax. With interspersed suggestion for diaphragmatic breathing, I described how she could tighten some muscles. For example, "that right knee can tighten while other muscles can spontaneously relax." During this 5-minute conversation, she spontaneously urinated.

TRAINING

This chapter provided an introductory sampling of principles and case reports of hypnotherapeutic approaches in nursing and health care. Practitioners find that these approaches ease their practice and their stress. Every patient encounter becomes more interesting when the nurse is aware of the possibilities hypnosis offers.

Nurses who want training in hypnosis should seek reputable training organizations that require a professional educational background and licensure for admission. Hypnosis is a powerful tool that can promote health and healing; however, it may do harm if misused (see nontherapeutic suggestions and countering measures). Hypnosis is a tool to be utilized within the auspices of one's profession; it is appropriate for trained nurses to utilize comfort-promoting and health-promoting hypnotherapeutic strategies.

REFERENCES

Bady SL: The best of both worlds: Integrating traditional and Ericksonian hypnosis. Presented at the Fifth International Congress on Ericksonian Approaches to Hypnosis and Psychotherapy, Phoenix, Arizona, December 1992

Barber J, Adrian C: Psychological approaches to the management of pain. New York, Brunner/Mazel, 1982

Benson H: Beyond the relaxation response. New York, Times Books, 1984

Benson H: The relaxation response. New York, William Morrow, 1975

Blankfield R: Suggestion, relaxation, and hypnosis as adjuncts in the care of surgery patients: A review of the literature. Am J Clin Hypn 33(3):172–186, 1991

Crowley R, Mills J: Therapeutic Metaphors for Children and the Child Within. New York, Bruner Mazel, 1986

Erickson M: An introduction to the study and application of hypnosis for pain control. In Erickson M and Rossi E (eds): Innovative Hypnotherapy. New York, Irvington, 1980, pp. 237–245

Erickson M: The Interspersal Hypnotic Technique for Symptom Correction and Pain Control. Am J Clin Hyp 3:198–209, 1966

Erickson M, Rossi E (eds): The Collected Papers of Milton H. Erickson. Vol. I, New York, Irvington, 1980, pp. 237–240

Erickson M, Rossi E, Rossi S: Hypnotic Realities. New York, Irvington, 1976

Ewin D: Relieving suffering—and pain—with hypnosis, Geriatrics 33(6):87–89, 1978

Finkelstein S, Howard M: Cancer prevention: A three year pilot study. Am J Clin Hypn 25(2–3):177–187, 1982

Gardner G, Lubner A: Hypnotherapy for children with cancer: Some current issues. Am J Clin Hypn 25(2–3):135–142, 1982

Hall H: Hypnosis and the immune system: A review with implications for cancer and the psychology of healing. Am J Clin Hypn 25(2–3):92–103, 1982

Hall M: Using relaxation imagery with children with malignancies: A developmental perspective. Am J Clin Hypn 25(2–3):143–149, 1982

Hammond C: Hypnotic suggestions and metaphors. New York, W.W. Norton, 1990

Hilgard E: Divided Consciousness: Multiple Controls in Human Thought and Action. New York, Wiley, 1977

Hilgard J, LeBaron S: Hypnotherapy of pain in children with cancer. Los Altos, California, William Kaufmann, Inc., 1984

Hoffman M: Hypnotic desensitization for the management of anticipatory emesis in chemotherapy. Am J Clin Hypn 25(2–3):173–176, 1982

Kiecolt-Glaser J, Glaser R, Williger D, et al: Psychosocial enhancement of immunocompetence in a geriatric population. Health Psychology 4(1):25–41, 1985

Larkin D: Metaphor, mythology and spiritual development. Addictions Nursing Network 2(4):11–13, 1990

Larkin D: Therapeutic suggestion. In Zahourek RP (ed): Relaxation and Imagery: Tools for Therapeutic Communication and Intervention. Philadelphia, W.B. Saunders Co., 1988, pp. 84–100

Levitan A: Hypnosis in the 1990's and beyond. Am J Clin Hypn 33(3):141–149, 1991

Levy S: Emotions and the progression of cancer: A review. Advances 1(1):10–15, 1984

Locke S, Hornig-Rohan M: Mind and Immunity: Behavioral Immunology. New York, Institute for Advancement of Health, 1983

Margolis C: Hypnotic imagery with cancer patients. Am J Clin Hypn 25(2–3):128–134, 1982

Meares A: A form of intensive meditation associated with the regression of cancer. Am J Clin Hypn 25(2–3):114–121, 1982

Melzack R, Wall P: Pain mechanisms: A new theory. Science Nov. 19:971–979, 1965

Newton B: Hypnosis and cancer. Am J Clin Hypn 25(2–3):89–91, 1982

Newton B: The use of hypnosis in the treatment of cancer patients. Am J Clin Hypn 25(2–3):104–113, 1982

Oliver G: A cancer patient and her family: A case study. Am J Clin Hypn 25(2–3):156–160, 1982

Olness K: Hypnosis: The power of attention. In Goleman D, Gurin J (eds): Mind Body Medicine. Yonkers, NY, Consumer Reports Books, 1993, pp. 277–290

Rapkin D, Straubing M, Holroyd J: Guided imagery, hypnosis, and recovery from head and neck cancer surgeries. Int J Clin Exp Hypn 39(4):215–226, 1991

Redd W, Rosenberger P, Hendler C: Controlling chemotherapy side effects. Am J Clin Hypn 25(2–3):161–172, 1982

Rogers M: Nursing science and the space age. Nurs Sci Quart 5:27–34, 1992

Rosen S: My Voice Will Go With You: The Teaching Tales of Milton H. Erickson. New York, W.W. Norton & Co, 1982, p. 82

Rosenberg S: Hypnosis in cancer care: Imagery to enhance the control of the physiological and psychological "side-effects" of cancer therapy. Am J Clin Hypn 25(2–3):122–127, 1982

Selye H: Stress without distress. New York, The New American Library, Inc., 1975

Spiegel D: Social support. In Goleman D, Gurin J (eds): Mind Body Medicine. Consumers Report Books, Yonkers, NY, 1993, pp. 331–350

Steggles S, Stam H, Fehr R: Hypnosis and cancer: An annotated bibliography 1960–1985. Am J Clin Hypn 29(4):281–290, 1985

Watkins J, Watkins H: Dissociation and displacement: Where goes the "Ouch"? Am J Clin Hypn 33(1):1–10, 1990

Yapko M: A comparative analysis of direct and indirect hypnotic communication styles. Am J Clin Hypn 25(1):270–276, 1983

Zahourek R: Clinical hypnosis and therapeutic suggestion in patient care. New York, Brunner/Mazel, 1990

14

Psychotherapy

Ann Damsbo

INTRODUCTION

Hypnosis is a useful tool in psychotherapy, and whether one actively uses hypnosis or not, it is valuable to have a basic understanding of its benefits and limitations. The therapist must always remember to get the patient's permission to manipulate symptoms. Also, the therapist must confer with attending physicians to let them know that symptoms may be masked or altered.

One patient who had been given the suggestion, in hypnosis, that he could experience a feeling of warmth and comfort instead of pain was seen on the weekend by a covering physician, not the doctor who had requested the hypnosis. When asked about his pain the patient replied that his knee just felt warm. The physician then ordered a series of tests to rule out infection!

A 35-year-old army major thought he might try hypnosis as a means of quitting smoking. His doctor agreed that it was a good idea and added that something might be done at the same time to diminish the pain the major was experiencing from a compound fracture of the tibia and fibula. The major had broken his leg in a parachute jump, the second in a series of three to qualify as a graduate of the army parachute school. The black humor about the school's students went like this: The first jump separated the men from the boys; the second separated the men from the idiots; and on the third, only the idiots jumped! The major was understandably reluctant to make the third jump with his leg bones pinned together with metal reinforcements.

The patient readily entered into hypnosis and was an excellent subject. Following the suggestion to quit smoking I casually gave the authoritative suggestion—without asking for ideomotor signal permission—"You *will* be able to walk back to your bed without crutches and without pain." The patient was able to walk back to the bed without support or pain.

Delighted with the seeming success of my suggestions, I returned that afternoon with the intent of reinforcing the suggestions and discovered the major smoking, with an ashtray overflowing with stubbed-out butts and ashes. He was resistant to re-enter hypnosis and was very angry without knowing why. It turned out that he unconsciously thought he needed the pain in his leg to avoid making the third and final jump, so he negated all the hypnotic suggestions. As soon as he learned that because of his leg injury and the internal fixation he would no longer be eligible for parachute duty, he no longer needed the pain. He fully recovered and was re-assigned to other duties and pursued hypnosis for smoking cessation.

This example illustrates the importance of using hypnosis only in your own field of expertise. My meager defense for this gross error in my judgment was that the major was only my fourth hypnosis patient, and I was still a physical therapist not yet fully trained as a psychologist. This situation also illustrates the importance of using a permissive approach. Substituting *"may"* for *"will"* makes a difference. Usually the patient will save himself from such lack of expertise, but it is not wise to count on it!

VARIOUS USES OF HYPNOSIS

In psychotherapy, hypnosis can be used for behavior modification. Many practitioners use hypnosis to help patients adhere to a diet or to quit smoking. Neufeld and Lynn (1988) report that hypnotic interventions in smoking cessation range from 0% to 94% and that their own 1985 study showed a 20% to 60% reported abstinence in a 5-year follow-up.

Andersen discovered a statistically significant positive association between hypnotic ability and weight loss. In a meta-analysis of hypnosis as an adjunct to psychotherapy for weight loss, Kirsch examined 18 studies, each comparing hypnotically prepared subjects with a control group. For all studies, with a follow-up ranging from 4 months to 2 years, the hypnosis clients lost more weight and kept it off longer than the patients who had behavioral–cognitive psychotherapy alone.

Some therapists make hypnosis audio tapes that clients can play at home, as often as necessary. The hypnotic suggestions for weight loss may include suggestions for specific eating habits (e.g., chew your food slowly, leave some food on your plate, eat only when you feel hungry, stop eating when you no longer feel hungry, don't eat standing up, don't eat in between meals, or don't eat after dinner) (Temes 1994).

Hypnosis can help alter sleep habits. Coe reported a case of a 16-year-old boy who had nightly episodes of night terrors, followed by violent behavior (Coe 1989). The patient was given posthypnotic suggestions that he would gradually become less aware of outside sounds

that had precipitated the night terrors. The terrors decreased with three episodes during the next 3 weeks, and then the patient was symptom free. On follow-up 3 months later, he had no further night terrors.

Hypnosis can be used to treat paraphilias. Polk reported successful treatment of a 38-year-old man who had a 14-year history of exhibitionism (Polk 1983). Hypnosis was employed during the 22-month court-appointed treatment period. Stava describes treatment of a man in his early twenties who admitted to molesting more than 20 different children, both male and female, over a period of 6 years. Stava combined hypnosis, induced dreams as described by Sacerdote (1967), and the affect bridge technique described by Watkins (1971), to successfully treat the patient as measured by penile tumescence.

Mac Hover describes four cases of successful treatment of post-traumatic stress disorder, using hypnosis for five to nine sessions. Length of treatment was positively correlated to length of time between trauma and treatment (Mac Hover 1985).

Somer describes a technique for a rape victim and her husband. Under hypnosis the husband imagined himself wrestling with the attacker and severely beating him, even though the attack occurred before the husband had met his wife. After the session, for the first time, the husband was able to be supportive of his wife (Somer 1990).

Muthe reported on a study using image rehearsal in hypnosis. Students became comfortable and familiar with newly acquired skills by rehearsing upcoming school situations. By rehearsing and visualizing a test situation while under hypnosis, students increased reading speed and comprehension during the actual examinations (Muthe 1967).

Psychotherapists can use hypnosis for peak performance. Callen compared runners who used autohypnosis with a control group. The trance group experienced hypnotic phenomena such as forgetting where they were, inability to recall events during the run, experiencing a floating sensation while running, forming mental pictures, counteracting unpleasant symptoms, and creativity at the 0.001 level of significance compared to the control group. Performance was improved (Callen 1983).

Pearson reported a first-hand report of a skull fracture from a falling brick in which he described his use of self-hypnosis to control pain and maintain consciousness (Pearson 1966).

Patients who have bulimia are easily hypnotized and usually dissociate more readily than do nonpatients or patients with other eating disorders (Kranhold 1992). Whether this is a contributing cause of their disease or an accompanying phenomenon is still under investigation. It is useful, however, to take advantage of their high hypnotizability and offer bulimics hypnotic suggestions for proper food intake.

Vanderlinden and Vandereycken used hypnosis in treating more than 50 female bulimic patients. Eating behavior was normalized, but at a fixed time and, if possible, at a fixed place. The patients were instructed to visualize themselves eating a normal meal. Under hypnosis they were given instructions to eat slowly and enjoy the taste of the food, pay attention to hunger and satiation cues, and relax after the meal by reading, watching a movie, or enjoying a pleasant daydream. The patients were instructed to plan binges—preferably with a nonfavorite food—and to follow with an activity. Often, suggesting binge eating has a paradoxical effect. Patients in this study showed changes in eating habits.

Hypnosis is often used to treat anxiety. A woman planning a honeymoon trip to Europe once witnessed a plane crash and was anxious about boarding a plane. The Stein Clenched Fist technique (discussed later) was used as part of the induction. Under hypnosis the patient was reminded that the plane she saw crash was not the one she would be on. She was told she could clasp the dominant fist any time she liked, in order to achieve calm relaxation. The woman reported that she had a pleasant flight.

I had the experience of once being on a plane when a woman asked to exchange her window seat with my aisle seat because she experienced anxiety on take-off and landing. I initiated a simple induction by asking her to stare at the "fasten seat belt" sign whenever it was lit. No mention was made of hypnosis, but the woman went into a light trance whenever she looked at the lit sign. At the conclusion of the trip she reported that it was her best flight ever.

Children who are well into adulthood may still hunger for parental approval. Hypnosis can create memories by enabling the patient to hear the approval that was usually withheld. Even after the parent's death, in hypnosis the patient can see that absent parent attending an important event that was missed in reality and hear the withheld praise.

Stein Clenched Fist Technique

The late Calvert Stein, MD, was an active member of the American Society of Clinical Hypnosis. He developed the clenched fist technique, and the description follows: After induction of hypnosis, Stein would ask a patient to listen for three pen taps and then recall a happy occasion. Then, the patient would be instructed to close the dominant hand into a fist. This action provided a safe haven for times when further therapy might become too threatening. Then, Stein would request the patient to listen for two taps and then remember an

unhappy experience. The patient was instructed to allow the distress, physical or emotional, to develop long enough for recognition, at which time the patient would have no further need for the physical or emotional discomfort. The patient could then displace the distress to the nondominant fist. Then the patient could neutralize the unpleasant memory by again squeezing the dominant fist while recalling the happy memory.

Stein combined the use of modeling clay with hypnosis in working with alcoholic patients. Under hypnosis the patient would permit his hands to freely model the clay after choosing a color to fit his mood. One patient was given hypnotic suggestions to alter his behavior without altering his drinking habits. Later, after altering his work, home, and driving activities, a casual suggestion was made to decrease by one drop the amount of alcohol in each drink. He soon tired of this and after using only one drop of alcohol in his ginger ale stopped using it at all. His drinking problems ceased, but hypnotherapy continued using the Stein Clenched Fist technique (Stein 1969).

Marital and Family Therapy

Hypnosis can be used to treat marital and family problems. Helping family members "walk a mile in each other's shoes" is an effective psychodrama method that can be enhanced with hypnosis. The protagonists can start to discuss the problem(s), while the therapist acts as director. When protagonists disagree, the director instructs them to switch roles and play the scene from their partner's viewpoint. When a crucial issue is reached, hypnosis can be used to bring the problem into focus and explore the psychodynamics involved. The psychotherapist can teach the clients to use an affect bridge to go into hypnosis and age regress to a time when an incident may have significant relevance to the current problem. This technique might uncover something as simple as a transference, where one spouse reminds the other of a disliked person.

A man complaining that his marriage was unsatisfactory entered into a psychodrama. He played the role of returning from an overnight trip. The "wife," not knowing the man's habits, stood ready to welcome him with a hug and a kiss. Instead, the protagonist devoted his first attention to his children and the family dog, ignoring his wife. When he was hypnotized and asked to switch roles he realized for the first time how slighted his wife felt.

A man separated from his wife and torn between her and his mistress was hypnotized and invited to project himself 5 years into the future with each of the women. He realized, for the first time, that he was repulsed by his wife's smoking.

The wife, seen separately, was eager to preserve her marriage; she was similarly invited to project herself into the future while under hypnosis and visualize her life with and without her husband. Knowing she was alienating her husband by smoking, she expressed a desire to stop. It was suggested that she could release endorphins with an ideomotor finger response that would give her a natural "high" far better than anything she could get from a cigarette. At last report she was not smoking. While the matter is not yet resolved, both are working toward reconciliation.

Ideomotor Responses

Ideomotor responses are often used during hypnosis sessions to help the psychotherapist understand what is going on with the patient. Pratt et al noted that a true ideomotor response is either slow and trembling or quick and jerky, while a voluntary movement is more rapid and smooth (Pratt 1984). Hilgard and Hilgard (1965) discovered the "hidden observer" phenomenon through ideomotor response. While conducting a demonstration of hypnotic deafness with a blind volunteer, E.R. Hilgard asked the hypnotically deaf student for an ideomotor finger response if some part of the individual could hear him. The student responded by raising a finger, and after coming out of hypnosis asked why his finger had lifted.

Using the Stein Clenched Fist technique with ideomotor finger signals is helpful in uncovering the cause of a psychogenic condition. An obese patient, much to her surprise, gave a negative ideomotor response to Dr. David Cheek's question, "Do you tend to dislike your present body image?" Further analysis revealed that she associated the obesity with health, having been underweight when she was ill (Cheek 1968).

A patient in her early forties had had several episodes of sudden onset of numbness and paralysis in her left upper extremity. She was referred for hypnotherapy. No paralysis was noted on arrival. She was instructed in the use of ideomotor responses and then asked the following questions:

Is there some psychological reason for this symptom?
Ideomotor response: Yes

Is it all right to learn what this reason is?
Ideomotor response: Yes

Is this symptom due to some inner conflict?
Ideomotor response: No

Are you punishing someone with this symptom?
Ideomotor response: Yes

Do you know whom?
Verbal response: My husband

Do you know why?
Verbal response: No
Ideomotor response: Yes

Please go back in time to the first time you suffered this condition and when you are there let your "Yes" finger rise.
(Pause) Ideomotor response: Yes

Now do you know why you have this symptom?
Verbal response: No
Ideomotor response: Yes

Squeeze your left fist on the count of three and something may pop into your mind that will help you know what this symptom means to you.
(Squeezes fist on count of three.)

What did you think of?
I just learned that my husband was cheating on me.

When your arm is paralyzed, who does the house work?
My husband (big smile). He waits on me too.

It seems a shame to put an end to all of that.
Right!

Isn't it inconvenient to have your arm paralyzed, especially when he isn't around?
Yes. It's hard to diaper a baby with one arm.

Would you like to learn to turn the symptom on and off at will?
Verbal response: Yes!
Ideomotor response: Yes

False Memories

Lay hypnotists have been especially successful in probing for and eliciting false memories. Some psychologists have also probed for sexual abuse using the type of leading questions that tend to implant false memories. It is true that when one is looking for something one is apt to find it, especially when using hypnosis to "enhance recall" without sufficient care to avoid confabulation.

A lay hypnotist hypnotized a young man and "discovered" that the man had been sexually abused by the late Cardinal Joseph Bernadine. When the highly respected Cardinal denied the charge, the accuser agreed to be seen by Dr. William Wester, an expert in forensic hypnosis and a highly successful psychologist and author. While working with Dr. Wester, the patient realized that it was a false memory and that no molestation had occurred. Unfortunately, the case made international headlines and Cardinal Bernadine suffered from the devastating notoriety.

Spontaneous Self-Hypnosis

Trauma, pain, and fright can produce a state of altered consciousness during which the patient is very receptive to hypnotic suggestion. An 11-year-old Taiwanese girl was having reconstructive surgery following polio. She had had her cast removed and the orthopedic surgeon was molding the ankle following a triple arthrodesis. The child looked as if she were asleep. When asked if she had had anesthesia, the surgeon replied, "No, but she certainly acts as though she had." I lifted one of the patient's arms and it remained in the catatonic posture. When I remarked that the child was in hypnosis, the surgeon said, "Whatever it is, it is helping because the procedure is usually very painful." Because I was new to Taiwan and did not yet speak Taiwanese, there was only nonverbal communication with the patient. Although she had no formal training in self-hypnosis, she intuitively used that altered state of consciousness to escape from pain.

HYPNOSIS AND SYSTEMATIC DESENSITIZATION

Phobias

Wolpe described systematic desensitization using a hierarchy of symptoms and starting with the least threatening factor and increasing to the most threatening, while gradually desensitizing the patient over a period of weeks (Wolpe 1969). With hypnosis, the process can be accelerated. When I worked with a claustrophobic navy submariner who would walk up three flights of stairs rather than take the elevator, I combined Stein's Clenched Fist technique, hypnosis, and Wolpe's systematic desensitization. In hypnosis the patient was asked to create a safe haven by closing his dominant fist and imagining himself in a place of his choosing, experiencing it with all his senses (seeing, hearing, smelling, tasting, and feeling). He was told he could return to his safe place anytime he felt the need simply by closing the hand he wrote with. He was asked to imagine the outside door of an elevator, grip his nondominant fist and experience the fear as long as needed. Then he was to drop the fear on the floor and close the dominant fist to experience the safe haven, and to conceal the fear on the floor. He was next asked to imagine himself stepping into the elevator but leaving the door open and to repeat the fist-closing sequence.

The patient was asked to visualize progressive scenes culminating in visualizing himself aboard the submarine and even shut in a closet in which his shipmates, upon learning of his claustrophobia, had once placed him. Each vision ended with him clenching his dominant fist and feeling safe.

At the end of the first session, the therapist accompanied the patient to the elevator for actual, rather than imagined, reinforcement practice. The patient did well until the third floor, where two corpsmen entered the elevator. One said, "I hope we don't get stuck here like we did yesterday!" The patient immediately closed his dominant right hand, and he stayed calm for the remainder of the ride.

At his second hypnotherapy session he reported improvement in his ability to remain calm on board the boat, even withstanding the harassment of his shipmates.

Bad Habits

Systematic desensitization can be used for stuttering, nail biting, hair pulling, as well as other compulsive behaviors. With any habit needing to be eradicated the patient can be age regressed by asking him to re-experience or see himself before the first episode of the habit. The patient is asked to close the nondominant fist on signal (a tap) and experience the emotions felt immediately before the first time he did the habit. He is asked to hold the emotion in his hand until he realizes these early emotions no longer have to be experienced in the present time. He then drops the emotions on the floor and closes the dominant fist to experience his safe haven. The patient is next asked to repeat the process for future episodes of the habit. The patient can continue to do this on his own for several minutes.

La Scala combines hypnosis with desensitization when he suggests there is nothing wrong with thumb-sucking as long as the child is "playing fair" (La Scala 1968). He explains that the child has 10 fingers, and the child admits he plays favorites with only one finger and is therefore not a good sport. In order to play fair, the child agrees to give equal time to each digit. With the child in hypnosis, La Scala then directs the child to start sucking his favorite finger and on the count of one move to the next, on the count of two, move to the next finger, and so on. His final suggestions can be "Now that's fine. All your fingers had the same amount of attention. You can suck them any time you like, but remember always to do it this way." After a few days of being fair and a good sport the child becomes bored and the follow-up appointment is usually canceled as the child no longer sucks his thumb.

Induction

The following induction is a typical, verbal hypnotic one, after which psychotherapeutic suggestions are given:

With your eyes closed, roll your eyeballs up as though you were looking at a spot on the inside of your forehead. Notice how stressful this is. Now relax your eyes and notice how much more comfortable this is. Let the comfort spread to your face and jaw so that your upper and lower teeth are not quite touching. Let the relaxation spread to your forehead, neck, shoulders, arms, forearms, and hands.

Take a deep breath and hold it for a slow count of five. Notice the tension, exhale, and notice the relaxation. Let it spread to your back, abdomen, pelvis, hips, thighs, and legs, all the way down to your toes.

Now, please think of a time when you were happy and comfortable. Imagine yourself in a very special place. It can be a real place or an imaginary place, a place you have been to before or a place you would like to go, indoors or out, or any combination of these.

Now, please close the hand that you write with into a gentle fist. You can enjoy thinking of your special place with all of your senses. See the beauty, notice the lighting, shadows, and colors, and hear the sounds—or if it is a quiet place—enjoy the silence; smell the fragrances and perhaps taste the tastes. Most importantly, feel the comfort. Because it is your own mental creation, it can be any temperature, any kind of weather, any season of the year. At any time you can go to this place of comfort and safety simply by closing your fist.

When you are in this state you have control over functions such as blood pressure, pulse, and heart rate and circulation. To prove this to yourself, imagine you can see the arteries of the index finger of your other hand. These arteries have muscles in the walls, and when these muscles relax the diameter of the artery is larger, permitting the blood to flow more freely, causing the finger to get warm. If we have a very sensitive thermometer we could measure the change in temperature. Your finger can signal this change in temperature by lifting up, seemingly all by itself in twitchy, jerky movements quite different from the way it lifts up when you do it on purpose.

Imagine yourself going down (or up) a flight of stairs, doubling your relaxation with each step. You can go into this state any time it is appropriate for you to do so simply by closing your eyes and closing your dominant hand and remembering how you feel right now. Each time you practice you will find you can go more deeply into hypnosis, more quickly and more comfortably.

After the induction, suggestions are given and then the patient is slowly guided back to the regular state.

PERSONAL USE OF HYPNOSIS

I was diagnosed with multiple sclerosis in 1958. I'd been having symptoms for 3 years, and I had no experience with hypnosis. I volunteered as a subject in a nurse's in-service demonstration on hypnosis. During my first hypnosis class, the instructor did not know about my multiple sclerosis and used an induction with an arm levitation technique. I had weakness in my right shoulder and hadn't been able to lift my arm above my head for quite some time. During the class, I sat with my weak right arm over my head for 20 minutes.

I was also using a cane, a short leg brace, and an eye patch because of double vision. I wanted to stay on duty as an Army physical therapist, but my symptoms were troubling, and, finally, I was medically evacuated to Letterman Army Hospital in San Francisco. There I saw a neurologist who said if I could rid myself of the brace, cane, and eye patch he would return me to active duty. I had the opportunity at this time to take classes in hypnosis from Dr. David Cheek and was able to use hypnosis to strengthen my weak muscles and do eye exercises to overcome the double vision—in spite of having been told that I was too old for improvement.

My doctor returned me to active duty where I served for 5 more years as a regular army officer. I opted for retirement after 15 years in the army and went on to get graduate degrees in psychology. My internship was in a burn unit, where I was recruited because of my ability to use hypnosis.

Shortly after graduation, I was on a cruise when I was struck by a severe headache. Because I had recently done a study on tension headaches (Damsbo 1979), I viewed this headache as an opportunity to practice what I had been using with my patients. This practice worked well for 3 days. On the fourth day I remembered that one should know the cause of a symptom before using hypnosis to mask it. Using self-hypnosis I determined that I had had such a headache before, when I was suffering from retrobulbar neuritis. I checked my vision and noted that the central vision in my left eye was gone. I didn't feel that I could trust the ship's doctor to know any more about my condition than I did, and I predicted that my neurologist would prescribe steroids to cool the optic nerve. With hypnosis, I reminded myself that my body could produce more steroids, so I visualized steroids the color of Pepto-Bismol coating my painful optic nerve. I experienced immediate relief of pain and 48 hours later my central vision had returned, though color vision was somewhat diminished. On returning to work I told my skeptical doctor of my experience. He remarked that retrobulbar neuritis couldn't clear up that quickly. I agreed that it never had before. Subsequent visual-evoked response tests indicated that I did have retrobulbar neuritis and that it did improve. My doctors were stunned. I continue to use hypnosis personally and professionally.

REFERENCES

Arnold MB: On the mechanism of suggestion and hypnosis. J Abn Psychol 41:107–128, 1946

Barber TX: Suggested ('hypnotic') behavior: The trance paradigm versus an alternative paradigm. *In* Fromm E, Shor RE (eds): Hypnosis: Research Developments and Perspectives. Chicago, Aldine Publishing, 1972

Callen KE: Auto-hypnosis in long distance running. Am J Clin Hypn 26(1):35–40, 1983

Capafono A, Amigo S: Emotional self-regulation therapy for smoking reduction. Int J Clin Exp Hypn 43(1):117–119, 1995

Cheek DB, LeCron M: Clinical Hypnotherapy. New York, Grune & Stratton, 1968

Chevreul J: De la Bafuette Divinatoire, du Pendule dit Exploratuer et dea Tables Tournantes au Point de Vue de l'Histoire de la Critique et de la Methode Experimental. Parie, Mallet-Richelieu, 1854

Choy DC: Syllabus on Hypnosis & Handbook of Therapeutic Suggestions. Des Plains, MI, American Society of Clinical Hypnosis Education and Research Foundation, 1973, p. 117

Damsbo AM: Clinical Hypnosis, A Case Management Approach. Cincinnati, Behavioral Sciences Center, Inc, 1987 Wm. Wester II Ed.

Damsbo AM: Tension headache treated with hypnosis. *In* Burrows GD, Collison DR, Dennerstein L (eds): Hypnosis. Amsterdam, Elsevier/North Holland, 1979

Damsbo AM: The Effect of Post Hypnotic Suggestion on Academic Achievement [unpublished PhD thesis]. School of Human Behavior, United States International University, 1974

Erickson MH: A special inquiry with Aldous Huxley into the nature and character of various states of consciousness. Am J Clin Hypn 8(1):14–33, 1965

Erickson MH: A Syllabus on Hypnosis and Handbook of Therapeutic Suggestions. American Society of Clinical Hypnosis–Education and Research Foundation, 1973, pp. 135–137

Erickson MH: Historical note on the hand levitation and other ideomotor techniques. Am J Clin Hypn IV:260–269, 1961

Erickson MH: Naturalistic techniques of hypnosis. Am J Clin Hypn 7:3–8, 1958

Erickson MH: Pediatric hypnotherapy. Am J Clin Hypn 1(1):25–29, 1958

Hartland J: The value of ego strengthening procedures prior to direct symptom removal under hypnosis. Am J Clin Hypn 2:89–93, 1953

Hilgard ER: Hypnosis in the Relief of Pain. New York, Wm Kaufmann, Inc., 1975

Hull CL: Hypnosis and Suggestibility, An Experimental Approach. New York, Appleton-Century-Crofts, 1933

Kirsch I, Montgomery G, Sapirstein G: Hypnosis as an adjunct to cognitive-behavioral psychotherapy. J Consult Clin Psychol 63:214–220, 1995

Koe GK: Hypnotic treatment of sleep terror disorder: A case report. Am J Clin Hypn 32(1):36–40, 1989

Kranhold C, Baumann U, Fichter M: Hypnotizability in bulimic patients and controls. Eur Arch Psychiatry Clin Neurosci 242(2–3): 72–76, 1992

Kroger WS: Clinical and Experimental Hypnosis, 2nd ed. New York, J.B. Lippincott, 1977

Loftus E: Reconstructing memory, the incredible eyewitness. Psychol Today 1974

Mac Hover FJ: Effects of hypnosis in the brief therapy of post-traumatic stress disorders. Int J Clin Exp Hypn 33(1):6–14, 1985

Meares A: A System of Medical Hypnosis. New York, W.B. Saunders Co., 1961

Mordey TR: The relationship between certain motives and suggestibility [unpublished master's thesis]. Roosevelt University, 1960

Muthe PHC: Increased reading comprehension through hypnosis. Am J Clin Hypn 9(4):262–266, 1967

Neufeld, S Lynn: A single session group self-hypnosis smoking cessation treatment. Int J Clin Exp Hypn 36(2):75–79, 1988a

Pearson RE: Communication and motivation. Am J Clin Hypn 9(1):18–25, 1966

Polk WM: Treatment of exhibitionism in an 18-year-old male by hypnotically assisted covert sensitization. Int J Clin Exp Hypn 31(3):132–138, 1983

Pratt GJ, Wood DP, Alman BM: A Clinical Hypnosis Primer. San Diego, Psychology and Consulting Associates Press, 1984

Schultz JH: Das Autogene Training. Stuttgart, George Thieme Verlag, 1932

Somer E: Brief simultaneous couple hypnotherapy with a rape victim and her husband. Int J Clin Exp Hypn 38(1):1–5, 1990

Stava L: The use of hypnotic uncovering techniques in the treatment of pedophilia, a brief communication. Int J Clin Exp Hypn 32(4):350–355, 1984

Stein C: Practical Psychotherapy in Nonpsychiatric Specialties. Springfield, Illinois, Charles C Thomas Publishers, 1969

Temes R: Hypnotic Suggestions for Controlling Your Food Intake. Brooklyn, 1994

Vanderlinden J, Vandereycken W: The use of hypnosis in the treatment of bulimia nervosa. Int J Clin Exp Hypn 38(2):101–111, 1990

Watkins N: The affect bridge, a hypnotherapy technique. Int J Clin Exp Hypn 19(1):25–30, 1971

Weitzenhoffer AM: General Techniques of Hypnotism. New York, Grune & Stratton, 1957

Wolpe J: The Practice of Behavioral Therapy. New York, Pergamon Press, 1969

Index

Note: Page numbers in *italics* refer to illustrations.

A

Abreaction, 25
Academic performance, anxiety related to, 89, 152
image rehearsal preparation for, 152
Adolescents, hypnotherapy for, 81
Adrenocortico-hypothalamo-pituitary axis, 44–45
Adrenocortico-sympatho-hypothalamic axis, 45
Adrenomedullo-sympatho-hypothalamic axis, 44–46
Aerosols, asthma therapy using, 117, 118
tonicity of, 118
Age regression, 12, 16
hypnosis role in, 12, 16
Airway, asthma effect on, 116–120
mechanical irritation of, 118
Alcohol abuse, hypnotherapy for, 152
pediatric, 90
Allergy, asthma triggered by, 116
hypersensitivity as, 35–36
immune response in, 34–36
Alpha waves, hypnosis effect on, 9
Amenorrhea, 73
causes of, 73
treatment of, 73
Ammonia, hypnotic susceptibility tested with, 80
trance-induced nonreactivity to, 80
Analgesia. See also *Anesthesia; Hypnosis; Pain.*
emergency room treatment using, 60
intravenous, 97–99, *98*
pharmacologic vs. nonpharmacologic, 97–99, *98*
radiology patient need for, 97–99, *98*
stress-induced, 45–46
Anemia, sickle cell disease with, 86–87
Anesthesia, 43–55. See also *Analgesia; Hypnosis.*
awareness during, 51–55
retrieval of in hypnosis, 12–13
suggestibility based on, 51–55
chemical, early history of, 28
dental, 132–133
emergency room, 59–64. See also *Emergency room.*
glove, 133
dental patient with, 133
hypnotic suggestion for, 2, 110, 133
oncology patient need for, 110
presurgical intervention effect on, 48–55
cost effectiveness of, 49–50
stress response produced by, 43–46, 53–55
tooth extraction hypnoanesthesia as, 133, 138
Animal magnetism, 23–25
Antidepressant drugs, quadriplegia therapy and, 86–87
Anxiety. See also *Fear.*
child with insect in ear and, 84
dental patient with, 131–132
immune response affected by, 34
neuroendocrine response to, 45–46
oncology patient with, 110–113

Anxiety (*Continued*)
presurgical intervention for, 49–55
procedure pain with, 82–84
radiology technique causing, 96–97, *98*
sleep disorder with, 88–89
stress response caused by, 46
surgery causing, 46, 51–55
test-related (academic), 89–90, 152
Arm levitation induction, 2, 133
Arm rub induction, 133
Artificial somnambulism, 25
Asthma, 115–125
allergy role in, 116
biology of, 116–118
causal factors of, 116–119
emergency room treatment of, 61–62
epidemiology of, 115–116
extrinsic vs. intrinsic, 116
hyperventilation in, 118
hypnotherapy in, 116–123
breathing retraining in, 122
induction method for, 122–123
literature review of, 117–120
nursing-based, 145–146
susceptibility related to, 121
symptom challenge technique in, 123
pediatric, 124–125
psychological factors in, 115–116, 118–122
relaxation therapy counterproductive in, 120–121
socioeconomic aspects of, 115–116
tape recording use in, 123
Atavistic phenomenon theory, 15
Athletics, hypnosis affecting, 8, 152
Atrial fibrillation, emergency room treatment of, 61
Attention, hypnosis definition related to, 1, 141
Attention deficit hyperactivity disorder, 90
hypnotherapy in, 90
Autoimmune disease, neuroendocrine effects in, 34
Automatic handwriting, dissociation relation to, 15
Autonomy, self-hypnosis effect on, 10
Avoiders, presurgical preparation of, 51
Awareness, anesthesia state and, 12–13
hypnosis definition related to, 1

B

Babinski reflex, age regression manifested in, 12, 16
Baquet, magnetic filings in, 24
Behavior, habitual, 155–156
hypnosis theory related to, 16
hypnotherapeutic modification of, 152–153, 155–156
Bleeding, hypnotherapeutic control of, 136, 146
Bleeding time, hypnosis effect on, 9
Blood pressure, hypnosis effect on, 9
Body image, hypnosis effect on, 10
Braid, James, 28

Brain, 16–17
hemispheres of, 16–17
function regions of, 16–17
hypnosis theory related to, 16–17
laterality of, 16–17
left, 17
right, 17
pain pathways in, 45
stress response pathways in, 45
Brain waves, hypnosis effect on, 9
Breathing rate, hypnosis effect on, 9
Breech presentation, 72
conversion of, 72
Broca's area, 16
Bronchoconstriction, asthma with, 116–119
Bruxism, hypnotherapy in, 135
Bulimia, hypnotherapy use in, 152–153
Burn injury, 62–64
emergency room treatment of, 62–64
pediatric patient affected by, 83–84
suggestions presented to the patient with, 62–64

C

Calm place imagery, 84, 86, 90
cultural differences affecting, 90
relaxation induction with, 84, 86, 90
Cancer. See *Oncology.*
Carbon dioxide, hyperventilation decrease of, 124
Catalepsy, hypnotic suggestion causing, 2
Catharsis, mesmerism use of, 25
CF (cystic fibrosis), 125
Chemotherapy, emesis anticipation due to, 111
relaxation therapy with, 110–113, 143–144
Chest pain, emergency room treatment of, 62
Child molester, hypnotherapy for, 152
Children. See *Pediatric patients.*
Chronic obstructive pulmonary disease (COPD), 123–124
Claustrophobia, desensitization for, 155
hypnotherapy for, 155
oncology patient with, 111–112
Clenched fist, hypnosis induction using, 153–156
Cognitive function, 80–82
atavistic phenomenon theory related to, 15
hypnosis effect on, 10–11
pediatric patient developmental stage and, 80–82
Coin drop induction, 133
Colles' fracture, emergency room treatment of, 61
Comfortable place imagery, 156
Communication, nonverbal, oncology patient and, 108
Conception, 76
stress effect on, 76
Conditioning, immune response modulated with, 33–36
taste stimulus used for, 33–34
Condyloma, venereal disease with, 75–76

Confusion, hypnosis induction using, 2
Consciousness, 14–15
  altered state of, definition of, 80
  special state of, hypnosis theory based
    on, 14
Convulsions, mesmeric, 25
COPD (chronic obstructive pulmonary
    disease), 123–124
Coping behavior, stress response and, 46,
    47–48
  surgery anticipation in, 46, 47–48
Cortisol, hypnosis effect on blood level
    of, 9
  stress response role of, 44–45
Costs, asthma treatment and, 115–116
  nursing hypnotherapy effectiveness and, 148
  presurgical preparation impact on, 49–50
  radiology hypnotherapy reduction of, 99
Coughing, chronic, 87–88
  "habit," 87
  hypnotherapy related to, 87–88
  pediatric patient with, 87–88
Crisis, mesmeric, 25
Cultural sensitivity, hypnosis and, 91
Cystic fibrosis (CF), 125

D

Daydreaming, imagery in, 11
Death and dying, oncology patient fear of,
    107, 113
Deformity, "silver fork", Colles' fracture
    with, 61
Delivery (pregnancy), 69–72
  training methods for, 69–72
Delta waves, hypnosis effect on, 9
Dentistry, 131–138
  anxiety aroused by, 131–132
  bruxism treatment in, 135
  gag reflex in, 135
  hypnotherapy used in, 131–138
    abnormal reaction to, 137–138
    induction methods for, 132–135
  pediatric, 136–137
  sedation in, 132–133
Depression, gunshot wound with, 86–87
  hypnotherapy for, 86–87
  immune response affected by, 34–35
Desensitization, claustrophobia treated by,
    155
  systematic, 155
Development, stage of, pediatric, 80–82
Diazepam, radiology patient sedated with,
    97–98, 98
Dietary management, early history of, 29
  eating habits and, 152
  hypnotism used for, 29, 152–153
Dislocation, shoulder, emergency room
    treatment of, 60–61
Dissociation, 15–16
  definition of, 15
  hypnosis theory related to, 15–16
  "laughing place" concept used in, 60–61
Distraction technique, pain management
    using, 82–83
Diving reflex, stress response role of, 44
Double-bind, definition of, 17
Dream catcher, 88
Dreaming, 14
  daydreaming, 11
  lucid, 14

Drug abuse, hypnotherapy for, 90
  pediatric, 90
Dysmenorrhea, 74
  hypnotherapy in, 74
Dysphagia, hypnotherapy for, 81

E

Ear, insect in, child with, 84
Earthquake, immune response affected by,
    37–38
Eating, binge, 152–153
  hypnotherapeutic modification of, 29,
    152–153
  tape recording related to, 152
Economic factors, asthma treatment and,
    115–116
  presurgical preparation impact on, 49–50
  radiology hypnotherapy reduction of, 99
Ego, hypnosis theory related to, 16
  strengthening of, 144
Electroencephalography (EEG), hypnosis
    effect on, 9
Emergency room, 59–64
  asthma in, 61–62, 145–146
  atrial fibrillation in, 61
  burn injury in, 62–64
  chest pain in, 62
  Colles' fracture in, 61
  dislocated shoulder in, 60–61
  hypnotherapy used in, 59–64
  lacerations in, 61
  nurse therapeutic suggestions in, 145–146
  staff emotional tone in, 59–60
  unintentional comments in, 59–60
Emesis, anticipatory, 111, 143
  chemotherapy with, 111, 143–144
  gag reflex hypersensitivity and, 135
  pregnancy causing, 66–67
Emotion. See also Anxiety; Fear.
  asthma triggered by, 116, 118
  hypnosis effect on, 11
Encopresis, hypnotherapy for, 89
  pediatric, 89
Endocrine system, stress response role of,
    43–46
Enuresis, 89
  hypnotherapy for, 89
  pediatric, 89
Eosinophilic granulomatous lung disease,
    86
  hypnotherapy for, 86
  pediatric patient with, 85–86
Erickson, Milton, his own child comforted
    by, 82–83
  hypnotic suggestion methods of, 2
Eroticism, hypnotic trance with, 15
Esdaile, James, 28
Estrogen, unopposed, 73
Evoked potentials, hypnosis effect on, 9
Examinations (academic), anxiety related
    to, 89, 152
  image rehearsal for, 152
Exhibitionism, hypnotherapy for, 152
Eye, retrobulbar neuritis affecting, 156–157
  white of, hypnotic induction profile based
    on, 2, 13
Eye-fixation induction method, 2
Eye-roll sign, 13
  hypnotic susceptibility and, 2, 13

F

Fainting, neurally-mediated, 89
Fallopian tube, conception and, 76
  spasm in, 76
False memory, hypnotic implantation of,
    154–155
Family problems, hypnotherapeutic
    approach to, 153–154
Fear. See also Anxiety.
  airplane flight causing, 153
  childbirth association with, 69
  dental procedure causing, 131–132
  fight-or-flight response to, 44
  pessimistic interpretations related
    to, 59
  radiology procedure causing, 96–98, 98
  trance-equivalent state induced by, 59–60
Feedback induction, 62
Feelings (emotion). See also Anxiety; Fear.
  asthma triggered by, 116, 118
  hypnosis effect on, 11
Fentanyl, radiology patient sedated with,
    97–98, 98
Fertility, 76
  stress effect on, 76
Fibrillation, atrial, emergency room
    treatment of, 61
Fight-or-flight response, mechanisms of, 44
Fractures, Colles', emergency room
    treatment of, 61
Freud, Sigmund, 30
  hypnotism rejected by, 30
Frontal lobes, hypnosis effect on, 9

G

Gag reflex, hypnosis control of, 135
Glove anesthesia, 2, 133
  dental patient with, 133
  hypnotic suggestion for, 2, 133
  oncology patient need for, 110
Granuloma, eosinophilic, 86
  hypnotherapy related to, 86
Gunshot wound, hypnotherapy related to,
    87
  pediatric patient affected by, 87
Gynecology, 72–78. See also Infertility;
    Menstruation; Sexually transmitted
    diseases.
  hypnotherapy used in, 72–78
  physician in practice of, 77–78

H

Habit behaviors, 155–156
  hypnotherapeutic modification of,
    152–153, 155–156
  undesirable, 155–156
Hair-pulling, hypnotherapy for, 155
Hallucination, asthmatic patient change as,
    120
  imagery intensity and, 11
  negative, 11
Hands together induction, 133
Handshake induction, 133

Handwriting, automatic, dissociation relation to, 15
Headache, assessment of, 85
  hypnotherapy for, 85, 156–157
  migraine, immune response role in, 37, 38
    juvenile, 37, 38
    mast cells and, 37, 38
  pediatric patient affected by, 84–85
  psychotherapist with, 156–157
Healing, dental patient imagery for, 136
  oncology patient imagery for, 112–113
  touch effectiveness in, 22, 108
Heart, hypnosis effect on, 9
Hemophilia, pain due to, 87
  pediatric, 87
Hemorrhage, hypnotherapy control of, 9, 136, 146
Herpes, genital, 75–76
Hidden observer phenomenon, ideomotor response due to, 154
History (of hypnosis), 21–31
  American investigators in, 28–29
  ancient, 21–23
  English investigators in, 27–28
  French investigators in, 25–27
  later developments in, 29–30
  Mesmer period in, 23–25
HIV infection, 75–76
Hormones, menstrual disorders related to, 72–74
  stress response role of, 43–46
Human papillomavirus, venereal warts due to, 75–76
Hyperactivity disorder, 89–90
  hypnotherapy for, 89–90
Hyperemesis, gag reflex hypersensitivity and, 135
  hypnotic control therapy for, 66–67
  pregnancy causing, 66–67
Hypermnesia, 12
Hypersensitivity, delayed cutaneous, 35
  hypnosis effect on, 35–36
  immune response role in, 35–36
  relaxation effect on, 35–36
  skin-testing for, 35
Hypersomnolence, pediatric, 88–89
Hypertension, pregnancy-induced, 68–69
Hyperventilation syndrome, 124
Hypnoreflexogenous technique, 69, 70
Hypnosis, 1–3. See also *Relaxation; Self-hypnosis.*
  anesthesia relation to, 12–13, 43–55. See also *Anesthesia.*
  asthma treated with, 116–123. See also *Asthma.*
  cautionary aspects of, 151–152, 154–155
  changes seen during, 7–13
    physiological, 7–13
    psychological, 10–12
  definition of, 1, 13–17, 80
  dentistry use of, 131–138. See also *Dentistry.*
  ease vs. difficulty of, 2
  emergency room use of, 59–64. See also *Emergency room.*
  experience of, 7–12, 141
  future research concerning, 17
  group, 144–145

Hypnosis (*Continued*)
  gynecology use of, 72–78. See also *Infertility; Menstruation; Sexually transmitted diseases.*
  history of, 21–31. See also *History (of hypnosis).*
  immune system modulation by, 33–39. See also *Immune response.*
  induction of, 2, 59–64
    arm levitation in, 2, 133
    arm rub in, 134
    basic, 2
    clenched fist, 153–156
    coin drop, 134
    confusional method for, 2
    eye-fixation in, 2
    feedback, 62
    guided imagery, 134–135
    handshake, 133
    hands-together, 134
    injured patient and, 60–64
    permissive, 2, 143
    rapid, 133–135
    verbal, 156
  neutral, 8, 10
  nursing utilization of, 142–148. See also *Nursing.*
  obstetrics use of, 65–72. See also *Pregnancy.*
  oncology use of, 107–113. See also *Oncology.*
  pediatrics use of, 79–91. See also *Pediatric patients.*
  psychotherapy using, 151–156. See also *Psychotherapy.*
  radiology use of, 95–104. See also *Radiology.*
  respiratory illness treated with, 115–125. See also *Respiratory illness.*
  scripts used during, 2, 102–103
  sensation and mentation during, 8–12
  signals from subject during, 2
    ideomotor, 2, 154
    movement, 2
  suggestions and instructions during, 2, 142–148, 152–156
    authoritative, 2
    catalepsy due to, 2
    direct, 2
    embedded, 2
    Ericksonian, 2
    glove anesthesia due to, 2, 133
    indirect, 2
    posthypnotic, 2, 136
    scripts for, 2, 102–103
  surgery preparation using, 46, 49–51, 136. See also *Surgery.*
  susceptibility to, 2, 80
    scales for measurement of, 80
  theory concerning, 13–17. See also *Theory (of hypnosis).*
  trance state of, 2, 10
Hypocapnia, bronchoconstriction triggered by, 118
Hypothalamo-pituitary-adrenocortical axis, 44–46
Hypothalamo-sympatho-adrenocortical axis, 45
Hypothalamo-sympatho-adrenomedullary axis, 44–46

I

Ideomotor signals, 2, 154
Image rehearsal, academic preparation using, 152
Imagery, brain hemisphere laterality and, 17
  cultural differences affecting, 90
  daydreaming, 11
  guided, dental hypnosis using, 134–135
  healing aspect of, 112–113, 136
  hypnotic state enhancement of, 11
  nursing hypnotherapy use of, 142–148
  oncology patient use of, 110–113
  place envisioned in, calm, 84, 86, 90, 134
    comfortable, 156
    laughing, 60–61
    peaceful, 142
    safe, 84, 86, 90
  psychotherapeutic induction using, 156
  radiology hypnotherapy use of, 101–104
  relaxation induction using, 60–61, 84, 86, 90, 134–135
  resistance to, 104
Imagination. See also *Imagery.*
  hypnosis effect on, 11
  mesmerism use of, 25
Immune response, 33–39
  behavior impacted by, 34
  conditioning role in, 33–36
  depression effect on, 34–35
  future research directions for, 38–39
  hypnosis effect on, 33–39
  migraine role of, 37
  neuroendocrine effects in, 34–35
  oncology patient stimulation of, 112–113
  pediatric studies on, 36–38
  relaxation affecting, 34–36
  self-modulation of, 35–39
  stress affecting, 34–35, 37–38
  warts remission and, 37
Incontinence, fecal, 89
  pediatric patient with, 89
  urinary, 89
Induction. See *Hypnosis, induction of.*
Infants. See also *Pediatric patients.*
  procedure-pain in, hypnotherapy for, 82
Infertility, 76
  hypnotherapy in, 76
  stress effect in, 76
Insomnia, pediatric, 88–89
Interspersal approach, 142
Irritable bowel syndrome, hypnotherapy for, 85–86
  pediatric patient with, 86
Intravenous (IV) therapy, child patient and, 147
  sedation administered in, 97–98, *98*

L

Labor (pregnancy), 69–72
  breech presentation in, 72
  contractions of, 69–72
  premature, 67–68
  training methods for, 69–72
Lacerations, emergency room treatment of, 61
Lamaze movement, 69

Laughing place, dissociation established by use of, 60–61
Laying on of hands, 22
Leading, dental hypnosis using, 132
   nurse utilization of, 142
Levitation, arm, hypnosis induction method using, 2, 133
Logic mechanisms, hypnotic trance effect on, 10–11, 14
Lung, chronic obstructive disease of, 123–124
   granulomatous disease of, 86
   hypnotherapy related to, 86, 123–124

M

Magnetism, 23–25
   animal, 23–25
   healing associated with, 22–25
   historical aspects of, 22–25
   Mesmer's use of, 23–25
Malpractice, obstetric-gynecology practice and, 77
   prevention of suit related to, 77
Mantra, 10
Marijuana use, pediatric, 90
Marital problems, hypnotherapeutic approach to, 153–154
Mast cells, migraine role of, 37, 38
Maxwell, William, 22
Meditation, hypnosis association with, 8, 10
Memory, "anesthesia awareness" as, 12–13
   false, implantation of, 154–155
   hypnosis interaction with, 12, 154–155
Menstruation, 72–74
   absence of, 73
   disorders of, 72–74
   excessive flow in, 73
   painful, 74
   premenstrual syndrome associated with, 73–74
Mentation, atavistic phenomenon theory related to, 15
   hypnosis effect on, 8–12
   pediatric patient developmental stage and, 80–82
Mesmer, Franz, 23–25
Mesmerism, 23–25
   crisis of, 25
   magnets used in, 23–25
Metabolism, hypnosis slowing-effect on, 9–10
   stress response affecting, 43–46
Metaphors. See also *Imagery.*
   therapeutic, 142
Metrorrhagia, 73
Midazolam, radiology patient sedated with, 97–98, *98*
Migraine. See also *Headache.*
   immune response role in, 37, 38
   juvenile, 37, 38
   mast cells and, 37, 38
Mimicry, hypnosis theory concerning, 16
Molester of children, hypnotherapy for, 152
Motor function, hypnosis affecting, 8
Movement, hypnosis affecting, 8
   signals from subject using, 2
Music, relaxation using, 76

N

Nail-biting, hypnotherapy for, 155
Narcotic medication, hypnosis reducing need for, 48, 49
   radiology patient need for, 97–98, *98*
Nausea, chemotherapy causing, 110–111, 143–144
   hypnotherapeutic control of, 66–67, 110–111, 143–144
   oncology patient with, 110–111
   pregnancy with, 66–67
Needles, child patient IV and, 147
   oncology patient fear of, 110
Neoplasia. See *Oncology.*
Nervous system, asthma provocation role of, 118
   stress response pathways of, 43–46
Neuritis, retrobulbar, hypnotherapy for, 156–157
Neuroimmunomodulation, 33–39. See also *Immune response.*
Neurypnology, 27
Neutral hypnosis, 8, 10
Neutrophils, relaxation modulation of, 36–37
   self-hypnosis effect on, 36–37
   stickiness of, 36–37
Night terrors, pediatric, 88–89
Numbness, glove anesthesia with, 2
   psychological, 154
Nursing, 141–149
   hypnotherapy used in, 141–149
      conversation including, 145–147
      cost effectiveness of, 148
      emergency room setting for, 145–146
      health promoted by, 142–143
      inductions and styles for, 142, 145–147
      negative suggestions counteracted by, 147–148
      pain management by, 143–144
      preoperative, 144
      training for, 148–149

O

Obstetrics, 65–72. See also *Pregnancy.*
   hypnotherapy used in, 65–72
   physician in practice of, 77–78
Oedipus complex, hypnosis theory based on, 15
Oncology, 107–113
   hypnotherapy used in, 107–113
      anxiety control by, 110–113
      approach to, 108–110
      beginning procedures for, 108–110
      claustrophobia counteracted by, 111–112
      death and dying in, 113
      imagery of healing in, 112–113
      nausea control in, 110–111
      negative suggestions blocked by, 109
      nonverbal communication place in, 108
      pain and needle phobia and, 110
      severity-of-problem scale used in, 110
      tape recording in, 109
Operating room, "anesthesia awareness" of patient in, 51–55
   personnel talking in, 51–55

Optic nerve, inflammation of, 156–157
Ovum, conception and, 76

P

Pacing, dental hypnosis use of, 132
   nursing utilization of, 142
Pain, chest, emergency room treatment of, 62
   childbirth association with, 69
   Colles' fracture with, 61
   dislocated shoulder with, 60–61
   eosinophilic granulomatous lung disease with, 86
   gunshot wound causing, 87
   hemophilia with, 87
   menstrual, 72–74
   neuroendocrine response to, 45–46
   nursing hypnotherapy management of, 143–144
   oncology patient fear of, 110, 113
   pediatric patient affected by, 82–85
   procedure-caused, distraction technique for, 82–83
   radiologic procedure with, 97–99
   sickle cell disease with, 86–87
   stress response caused by, 45–46
   trance-equivalent state induced by, 59–60
Panic attack, radiology procedure causing, 96–97
Papillomavirus, venereal warts due to, 75–76
Paralysis, psychological, 154
Parasympathetic nervous system, stress response role of, 44
Parturition, 69–72
   breech presentation in, 72
   contractions of, 69–72
   premature, 67–68
   training methods for, 69–72
Pediatric patients, 79–91
   asthma affecting, 124–125
   attention deficit hyperactivity disorder in, 90
   burn injury in, 83–84
   chronic coughing by, 87–88
   cystic fibrosis in, 125
   dental procedures in, 136–137
   developmental stage of, 80–82
   encopresis in, 89
   enuresis in, 89
   eosinophilic granulomatous lung disease in, 86
   gunshot wound affecting, 87
   headache affecting, 85
   hemophilia in, 86
   hypnotherapy for, 79–91
      cultural sensitivity and, 91
   immune response studies in, 36–38
   irritable bowel syndrome in, 85–86
   migraine in, 37, 38
   pain management for, 82–85
      acute pain in, 83–84
      chronic pain in, 85
      procedure pain in, 82–83
   sickle cell disease in, 86–87
   sleep disorder in, 88–89
   substance abuse in, 90–91
   sycope in, neurally-mediated, 90
   test anxiety in, 89–90
   warts in, 37
Pessimism, fear related to, 59
Phobias, hypnotherapeutic treatment of, 155

Physicians, burn out affecting, 77–78
  emergency room, 59–60
  obstetric-gynecological, 77–78
Piaget stages, 80–82
Pituitary-hypothalamo-adrenocortical axis,
    44–45
Posthypnotic suggestion, 2
  method for establishment of, 2
Post-traumatic stress disorder,
    hypnotherapy for, 152
Prausnitz-Küstner reaction, 35
Pregnancy, 65–72
  false, 73
  hypertension induced by, 68–69
  hypnosis use during, 65–72
  labor and delivery phase of, 69–72
  nausea during, 66–67
  premature labor affecting, 67–68
  vomiting during, 66–67
Premenstrual syndrome, 73–74
  hypnotherapy for, 73–74
  physiology of, 73–74
Procedure pain, pediatric patient affected
    by, 82–83
  radiology patient with, 97–99
Pseudocyesis, 73
Psychoanalysis, hypnosis theory related
    to, 15
Psychodrama, marital and family therapy
    using, 153–154
Psychological factors. See also
    Psychotherapy.
  abnormal reaction to hypnosis due to,
    137–138
  asthma and, 115–116, 118–122
  attention deficit hyperactivity disorder
    with, 89–90
  chronic cough associated with, 87–88
  numbness and paralysis due to, 154
Psychoneuroimmunology, 33–39. See also
    Immune response.
  organizations and resources for, 38–39
Psychotherapy, 151–157
  hypnosis used in, 151–157
    cautionary aspects of, 151–152,
      154–155
    false memories implanted by, 154–155
    habitual behaviors treated with,
      155–156
    induction of, 153, 156
      clenched fist, 153
      verbal, 156
    marital and family problems and,
      153–154
    personal use of, 156
    phobia therapy with, 155
    variety of symptoms treated with,
      152–153, 155–156

R

Radiology, 95–104
  analgesia need related to, 97
  anxiolysis need related to, 97
  hypnotherapy used in, 98–104
    concept of, 99
    economic factors of, 99
    imagery with, 101–104
    methodology for, 99–104
    personnel rapport skills in, 100
    potential of, 98–99

Radiology (*Continued*)
    relaxation with, 101–104
    script for, 102–103
    self-hypnosis as, 101–104
    suggestibility aiding in, 100–101
  office setting for, 95–96
  patients' perceptions of, 96–97
  pharmacologic sedation need in,
    97–98, *98*
  procedure pain of, 97–99
Rapport skills, radiology hypnotherapy use
    of, 100
Recollection, anesthesia awareness in,
    12–13
  false, implantation of, 154–155
  hypnosis interaction with, 12, 154–155
Reduction, Colles' fracture, 61
  dislocated shoulder, 60–61
Reframing, definition of, 17
  nursing hypnotherapy use of, 142
Relaxation. See also *Hypnosis; Self-
    hypnosis.*
  asthma not to be treated with, 120–121
  chemotherapy eased by, 110–113,
    143–144
  difficult gynecologic patient and, 76
  emergency room use of, 60–64
  hypnosis association with, 8–10
  immune response affected by, 34–36
  nursing hypnotherapy use of, 142–148
  oncology patient use of, 110–113
  pediatric patient treated with, 79–91
  radiology patient in, 101–104
  script for, 102–103
Religion, hypnotherapy proscribed by, 80
Respiration rate, hypnosis effect on, 9
Respiratory illness, 115–125
  asthma as, 61–62, 115–123. See also
    Asthma.
  COPD as, 123–124
  earthquake stress affecting, 37–38
  hyperventilatory, 124
  pediatric, 124–125
Royal touch, 22

S

Safe place imagery, cultural differences
    affecting, 90
  relaxation induction using, 84, 86, 90
Saliva, immunoglobulins in, self-hypnosis
    effect on, 36
Scripts, hypnotic trance management
    using, 2
  relaxation technique using, 102–103
Sedation. See also *Analgesia.*
  dental patient given, 132–133
  intravenous, 97–98, *98*
  radiology patient need for, 97–98, *98*
Self-hypnosis. See also *Hypnosis;
    Relaxation.*
  autonomy increased during, 10
  immune response modulation with, 35–39
  menstrual disorders treated with, 73–74
  migraine remittance by, 37
  neutral, 10
  oncology patient use of, 109–110
  psychotherapist using, 156
  radiology patient use of, 101–104
  relaxation associated with, 8
  resistance to, 104

Self-hypnosis (*Continued*)
    salivary immunoglobulins modulated
      by, 36
    spontaneous, 155
    white cell stickiness modulated by,
      36–37
Sensory function, hypnosis-caused changes
    in, 8, 11–13
Sentinel points, during sleep, 14
Sexual dysfunction, female, 74–75
Sexually transmitted diseases, 75–76
Shoulder, dislocation of, emergency
    treatment of, 60–61
Sickle cell disease, 86–87
  hypnotherapy for, 86–87
  pain due to, 86–87
Signals, hypnotic trance monitored by, 2
"Silver fork" deformity, Colles' fracture
    with, 61
Skin-testing, hypersensitivity and, 35
  hypnosis effect on, 35–36
Sleep, 13–14
  hypnosis theory related to, 13–14
  physiologic state of, 13–14
  "sentinel points" during, 14
Sleep disorder, hypnotherapy for,
    88–89
  pediatric, 88–89
Smoking, 29, 90, 152
  cessation of, 29, 152
    early history of, 29
    hypnotism used for, 29, 152
    pediatric, 90
Socioeconomic factors. See also *Costs.*
  asthma treatment and, 115–116
Somnambulism, 25–26
  artificial, 25
  early hypnosis studies and, 25–26
Sophrology, 28
Speech, brain hemispheric laterality and,
    16–17
Staring, hypnosis induction using, 2
Stein clenched fist technique, 153–156
Stimulus, taste, conditioning accomplished
    using, 33–34
Storytelling. See also *Imagery.*
  therapeutic, 142
Stress response, 43–46
  analgesia induction as, 45–46
  anxiety as cause of, 46
  earthquake causing, 37–38
  fertility affected by, 76
  fight-or-flight response to, 44
  hypnosis effect on, 46, 50–51
  hypothalamo-pituitary-adrenocortical axis
    in, 44–46
  hypothalamo-sympatho-adrenocortical
    axis in, 45
  hypothalamo-sympatho-adrenomedullary
    axis in, 44–46
  immune response affected by, 34–35,
    37–38
  pain as cause of, 45–46
  physiology of, 34–35, 43–46
  presurgical intervention for, 48–55
  surgical procedures causing, 43–55
Stuttering, hypnotherapy for, 155
Substance abuse, hypnotherapy for, 91
  pediatric, 90–91
Suggestibility, 2
  anesthesia "awareness" marked by,
    51–55
  burn injury therapy and, 62–64

Suggestibility (*Continued*)
  negative comments acting on, 100–101, 109, 147–148
  radiology hypnotherapy use of, 100–101
Suicidal ideation, hypnotherapy related to, 86–87
  quadriplegic patient with, 86–87
Surgery, 43–55
  anticipation of, 46, 47–48, 50–55
  anxiety related to, 43–46, 51–55
  coping behavior related to, 46, 47–48
  gynecologic, 75
  hypnosis used with, 46, 49–51
    early history of, 27–29
    intraoperative, 51–55
    postoperative, 54–55
    preoperative, 46, 49–51, 75, 144
  interventions in preparation for, 48–55
    cost effectiveness of, 49–50
  stress response associated with, 43–46
Susceptibility, 2, 80
  hypnotic, 2, 80
  scales for measurement of, 2, 80
Swallowing, dysfunctional, hypnotherapy for, 81
Sympatho-hypothalamo-adrenocortical axis, 45
Sympatho-hypothalamo-adrenomedullary axis, 44–46
Syncope, neurally-mediated, 90

T

Tape recording, asthma therapy using, 123
  eating habits directed by, 152
  oncology hypnotherapy use of, 109
Taste stimulus, conditioning accomplished using, 33–34

Teeth, extraction of, hypnoanesthesia for, 133
  grinding or clenching of, 135
Tests (academic), anxiety related to, 89–90, 152
  image rehearsal for, 152
Theory (of hypnosis), 13–17
  atavistic phenomenon, 15
  behavioral, 16
  dissociative state, 15–16
  ego state, 16
  hemispheric laterality, 16–17
  psychoanalytically oriented, 15
  sleep state, 13–14
  special consciousness, 14
Theta waves, hypnosis effect on, 9
Thinking, atavistic phenomenon theory related to, 15
  hypnosis effect on, 10–11
  pediatric patient developmental stage and, 80–82
Thumb-sucking, hypnotherapy for, 155–156
Time, hypnosis effect on sense of, 10, 112, 137
Tobacco use, 29, 90, 152
  cessation of, 29, 152
    early history of, 29
    hypnotism used for, 29, 152
  pediatric, 90
Touch, healing aspects of, 22
  oncology patient and, 108
  royal, 22
Tourniquet, time limit for extended by hypnosis, 61
Trance state, 2, 10
  logic mechanisms affected by, 10–11, 14
  meditative, 10
Trance-equivalent state, 59–60
Transference, hypnosis theory based on, 15
  mesmeric, 25

U

Utilization, 2
  dental hypnosis strategy using, 132
  nursing hypnotherapy strategy using, 141

V

Venereal diseases, 75–76
Vision, double, hypnotherapy for, 156–157
Visualization. See *Imagery.*
Vital spirit, 22
Vomiting, chemotherapy-related, 111, 143–144
  gag reflex hypersensitivity and, 135
  hypnotic control therapy for, 66–67
  pregnancy causing, 66–67

W

Warts, immune response remission of, 37
  self-hypnosis and, 37
  venereal, 75–76
Weight loss, 152–153
Wernicke's area, 16
White cells, relaxation modulation of, 36–37
  self-hypnosis effect on, 36–37
  stickiness of, 36–37
Wound, gunshot, 87
Writing, automatic, dissociation related to, 15